THE
LEAN BODY
SOLUTION

A Revolutionary Approach to Getting in
Amazing Shape without Absurd Dieting or
Spending Countless Hours in the Gym

Michael Hermann & Dylan Jones

ISBN 979-8-35093-977-4

All Rights Reserved

Copyright © 2023 Performance Revolution Pty Ltd.
All rights reserved. No part of this publication may be copied, shared, stored within a database or retrieval system, or distributed in any format or media (electronic or mechanical) without the express written consent of Performance Revolution Pty Ltd. You do not have the right under any circumstances to reprint, resell, redistribute, or auction *The Lean Body Solution*.

For all product inquiries, contact
info@performancerevolution.com.au

Photography credits:
iStock: pages 13, 42, 57, 63, 70, 84, 101, 120, 121, 331

Disclaimer

The authors are not licensed medical practitioners or physicians and do not offer medical diagnoses, treatments, suggestions, or counselling. Although adhering to many of the Australian Dietary Guidelines, the information presented within this publication has not been evaluated by the Australian Government Department of Health or National Health and Medical Research Council (NHMRC) and is not intended to diagnose, treat, cure, or prevent any disease. More information about these relevant bodies and proposed guidelines can be found by visiting: **www.eatforhealth.gov.au**.

The nutritional values represented in this publication are estimates and should not be solely relied upon for your dietary strategy.

Full medical clearance from a licensed medical practitioner or physician should be obtained before commencing or modifying any nutritional or lifestyle program with full disclosure of the nutritional changes being sought.

The authors claim no responsibility to any person or entity for any loss, liability, or damage caused or alleged to be caused both directly and indirectly as a result of the interpretation, application, or use of the information contained herein this publication.

Contents

Introduction	7
Getting the Most Out of This	10
Travelling the Road Less Stupid	12
Beyond Calorie Counting	16
Making Macros Matter	27
Finding Good Macronutrient Sources and Substitutions	32
Determining Your Body-Composition Goals	38
Measuring Your Progress	40
Designing Your Lean Body Nutrition Plan	46
Calculating Your Lean Body Nutritional Requirements	54
Structuring Your Lean Body Plan	61
Troubleshooting Nutrition and Overcoming Stagnation	66
Framing Fibre	80
Choosing Leaner Beverages	86
Getting Your Water Intake Right	92
Understanding Alcohol	96

THE LEAN BODY KITCHEN — 107

Kitchen Equipment Essentials	108
Preparing, Packing, and Storing Your Meals	110
Principles for Making Your Own Lean Body Recipes	114
4 Steps to Making Nutritious Shakes and Smoothies	115
5 Steps to Making Tasty, Clean, and Lean Sandwiches	121
4 Simple Steps to Super Soups and Stews	126
10 Tips to Lean and Delicious Salads from Start to Finish	131
Super Sides for Complete Meals	138
Leaner Snack Alternatives and Ideas	140
A Brief Word on Supplements	141

CONTENTS

THE LEAN BODY RECIPES — 143

Breakfast	145
Post-Workout Shakes and Snacks	171
Lunch and Dinner	183
Dessert	215
Snacks and Dips	233
Sides	243
Sauces, Dressings, and Condiments	259
Better than Fast Food	271
Treats	308

THE LEAN BODY WAY — 323

The Great Disparity and Ensuring Your Success	324
Closing Thoughts	327
Our One Request	329
Where to Next	330

Recipe Index	332

About the Authors	336

"PROGRESS LIES NOT IN ENHANCING WHAT IS, BUT IN ADVANCING TOWARD WHAT WILL BE".

Introduction

We live in a time of rapid progress and accelerating technological advancement.

It's a world where once seemingly far-reaching fantasies are soon becoming tangible realities in a very short period of time.

Many challenges that were once prevalent in common everyday lifestyles have been reduced (and even removed) with scientific development.

People now, more than ever before, have access to more resources and information. Yet despite all of the development and accelerated improvements, it seems like in many areas we are a long way behind.

With all the breakthroughs in medicine, healthcare, technology, and communication, it's ironic that as a society, we are fatter and unhealthier than ever before.

With so much information at our fingertips, we are for the most part lost as to why we can't get in shape and stay in shape.

There also seems to be no shortage of people conjuring up their own unique solutions and offering compelling answers to this age-old problem.

There are more results-promising weight-loss programs and fitness regimes than ever before.

There are more experts imparting their wisdom and life advice than ever before. There are more health-claiming dietary supplements and well-being products than ever before.

And let's not forget the countless social media influencers also offering their secret methods, hacks, and formulas to a leaner waistline.

If that's not enough, the food itself is also talking to us all of the time, too! Countless food products are decorated with labels claiming that they're full of 'XYZ' and how good the product will be for our waistline and our health.

Yet here we are. For all the noise and discourse, for the most part we as a people are a bunch of overweight and unhealthy sad sacks who are bulking out the atmosphere.

INTRODUCTION

With more information about nutrition and getting in shape than ever before, people are more confused and ambivalent than ever before.

And to further muddy the waters, many who work in the relevant areas of health are either dumbfounded or constantly squabbling amongst themselves as to what is right and what is wrong.

It is our undertaking in this text to not add more dirt to muddied waters, or to make an entangled web even more intricate.

What we are suggesting in this text is not another variation on a theme, but rather a complete paradigm shift.

Why? What is currently in place has produced meagre results at best.

And this is for good reason. As you will soon discover, the prevalent theories and underpinnings we're so heavily relying upon are fundamentally flawed at their foundations.

How can one be sure of this? Simply look around you—what is currently established is not working. In fact, you could argue it's making us worse!

And it's likely you can very personally relate?

Perhaps you have read every nutrition book, listened to every healthy eating podcast, and followed every diet hack and strategy to no avail!

Maybe you have tried counting Calories[1], restricting various food groups, observing strict fasting periods, or followed popular diets only to get nowhere—or worse yet—rebounded back to a worse place than where you started!

This should come as no surprise though (as you will soon learn). We the authors have seen A LOT of this first-hand in dealing with MANY people from all walks of life.

Many different people with the same fundamental problems going unchecked.

In this text, we will address why you likely had limited success with the common aforementioned measures and question the highly and widely held assumptions that underpin them.

Further, we will seriously shake and dismantle the underlying theories and ideologies at the centre of most conventional dietary

---

1. Calories: To simplify the communication of the energy content in foods, nutritional information labels list caloric values. These values are actually kilocalories and should be denoted by using 'kcal' or an upper case 'C' when referring to 'Calories'. For instance, one thousand calories is equivalent to 1 kcal or 1 Calorie. With this fact in mind, we will be using the kilocalorie measure that is denoted by the word Calorie/s throughout this text.

INTRODUCTION

advice and the proposed methodologies that accompany them. We will show you an alternative approach that we have seen produce sustainable results for many of our clients time and time again without recourse.

If you have constantly struggled to get in good shape, if you have tried every diet imaginable, if you've taken every supplement or pill, and you have tried every fitness program on the highly saturated market, then you're about to discover the answers you have been searching for!

This is not some cheesy, feel-good book that was put together without cogent thought. We have put several YEARS into testing, tweaking, and verifying the results over a long span of time with a large client database. We have also considered all the relevant research and scientific studies and carefully evaluated these for their veracity.

Our primary goal is not a book that will be a good read (though we're certain it will accomplish that). No, our goal is a resource that changes people's lives for the better in a BIG way. We're confident you will use this text as a reference tool for many years to come. We value your time and your attention and it is with this in mind that we have created the best book possible for you.

But don't take our word for it—apply it for yourself. Examine it under your own microscope, grapple with the ideas, and put it to the test. And if you're uncertain about whether you should attempt to do any of that, ask yourself "Why not?" Most of what we currently have is not working and you have nothing to lose in employing this alternative (apart from a lot of body fat).

Whether you're really out of shape with lots of clothing sizes to drop, or you're on a leaner trajectory and you're determined to finally start seeing visible abs, we can assure that the answers are within this text.

It doesn't matter if you're a full-time mum, a competitive athlete, or corporate desk jockey. We're confident this resource will enable you to finally get long-lasting, life-changing, body-altering results!

Are you ready? If so, the first step is to know how to properly digest everything you're about to learn.

Getting the Most Out of This

"DON'T TAKE CONTENT FROM CONTEXT".
ANONYMOUS

We have put this resource together with one particular word in mind: relevancy. The information you will find within this resource is not only concise and accurate, it is also based on years of experimentation with real-life clients with real results. We have endeavoured to make the concepts as simple as possible to understand and we will not waste your time with information that has no practical application.

For this reason, we can say with conviction that all the information in this book is important and should not be skipped-over or cherry-picked. We encourage you to read this text from start to finish to not only get all the necessary information, but also to ensure you read it in a context that makes sense. We have structured the information in the order we have for good reason: you must understand the fundamentals in the prior sections before you can move onto the subsequent sections.

We promise it will all make sense, and that you will eliminate a lot of questions and doubts that you may have by simply reading this book in its entirety, in an orderly manner. Once you have read the text in full, then you can jump back to places and use it as a reference.

The first half of this text will deal with the principles of nutrition for lean and healthy eating and how a person can formulate their own plan to reach their goals. The second half of this text is dedicated to the recipes we have used with clients over the years to help them achieve great results with their body and their health.

GETTING THE MOST OUT OF THIS

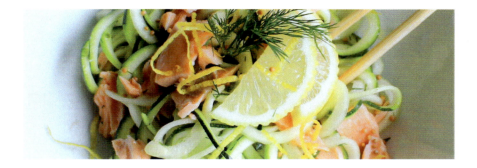

In regard to our recipes, we have spent a lot of time experimenting and tweaking to get them just right. The ones we've included have three major attributes that warrant their inclusion in this text:

1. They provide great nutritional quality.

2. They are relatively simple to make and not time-consuming.

3. They taste great! We have tested a plethora of recipes on a large sample size of clients and only the best voted ones have made the cut!

As a bonus, too, we have also included some recipes that are a far better alternative version of some common not-so-lean-and-healthy foods that many of us are often tempted to indulge in.

We also realise that you may travel from time to time and often don't have access to your kitchen. For this reason, we provide not only portability measures within this text, but also nutrition principles you can take wherever you go. This will ensure that you can consume meals that are consistent with your goals no matter the circumstance you find yourself in.

When it comes to nutrition (and most things worthwhile), application is where the greatest amount of learning and results will occur. Eating to be leaner and healthier is relatively simple: we make it hard for ourselves by making excuses and blaming other people and circumstances around us. Not sticking to good habits, or by applying some principles and not others within your nutritional plan, WILL NOT yield results. You don't go to a doctor to write your own 'scripts, nor should you invest in a nutrition resource only to follow your own nutritional rationalisations and urges.

We want you to enjoy your food. However, there is a smart way about this, and there is a dumb way: we will show you the smart way.

THE LEAN BODY SOLUTION

Travelling the Road Less Stupid

> "I DON'T NEED TO DO MORE SMART THINGS. I JUST NEED TO DO FEWER DUMB THINGS".
>
> KEITH CUNNINGHAM

You will likely find it intriguing that a book dedicated to leaning down will have very little to say about exercise. This is certainly not because we are anti-exercise or we don't believe it has any place. Exercise definitely has a place in longer-term body composition and health goals.

The problem we find, however, is that no matter what program people are looking to pursue, most put this component in too high a place. Essentially, they become fixated on addressing the symptoms, and not the underlying problem (i.e. the real reason that they're not in shape).

When we ask most prospective clients why they aren't where they should be with their body and their health, they often answer with "Because I'm not exercising enough and I'm carrying too much fat".

If this sounds like you too, then you have a problem in your thinking that needs addressing. "Not exercising enough and carrying too much fat" are symptoms and not the real problem. Sure, these things indicate that something's wrong—but they don't reveal what.

The author of the opening quote (whose book bears the same title as this chapter) puts it best: "We mistakenly believe that we know what the problem is because we can easily identify the places that we don't 'have' what we want (the symptoms)".

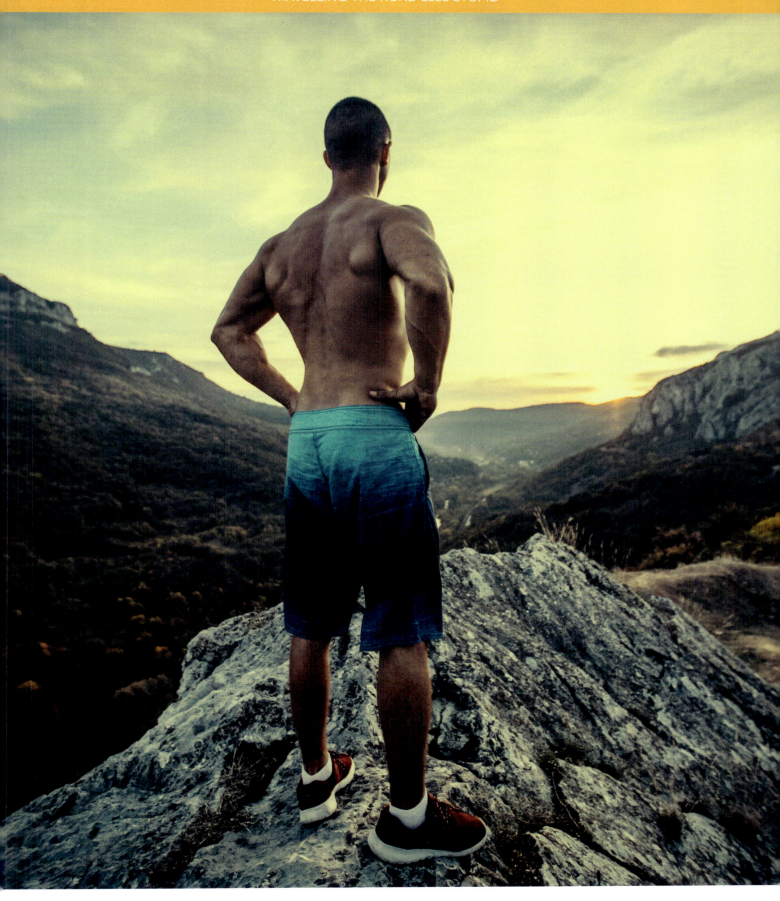

People easily associate problems with things they don't have and they mistakenly think that they just have to 'do something' so the symptoms will go away. The problem, however, is not the symptoms that are in a person's line of sight, but rather the present obstacles that are preventing the person from getting in shape—in this case it's poor nutritional habits.

It's the difference between asking oneself, "What can I do to lose all of this excess fat?" instead of "Why am I so badly out of shape?"

Due to this incorrect thought process, many wrongly believe that exercise alone will make them lean and then dedicate hours upon hours to training with very little to show for it.

The problem, however, is excessive consumption of the wrong type of foods that puts on excess body fat (the symptom). Only a dedicated focus to rectifying the poor nutritional habits will thus eliminate the excess fat.

We are astounded by the number of people who try and out-train a poor diet. They misdirect so much energy and effort into doing all types of fanciful 'fat-burning workouts' when they have no control of any of the input variables and the root cause of their problem (i.e. what they throw down their neck!).

If you're out of shape and have exercise equipment that is gathering dust (or a gym membership that hasn't been used in a while), you can attest that these measures failed to resolve your problem and were instead attempts wrongly aimed at your symptoms.

By saying this, we certainly are not trying to deter anyone from moving more or working out regularly. No; we just want the emphasis and focus to be where it is lacking for most people—nutrition!

To put it bluntly: exercise has numerous health benefits, but if you have to exercise to maintain your body fat level within a healthy range, then your diet needs work.

For those who have fat to lose and want to keep it off longer term, the solution to their problem undeniably lies in what they push down their throat.

We are often approached by people wanting to lose fat or build muscle by focusing on just exercise and no dietary intervention. These people are quickly met with, "We are sorry, but we cannot help you". We don't say this to be hardlined—we actually cannot possibly help them without nutrition in the equation.

Knowing what you know now, your thought process should be similar for any kind of program that promises improved body composition without adequate dietary intervention. Focus on the food, and you will be surprised with how little training is actually required for a leaner and healthier body... not to mention how much time and heartache you will save yourself in the process.

A great example of what we're referring to is one of our Lean Body Program clients Jane. Jane used to do endless amounts of cardio, eat very little, and drink wine like it was about to go out of fashion. When Jane came to us, she followed our nutrition advice as prescribed in 'The Principled Approach' section of this guide. Because Jane had these habits ingrained, we were able to double the amount of food she was eating, stop the crazy daily cardio and drinking, and give her three short and targeted weights sessions per week.

As a result of her new approach to her nutrition, Jane was able to build lean muscle, sculpt her trouble areas (stomach, butt, and thighs), and create a higher resting metabolic rate (RMR) that demanded more from her body at rest. Jane's results were stunning: she dropped more than 10 kg of stubborn fat and built 2 kg of lean muscle in a matter of months! She sculpted a lean body that every other 47-year-old envied! (You can check out Jane's video testimonial at **https://performancerevolution.com.au/#success-stories**.) The most admirable part of Jane's story was that she transformed her nutrition while being a single mum of two kids, working as an executive manager for a large bank, and studying a master's degree all at the same time!

Jane's story illustrates what is possible if you pay attention to what you consume, rid yourself of excuses, and apply yourself to the few key areas that will deliver highly leveraged returns for the time and effort invested.

Now that you're clear on the importance of nutrition and the order of operation, it's time to develop a fundamental understanding of what actually happens when you push nutrients down your neck. The first consideration is clarification of a concept that is emphatically propagated but heavily misappropriated when it comes to human metabolism and body composition change: 'energy balance'.

Beyond Calorie Counting

> "ALMOST EVERY SIGNIFICANT BREAK-THROUGH IS THE RESULT OF A BREAK-WITH TRADITIONAL WAYS OF THINKING".
> STEPHEN R. COVEY

As you read this text you will soon notice that there is very little preoccupation on 'Calories'. This is for good reason and you will soon learn why.

It has been widely assumed for some time that the fundamental cause of weight gain is an energy imbalance between Calories consumed and Calories expended (i.e. Energy Balance Theory).

Energy Balance Theory

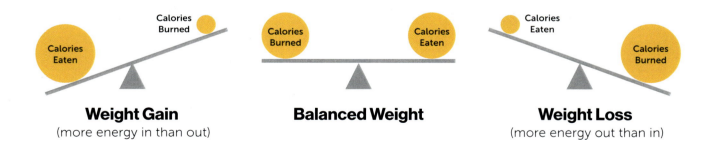

Weight Gain
(more energy in than out)

Balanced Weight

Weight Loss
(more energy out than in)

Adopting this premise, the only way a person can lose weight and body fat is to consume fewer Calories than they expend or expend more Calories than they consume: Calories In, Calories Out (or CICO for short). However, this premise has a number of innate errors, which you will soon come to realise.

Before discussing the topic of energy balance and Calories further, let's first get clear on what a 'Calorie' actually is. Calories are not a measure of energy but rather a measure of a *particular type of energy*—heat energy to be exact.

The traditional method to find the amount of Calories in a given substance (in this instance, food) is to place a sample inside a bomb calorimeter as shown below:

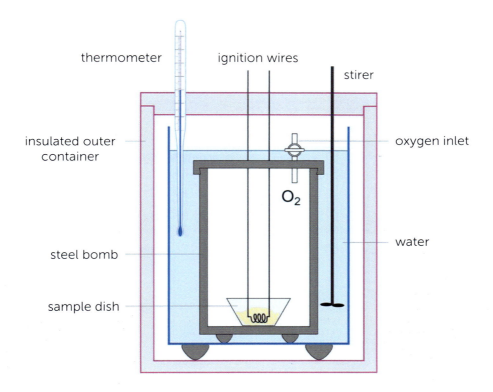

The food is then ignited and the amount of Calories it contains is derived from measuring the temperature of the water outside the bomb as shown (heat transfers from warmer bodies to colder bodies). A Calorie is the amount of heat energy required to raise 1 kilogram (or 1 L) of water by 1°C.

As you have likely seen on food labels, foods are attributed Caloric energy values based on predominantly their macronutrient composition: 1 gram of fat equals 9 Calories; 1 gram of protein equals 4 Calories; 1 gram of carbs equals 4 Calories, etc.

The sum of these Calories consumed is then often used to determine daily intake targets to lose weight, gain weight, or maintain weight, depending on the person's goals.

BEYOND CALORIE COUNTING

So what's the problem with measuring foods in Caloric terms and manipulating one's energy intake to influence body composition? There are quite a few. The first issue is that your body is not an enclosed bomb calorimeter. It's vastly different and more complex: the fact that you're breathing in and out right now proves it.

A bomb calorimeter is what is called a closed thermodynamic system. This means that energy can flow in and out of the system but there is no exchange of matter (mass) between the system and its surroundings during the combustion process. You, on the other hand, are an open thermodynamic system: you breathe, you eat, you sweat, you poop, and you initiate a number of mass exchanges with your environment as illustrated below:

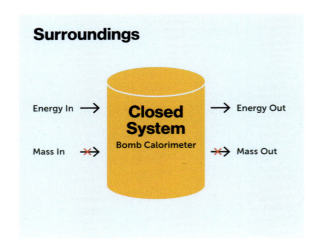 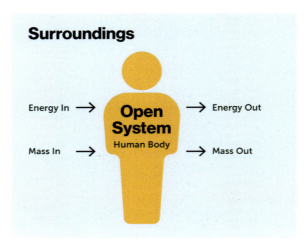

Here is a simple experiment for you: fill up a mug with boiling water. Put your hand on the wall of the mug and notice how the mug is quite warm. Now tip the water out of the mug and replace it with the same amount of water that is room temperature. The mug should soon feel a lot cooler to touch. In this scenario, the energy content going into the mug (heat) decreased, but the mass of water remained the same. In the same way, you can have a negative energy balance (fewer Calories in than Calories out) but still maintain the same body mass.

This is because Calories represent the heat released upon food oxidation and therefore have no impact on body mass. When you stand on a bathroom scale, the reading does not measure your Calories. The scales measure your body mass (and of course the force exerted on it by gravity). Energy has no mass at all, so energy balance has no relevance to your weight or body mass.

Thus, the only property of food that can alter your body mass is its nutrient mass, not its energy content.

Mass Balance Model

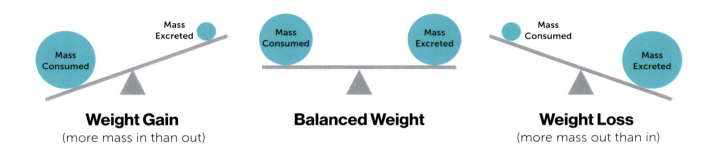

Weight Gain
(more mass in than out)

Balanced Weight

Weight Loss
(more mass out than in)

If you have been frustrated with a lack of weight loss by fervently reducing your Caloric intake (a 'Calorie deficit'), you can now understand why.

Energy balance and mass balance are separate balances in the human body and both can go in different directions. This also explains how someone might have had success losing weight whilst following a Low-Calorie diet or imposing a 'Caloric deficit'—in these instances, both net energy and mass balance were negative, and the weight loss was the result of the underlying mass imbalance.

What determines your body mass is not energy flow (Calories in versus Calories out) but mass flow: mass in versus mass out. Hence, to be in mass balance for a particular nutrient, a person must be consuming the same amount of that nutrient as they are losing or excreting. Each day we experience a mass change: mass in versus mass out.

'Mass in' refers to the daily absorbed nutrients via the diet, while 'mass out' refers to the nutrients lost via nutrient oxidation and excretion (CO_2, water, urea, etc). 'Mass out' is NOT a consequence of the heat release via nutrient combustion (i.e. daily energy expenditure).

Whether it's the absorption of 1 g of fat, protein, or carbohydrate (mass in), body mass increases by exactly 1 g independent of the substrate's Calories (as you will see in specific examples later on).

An absorbed nutrient contributes to a person's total body mass as long as it remains within their body. How the body stores, utilises, and discards various different nutrients is a very interesting and important topic that will be discussed in later sections of this text.

Mass balance equations typically only consider essential nutrients, vitamins, and minerals. These are the nutrients that the body needs that have to be obtained from the diet in sufficient quantities to prevent deficiencies and maintain health. Non-essential nutrients like carbohydrates, for example, are still important for providing energy to the body, but they are not considered in many mass balance equations because the body can synthesise this substrate from other nutrients or convert them from storage forms (e.g. body fat).

However, carbohydrates can have a role in fuelling high-intensity exercise modalities. We recommend resistance training and other forms of high-intensity training to our own clients, and thus have included carbohydrates in our mass balance equations.

It is the 'mass in' part of the mass balance equation that most people have difficulty with, and this will be the largest part of the discussion throughout this text.

Mass intake can also be divided into the following groups:

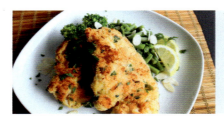

Energy-providing mass: The daily mass intake of fat, protein, carbohydrate, soluble fibre, and alcohol.

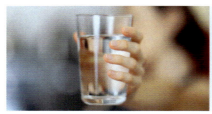

Non-energy-providing mass: The daily mass intake of insoluble fibre, vitamins, minerals, and water.

It bears repeating here that Calories have no impact on body mass!

We also do not consume or eat Calories. Calories are heat, and heat is not used for metabolic processes. Instead, we eat food, and different foods have differing amounts of chemical potential energy, which can be released as a food is metabolised.

The chemical energy stored in your food is converted into work, thermal energy, and/or stored (yes, that includes your fat tissue). This is an important factor to remember and we will be exploring this more in depth later on.

Another issue to consider is the erroneous acceptance of the CICO premise that the same outcome will ensue from ingesting equal Caloric amounts of differing foods without consideration of their mass composition. Your body does not combust foods in the same rapid way as a bomb calorimeter, and it also combusts different foods differently (it actually metabolises foods, to be fair).

Not only does the body metabolise (rather than 'burn') various foods differently, different people will metabolise foods at varying metabolic rates.

Unlike the innate presumptions under the energy balance theory, the mass balance model does not predicate having any type of mass from any type of food to influence weight change. The degree of daily food intake (mass in) is influenced by the interplay between the surroundings, the body's innate makeup, and by how the underlying biochemistry of various foods relate to satiety.

When it comes to how various foods will react in your body, there are important factors to consider that are not accounted for by Caloric values. This includes a food's effects on inflammation, the endocrine system, the digestive system, the nervous system, and more. These effects are all dependent on a food's mass makeup. Framing fat loss and body composition change as simply an equation of 'Calories in, Calories out' is both myopic and misleading.

The human body is much more complex than a calorimeter, and there are many factors that can affect the way in which the body metabolises and utilises food. This is based not only on the type and quality of a food but also the other foods that may be consumed at the same time and how they're interacting with each other and the body.

Energy content is not the determining factor in body composition change or overall health. Calories can give us an idea of the energy content of food, but they do not give us clarity on how much energy is actually derivable for the human body from a given portion of food.

Available Energy vs Effective Energy

Establishing Caloric values can give an indication of the total available energy content of foods, but it cannot give an indication of the effective energy of foods.

What does this mean? A food's Caloric value accounts for all forms of digestible and indigestible nutrients, but it does not factor in what your body actually utilises for energy and what it does not absorb or discards.

Some of a food's energy can be lost as waste during digestion, and some can be used up by the body in processing the food. The available energy is the total energy consumed, whereas the effective energy is the energy that is left over and ready for the body to actually utilise.

For example, foods containing higher amounts of fibre can slow down the digestion and absorption of carbohydrates and fat, leading to less energy being absorbed from a food and a more gradual release of effective energy. Hence, fibre can reduce the likelihood of fat storage while also helping to promote satiety. Fibre can also bind to fats in the digestive tract, which can reduce their absorption and result in a lower effective energy value of the food being consumed.

Under the CICO premise, what dictates body composition change is overall energy balance. Thus all Calories amount to the same, regardless of where they are derived from. However, ingesting protein is not the same as ingesting the equivalent amount of fat or carbohydrate (even if the nutritional package says it has

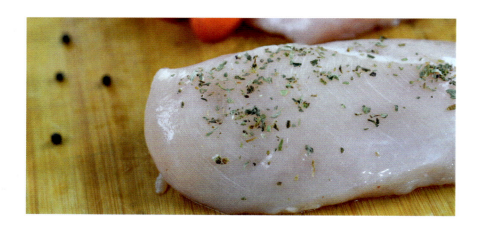

the same amount of 'Calories' or energy). Protein is preferentially allocated towards repairing lean tissue, but it is not the body's primary choice as a fuel source.

Protein also has a higher TEF or thermic effect of food. The TEF is the energy demand required above the body's resting metabolic rate for digestion, absorption, and disposal of ingested nutrients. Although not all sources agree on exact figures, it is clear that protein has a much higher thermic effect (20–30%) compared to that of carbohydrates (5–10%) and fat (0–5%). To help bring this home, let's use a practical example:

> *All other things being equal, let's say you were given an extra 70 g of pure protein each day, on top of your average nutritional intake, for seven days. Then, on a separate occasion, you were given an extra 70 g of pure sugar (same Caloric value) each day, on top of your average nutritional intake, for seven days. Which scenario do you think will result in the most fat gain?*

You can bet with confidence that the sugar scenario will add more fat mass to your frame.

Why is this so? One major reason is the TEF. The other, as previously mentioned, is the preferential allocation of the protein towards lean tissue repair. The amino acids in protein are usually incorporated into bodily structures and are not preferentially oxidised for energy (as opposed to carbohydrates). The body clearly preferences fats and carbohydrates for energy production more so than protein. However, if energy utilisation is all about CICO and you were to have a meal with exactly half protein and half carbohydrate, you're apparently going to have the same amount of effective energy after consuming both. This is clearly not the case.

And no, the answer to getting leaner is not eating a diet of just pure protein with no carbs or fat. Protein is not a great fuel source and a person needs enough of the other essential nutrients (such as fatty acids) to function properly. A diet with enough protein rather than excessive protein is warranted.

The argument against relying on nutritional Caloric values to lose fat doesn't end there though. Let's now talk briefly about food bioavailability and micronutrient density.

The Importance of Bioavailability and Micronutrient Composition

Not only does the macronutrient composition of your food matter (the portion of carbohydrate, fat, and protein), there is a lot to be said for bioavailability and micronutrient composition of your food too for your longer term health, body composition, and performance.

Food bioavailability is the proportion of a food's nutrients that are absorbed by the body and made available for use after being ingested. For example, some nutrients like iron are more bioavailable from animal sources than from plant sources. Food bioavailability can be influenced by a variety of factors, including the form in which a food is consumed, the presence of other foods or nutrients that can interact, and the health and function of a person's digestive system. Cooking methods, food processing, food storage, and the presence of certain compounds in a food can also inhibit or enhance a food's absorption and, thus, can affect the bioavailability of certain nutrients.

Micronutrient-rich foods (those that include more vitamins, minerals, etc.) not only offer more for your longer-term health, but these also assist with proper functioning of the digestive, musculoskeletal, cardiovascular, and other systems of the body, which are, again, often not equated for under the CICO premise. These types of nutrient-rich foods are contained in the 'Finding Good Macronutrient Sources and Substitutions' section of this text.

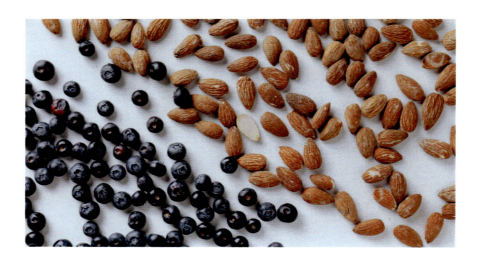

Exercise Estimations Won't Save You

It's not just the 'Calories in' part of the energy balance equation that has serious limitations, the 'Calories out' side also has its pitfalls.

If you're thinking that certain fitness apps and devices that measure 'Calories burned' during activity will serve justice for you body-composition goals—think again. Most of these are by no means an accurate guide to how much energy you're really expending. Even if these tools are more accurate (as some higher-quality heart-rate monitors boast), they do not differentiate between and account for the substrate being utilised for energy (e.g. glucose or fat). Most of these devices only account for overall energy output during an activity (expressed as 'Calories burned') and often fail to account for the differences in the recovery cycles of various different activities and the subsequent substrates being utilised.

For instance, activities performed at a lower intensity such as walking will predominantly rely on fat as the main fuel source. However, higher-intensity activities like resistance training will predominantly use the most readily available fuel source (glucose) for energy. Also, in the days following a high-intensity activity such as weight training, the body has a higher metabolic rate as it continues to expend energy and demand more protein for repairing and rebuilding muscle tissue. This is not accounted for by most consumer fitness apps and devices that simply express 'Calories burned' as the overarching dynamic.

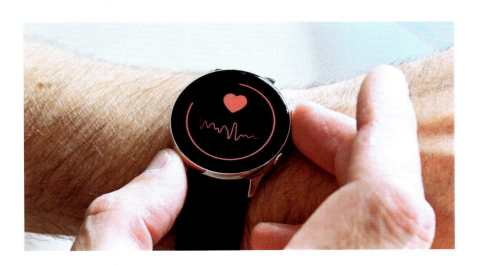

If Not Calories, Then What?

As you can see, focusing on Calories as the means of changing one's body composition and health status has some serious limitations. The amount of energy utilised, stored, or lost depends on multiple factors such as the nutrient type, the quantity of food consumed, the nutritional quality, and the type and level of physical activity, to name a few.

Calories are not a great appropriation for human metabolism and are mostly irrelevant (and often heavily misapplied) when it comes to influencing body composition change.

The common cliches "fat loss is all about being in a Calorie deficit" and "you can eat whatever you want as long as it fits your macros and Calorie targets" is terrible advice and should be met with rejection.

With all these factors to consider, you're probably now wondering, how on earth a person knows how much to eat and the types of foods they should be consuming? Furthermore, how does one keep track of everything and assess it if not for Calorie tracking? We will cover this later on and provide a longer-term solution that does not require food tracking (especially Calorie tracking).

The amount of food you consume matters, however, you cannot rely on Caloric values for determining your nutritional requirements and your lean-body outcomes. Also, there is often way too much misdirected preoccupation on the ill-informed quantitative aspects of food and too little emphasis on the underappreciated qualitative aspects of food when trying to promote a leaner and healthier body composition.

Instead of questioning "How many calories are in a given food?", some better questions to ask yourself about your food are: "How will a given food affect my appetite and energy levels?" and "What is the quality or nutritional value of a given food?", and "How will a given food affect my overall mass?" Answer these questions regularly and you will be well on your way to a leaner and healthier body without the CICO OCD.

When you understand and acknowledge the composition of your food, it becomes far easier to get the quantity right.

Making Macros Matter

> "THE TRUE BEAUTY AND ESSENCE OF THINGS LIE IN THEIR COMPOSITION. IT IS THROUGH UNDERSTANDING THE INTRICATE INTERPLAY OF ELEMENTS THAT WE GAIN A DEEPER APPRECIATION OF THEIR TRUE VALUE".
>
> ANONYMOUS

You have probably heard the term 'macros' thrown around in the fitness and nutrition space quite a lot. Macros refers to the three major macronutrients that make up the majority of a person's diet: protein, fat, and carbohydrates. The manipulation or preferencing of macros is behind many popular nutrition plans like low-fat and low-carb/ketogenic diets.

Some nutrition plans also do this in terms of expressing percentage ratios such as a 40/30/30 macro split diet, where 40% of the energy comes from carbs, and 30% comes from each fat and protein.

But before getting hung up on specific percentages or ratios for macronutrients, it would be wise to first consider what your own personal requirements are for essential amino acids (protein), essential fatty acids, as well as how many carbohydrates might be required to fuel your activities.

Protein

Protein is an essential macronutrient that plays numerous structural and functional roles in the body. Protein is required for building and repairing tissues of the body such skin, hair, nails, organs and, of course, muscle. Protein also assists with many vital roles in the body, including immune function, hormone production, and

MAKING MACROS MATTER

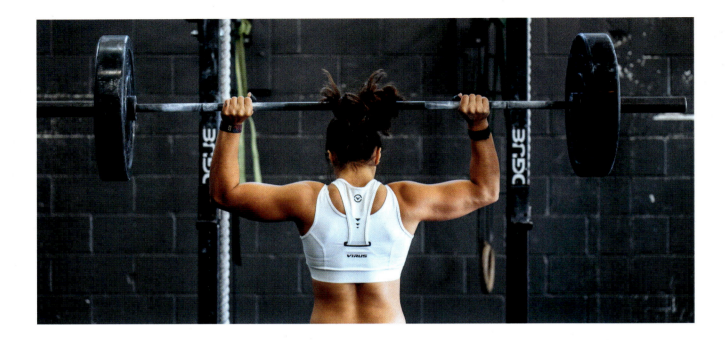

enzymatic function. Protein intake requirements remain relatively stable, regardless of changes in carbohydrate or fat consumption.

Getting enough protein is essential for maintaining your muscle tissue—especially if you're doing resistance training (as we advise our own clients doing our Lean Body Program). Doing resistance exercise increases muscle tissue breakdown (protein mass out) and will require more protein for tissue turnover, growth, and repair (protein mass in). Around 2.2 g of protein per kilogram (or 1.0 g of protein per pound) of bodyweight is a good starting point for protein if you're engaging in high-intensity forms of exercise like weight training.

For practicality and mathematical ease, we will use 2 g of protein per kilogram of bodyweight as an intake target throughout this text.

Unlike excess carbohydrate and fat, the body does not store excess protein as body fat. Protein tissue turnover needs to be met with a regular intake of adequate amino acids from the diet to facilitate what the body needs. If there is insufficient dietary protein intake, the body may not have enough amino acids available to support protein synthesis and maintenance. This can lead to negative nitrogen balance, where the rate of protein breakdown exceeds the rate of protein synthesis. This leads to a breakdown of your lean tissue and is not a good situation for your body in general.

On the flipside, excess protein intake beyond the body's needs will not be stored as body fat. Instead, it is processed by the kidneys and excreted via the urine. In some cases, excess protein can be metabolised and used for energy by the body, but protein is not the body's preferred fuel source. Sufficient protein rather than excessive protein is what's required. Also, if you have existing kidney problems, a diet too high in protein can cause further damage and is not advised.

If better body composition is the goal, consuming solely protein is not good practice, either. If there is inadequate carbohydrate or fat in the diet to meet energy demands, the body can begin to break down protein and muscle tissue for fuel (not ideal). This is one of the reasons why we suggest feeding the body every few hours and why we do not generally recommend prolonged periods of fasting.

Carbohydrates

Although exogenous carbohydrates are not essential for survival (the body can make glucose from other sources like protein and fats via processes such as gluconeogenesis), they are the body's most readily available fuel source for high-intensity exercise and replenishing glycogen stores thereafter. The rate at which carbohydrates can be broken down and utilised by the body as energy is faster than the rate at which fats or proteins can be utilised. Hence, carbohydrates can be used to support performance and muscle growth associated with high-intensity activities.

Determining carbohydrate intake, therefore, has a lot to do with the amount of high-intensity training a person is looking to engage in and the body size they're looking to attain. Out of all the macronutrients, carbs usually have the greatest effect on body mass. Thus, if fat loss is stagnating, carbs can be lowered, if required.

To maintain carbohydrate mass balance, carbohydrate intake needs to be balanced with the energy expenditure from carbohydrate oxidation.

All carbohydrates are eventually get broken down into glucose within the body. Any excess glucose beyond what your body requires for immediate energy is stored in the form of glycogen in the liver and the muscles. In the average-sized person, the liver can store between 70–100 grams of glycogen and the muscles can store around 400–500 grams. Once these glycogen stores are full, any additional carbohydrates consumed can be converted into body fat.

As previously alluded to, carbohydrates (along with dietary fat) are protein-sparing and their presence reduces the likelihood of protein being broken down for fuel by the body.

Fat

Fat is an essential macronutrient. It is required for the production of hormones that play vital roles in various bodily functions such as metabolism, growth, and reproduction. Adequate dietary fat intake is required to support healthy cell function and the overall health of the body's tissues and organs. Fat is also necessary for the absorption of various fat-soluble vitamins and certain antioxidants. Sufficient fat intake increases satiety as this macronutrient takes longer to digest than carbohydrates or protein. Fat is also the most energy-dense macronutrient (9 Calories per gram) and the body's preferred fuel source for prolonged endurance exercise and low- to moderate-intensity activities.

When the intensity of physical activity is lower, the body can efficiently utilise fat stores to provide the necessary energy. The body breaks down stored fat into fatty acids, which are then transported to the muscles and other tissues to be used as fuel (a process known as lipolysis). Interestingly, high-carbohydrates diets increase insulin levels and favour fat storage while inhibiting lipolysis—an interesting point to consider if you're wondering why you might not be getting leaner whilst trying to restrict 'Calories' on a diet consisting predominantly of carbohydrates.

About 1–2 g of fat per kilogram (or ~0.5 g–1.0 g of fat per pound) per day is the general recommendation to avoid essential fatty acid deficiency. In the presence of more carbs, it's usually sensible to keep fat to the minimum (1 g per kilogram of bodyweight) as high sugar and high fat over time can be a dangerous mix for one's health.

NOTE: Basing recommended amounts of macronutrients on a person's lean mass is slightly more accurate. However, using bodyweight is more practical and includes a wider range of

people who may not have access to more accurate methods of determining body composition.

Since dietary fat is highly satiating and good at suppressing hunger, ketogenic (high-fat, very low-carb) diets can be an effective approach and fat-loss solution for some people who struggle to lose fat (especially if they're not engaging in much high-intensity exercise). In a ketogenic diet, dietary fat is increased, protein intake is kept the same, while carbohydrate intake is very low (typically as close to zero as possible). Not only are ketogenic diets quite effective for losing fat via fat oxidation, fat can also be lost via the excretion of fatty acid derivatives when the body is in a state of ketosis.

Hence, when the body is utilising predominantly fat for energy, the 'mass out' part of the mass balance equation can be greater than otherwise due to hormonal changes that occur on lower carb diets. With that said, although it is easier to attain negative mass balance on a ketogenic diet (as you will later see), there still needs to be less mass in than out. One can't simply eat as much fat and protein as they like on a low-carb diet without putting on excess body fat at some stage.

The increased fat allowance with lowered sugar levels also allows for more fattier meats to also be consumed on ketogenic diets.

It's worth noting too that when the body shifts to a ketogenic diet, it also tends to release more water, as opposed to storing it. There are a couple of possible reasons for this. Firstly, glycogen is 3-4 parts water. When consuming fewer carbohydrates than usual, the body's glycogen stores become depleted, leading to water loss. Secondly, consuming less carbohydrates on a ketogenic diet also means the body produces less insulin. This decrease in insulin can signal the kidneys to excrete more water and retain less. Because body water carries electrolytes, any fluid loss usually results in the kidneys excreting more essential electrolytes too, particularly sodium, potassium, and magnesium. It should be noted that the extent of water and electrolyte loss on a ketogenic diet can vary greatly from person to person. The relationship between insulin levels and kidney function is complex and can be influenced by many factors.

Hence, when considering ketogenic dietary approaches, it would be prudent to first consult a relevant health professional or physician to make any necessary micronutrient adjustments.

Finding Good Macronutrient Sources and Substitutions

"YOU CAN'T POLISH A TURD".
AUSTRALIAN PROVERB

There are some great foods for getting leaner and healthier, and there are others that are not. We have included some lists below of foods with higher nutrient value that are segregated under each macronutrient. Food intolerances and personal medical provisions aside, consider including these foods when designing your own lean body nutrition plan. These lists are very handy for when you want to (or need to) substitute one food for another in your recipes and or daily nutrition plan. Boredom, variety, and availability are the usual factors that influence substitution. Getting leaner and healthier will likely not be a struggle if you stick to the following foods the majority of the time as outlined.

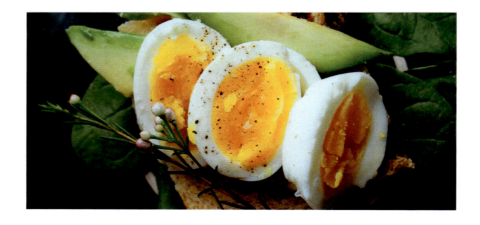

Good Sources of Protein

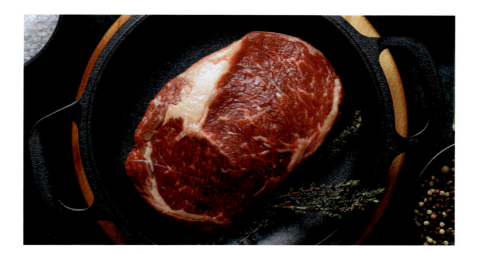

Animal sources:

- Poultry (whole cuts or ground)
- Red meat (whole cuts or ground)
- Eggs/egg whites (omega-3 and free-range preferred)
- Whey and other lean sources of protein powder (caseinate, egg white, etc.)
- Pork (whole cuts or ground)
- Game meats (venison, kangaroo, ostrich, etc.)
- Cottage cheese
- Plain Greek yoghurt
- Canned fish/seafood (e.g. salmon, tuna, sardines, etc.)
- Most fresh fish/seafood

Plant sources:

- Legumes: chickpeas, soybeans, lentils, black beans, pinto beans, etc.
- Protein powders: rice, pea, hemp, pumpkin
- Tempeh
- Tofu
- Seitan

NOTE: It must be noted here that plant sources are included for those who prescribe to this way of eating. However, plant sources of protein are naturally less bioavailable and contain incomplete proteins (not all amino acids are present).

Good Sources of Fat

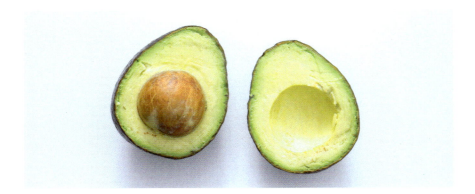

- Oils: fish, flaxseed, olive, perilla, sesame, coconut, and chia
- Seeds: sunflower, flax/linseed, hemp, chia, and pumpkin seeds
- Nuts: walnuts, Brazil nuts, almonds, pecans, pistachios, etc.
- Butters: ghee/clarified butter, almond and natural peanut butter
- Avocados

Good Sources of Carbohydrates

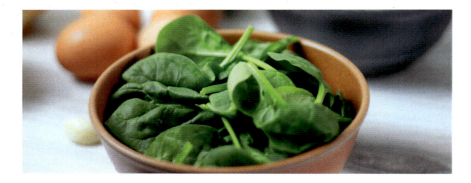

The following carb sources are arranged on a continuum of carbohydrate density and what should be consumed most versus least for attaining lean body goals:

Consumable at most times of the day:

- Leafy vegetables: spinach, kale, bok choy, cabbage varieties, lettuce varieties, etc

- Low-moderate starch vegetables: broccoli, cauliflower, green beans, asparagus, celery, radish, mushrooms, eggplant, cucumber, zucchini, onion, capsicum (bell pepper) varieties, carrots, peas, parsnips, squash, and pumpkin varieties

Consumable at some times of the day:

- Oats: whole, steel-cut, or rolled ('whole rolled oats' or 'old-fashioned oats')
- Fruits: citrus fruits, cantaloupe, berries, cherries, apples, pears, peaches, plums, apricots, kiwi fruit, papaya, bananas etc.
- Quinoa
- High-starch vegetables: potatoes, yams, sweet potatoes
- Legumes and beans: lentils, chickpeas, peas, Black beans, kidney beans, navy beans, pinto beans, soybeans, etc.
- Rice: non-white coloured forms such as brown, black, and wild rice varieties (minimally processed)

Best consumed within workout window:

- Wholegrain breads, cereals, and pastas (minimally processed)
- Dried and sugary fruits: dates, sultanas, raisins, etc.

The recipes you will find in the latter half of this book all incorporate ingredients from the macronutrient sources above. Beverages, condiments, flavourings, and other components that don't make up the bulk of one's diet will be addressed later on in this text. If you're wondering how macronutrient requirements can be calculated fully, this will also be addressed at a later stage. Although the macronutrient sources above are very nutritious and healthy, you can have too much of a good thing.

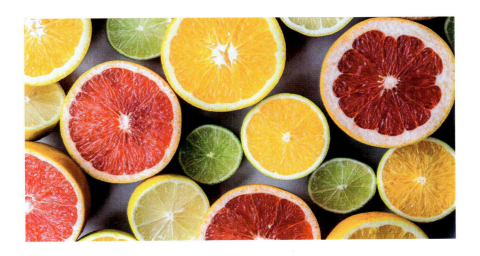

Eating Healthy?

"But I eat healthy" is a common objection we get from many people when questioning their nutrition, and promoting a leaner and healthier body composition to them. We can say with confidence that if you're not in a healthy body composition range, your diet is not 'healthy' and needs some work. This may come as a surprise to you but 'eating lean' is not the same as 'eating healthy'. We are not saying you should avoid healthy foods—what we are saying is that it's all a matter of context.

Although eating foods with better nutritional quality makes getting leaner far easier and more sustainable, you can still eat too many 'healthy' foods and be overweight (an 'unhealthy' trap many people fall into). The key word in the previous statement is 'too many'. As per the mass balance equation, if you're consuming too much mass relative to what you're excreting, you will naturally gain weight (and usually in the less desirable form of body fat).

And no, the answer is not to starve yourself, either. Our goal with this text is to help you get leaner while consuming wholesome food that tastes great!... without leaving you feeling like you're starving yourself. Looking one's best shouldn't come at the detriment of not feeling one's best.

We want you to eat to be lean and, at the same time, help you tick as many boxes that you can for your longer term health (including your mental health!). We can assume that by picking up this resource, that you're not only looking to get lean, but that you're also looking to STAY lean longer term. This book will help you do exactly that! It will also show you how you can pivot and adapt your own nutrition based on your evolving goals, life circumstances, and challenges.

The problem with most diet-based plans is that they don't give longer-term solutions to the person once the diet stops working or has run its course. Often, this happens for three main reasons.

1. The person doesn't get the desired body composition results from following the plan.

2. The person does not feel energised on the diet and begrudgingly eats the foods on the diet out of willpower. When the willpower taps out, the person reverts back to the foods they were eating previously, and there is no longer- term

FINDING GOOD MACRONUTRIENT SOURCES AND SUBSTITUTIONS

continuity of the diet they just invested themselves in (not just timewise and financially, but more so EMOTIONALLY).

3 Third, the person gets bored with eating the same foods all the time. Although the diet may produce positive body-composition results, the recipes and foods are repetitive, bland, and tasteless. The average Joe or Jane usually has a whole other lifestyle and set of circumstances that are not synonymous to that of an atypical meathead who sticks to the un-coveted chicken and broccoli six times per day.

We will soon show you how you can design your own plan, prepare your own tasty foods, eat on the run, substitute your foods, and determine how to make great food choices (even during the times you feel like you don't have control).

Oh, and if you ever ask yourself the question, "Why eat this particular food?", we have also highlighted the nutritional perks of the main ingredients in all of our recipes.

We don't just tell you how to make our recipes either—we show you, too! All our recipes come with pictures and many also have a video link within (ebook version) to demonstrate how simple and easy these are to create.

A lot of recipes on the market involve using a plethora of exotic ingredients, elaborate cooking techniques, and tons of time. Our methods, on the other hand, are time-efficient, easy to follow, and include ingredients you can source just about anywhere.

We will show you how to set up your kitchen and present you with the most proficient ways to prepare your food. With that said, we can't do it all for you, either—you will need to learn some basic life skills if they're lacking and chop your own carrots, so to speak.

You're going to make a lot of mistakes along the way, too, but you shouldn't let these deter you. Heck, we made ample errors while designing and refining many of the recipes in this book! Mistakes are part of the learning process and you will learn far more from your failures than you ever will from your successes. Something is only ever a true mistake if you don't learn from it. So get your hands dirty and do the work—it will be one the best decisions you ever make!

Before jumping into the kitchen, though, you will first need to determine where you're currently at and where you need to go with your body composition so you can develop a plan for getting there accordingly.

THE LEAN BODY SOLUTION

Determining Your Body-Composition Goals

"WHAT GETS MEASURED, GETS MANAGED".
PETER DRUCKER

Oftentimes, we want to go places without first determining where we are currently at and how to measure the distance in between. Before looking to change your body, it's wise to determine what it is currently composed of. The simplest definition of body composition is the amount of lean mass versus fat mass your body is made up of.

To find your body composition, you will need to know your body-fat percentage. This can be determined via various body scans or via calipers with an experienced health professional (more on these measurement tools below). Once you know your body composition, this can be a good way of directing your goals.

For instance, if you find that your body fat percentage is too high, you can lower your mass intake over time to get into a leaner range. If you are too lean or need to gain some muscle mass, you can increase your mass intake and/or decrease your mass expenditure. See the table below for the various body fat ranges:

Body fat percentages for various age ranges

Age	Men 20-29	Men 30-39	Men 40-49	Men 50-59	Men 60-69	Women 20-29	Women 30-39	Women 40-49	Women 50-59	Women 60-69
Unsustainably Low	<8%	<11%	<12%	<13%	<14%	<14%	<18%	<20%	<21%	<22%
Very Lean	8-11%	11-14%	12-17%	13-19%	14-20%	14-16%	18-21%	20-23%	21-25%	22-26%
Lean	11-15%	14-18%	17-21%	19-22%	20-23%	16-19%	21-24%	23-27%	25-29%	26-30%
Fair	15-19%	18-21%	21-23%	22-25%	23-25%	19-23%	24-27%	27-29%	29-32%	30-33%
High Fat	19-23%	21-25%	23-26%	25-28%	25-29%	23-27%	27-29%	29-31%	32-34%	33-36%
Dangerously High	23%>	25%>	26%>	28%>	29%>	27%>	29%>	31%>	34%>	36%>

The above table does not factor in variances in race or body type, but offers good general guidelines. As represented, it is generally not advised to sit at the extreme ends of the spectrum for body fat long term. It is also important to consider performance and that maintaining too low or too high of a body fat level can significantly affect recovery and overall long-term progress. In consideration of these factors, you should establish realistic outcome goals for your desired body fat levels.

If you are unsure of how to do this, then consult a qualified health professional in this area or simply send us a message at performancerevolution.com.au/#contact, stating your goals and current body-composition measurements.

Measuring Your Progress

"MEASURE YOUR PROGRESS IN INCREMENTS, CELEBRATE EVERY STEP FORWARD, AND EMBRACE EVERY OBSTACLE AS MERELY A CHALLENGE TO OVERCOME".

MARIE FORLEO

It's difficult to get any kind of results (and keep yourself accountable) if you're not measuring your progress regularly. When it comes to attaining your lean body goals, there are a number of tools you can use depending on the stage you are currently at in your lean body quest.

Before proceeding, it's worth mentioning that you should not get hung up emotionally on the body measuring tools that are about to be introduced. You're going to need a measurement of where you're at to determine your progress, while also being able to provide accurate data to make adjustments. This way you can better avoid stagnation and keep getting results on a more consistent basis going forwards.

We already hear some of you saying, "but getting on the scale gives me anxiety". That might be the case, but laying on a hospital bed one day in the future with many things jammed up every orifice of your body will cause you a great deal more anxiety. To prevent this, you need to take actions right NOW! This might be difficult to accept, but it's a lot easier to stomach when you remember that you're committed to changing your current predicament and you're taking the necessary steps to do so. You can take your measurements knowing that not all these tools will warrant eternal use and they will likely be required less once you have reached (and are maintaining) your desired body composition.

Below are the various measurement tools you can use, followed by guidelines based on the stage of the progress you're at. Be sure to download our bonus resources via the following link too - these include guidelines for how to measure your progress accurately and pick the right kind of implements to use.

VISIT LEANBODYSOLUTIONRESOURCES.GR8.COM FOR BONUS RESOURCES

Weight
(TAKEN DAILY, AVERAGED WEEKLY)

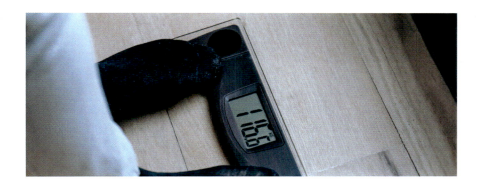

There are many factors affecting body weight and its trajectory is rarely ever linear. Sleep, dehydration and water intake, fatigue, time of the day, and a lot of other metabolic functions contribute to fluctuations in body weight.

Hence, the best time to take your weight is as soon as you wake up (if not, at another time of the day that is similar each time and relative to your meals). Do this each day of the week and divide the total by seven to get your average weekly weight. Again, don't get hung up with any day-to-day fluctuations on the scale. Weight is not the issue—it's what your weight is made up of that is!

Remember that most scale fluctuations are to do with changes in water weight (more than 60% of a person's mass). Also remember with weight we are looking for the trend of your average weekly weight scores going in the right direction over time. Recording your weight is necessary to make sense of your caliper measurements and determining some hard numbers around how much of your mass is lean vs fat mass.

Photographs
(TAKEN ONCE PER WEEK)

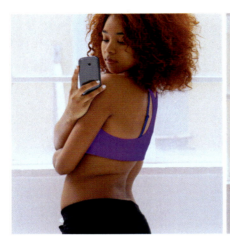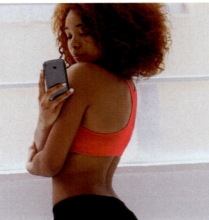

Photos are an excellent tool for tracking body composition changes. Great progress pictures are all about one thing—uniformity. Front, side, and rear photos taken at the same distance with similar attire and lighting are essential. If you haven't done so already, download our 'Perfect Progress Photo Taking Guide' via the link above so you can save time and get your photos right each and every time.

Photographs are usually the most emotionally profound way of actually 'seeing' your changes and keeping motivated towards your goal. If you have resistance to taking photos, simply ask yourself whether you get more motivated by seeing your numbers like your weight go down, or more so when a friend who hasn't seen you in a little while remarks that you're looking leaner? We bet it's the latter by a long way! You might brush your teeth in the mirror each day, but you're unlikely to see the small changes that compound over time.

And if you want some more encouragement and motivation to take photos, send them to us (**info@performancerevolution.com.au**) and we can give you some feedback on your progress. To minimise variability, it's best to take your photos at the same time of day each time (first thing in the morning when you wake up preferably). Remember, always take your progress photos! Even if you don't feel you're making progress. When taken properly, they're the best way to measure progress and can be a more profound guide than body-composition measures such as skinfold and scans.

Girths
(EVERY FORTNIGHT)

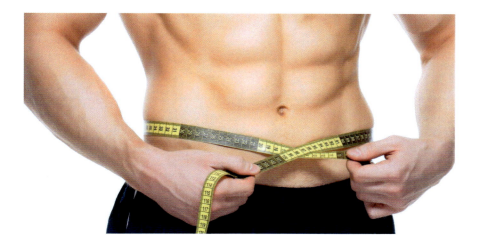

Measuring your girths with a tape measure is good for determining which areas of the body are becoming smaller or larger relative to others while also giving you a great indication for the clothing sizes you are aiming for. Using a tape measure can also highlight where you may be disproportionate in size relative to other body parts. Again, doing these first thing upon waking up in the morning is preferable. If not, at the same time of day each occasion.

Skinfolds
(FORTNIGHTLY)

Girths can tell us which areas of the body are enlarging or shrinking but they don't tell us exactly what those areas are composed of (i.e. how much is muscle versus fat). This is where calipers come into play. Calipers will help you determine where you're storing the most fat and which aspects of your physique are leaner relative to others. If possible, have someone else (preferably someone trained and experienced) take your girth measurements and skinfolds regularly. Also make sure it is the same person taking these each time so you can have consistency with your measurements.

DEXA scan
(EVERY FEW MONTHS)

Like calipers, DEXA scans are very handy for determining whether you're losing or gaining muscle mass or fat mass. Although not essential for the body-composition metrics just mentioned (if you're using calipers and girths), DEXA scans are more accurate and can also be beneficial for measuring bone density and helping assess one's risk of bone diseases like osteoporosis. DEXA scans can be booked at most radiology clinics for a small fee.

Each of the measurement tools above will be more or less relevant depending on where you're at with your body composition goals and how much fat you have to lose. Below are some guidelines for determining which stage you are currently at and which measurements should be given priority:

Stage 1: More fat to lose ('dangerously high' category)

Daily weight (averaged weekly), weekly photographs, and fortnightly girths will usually suffice for this group. You have a lot of fat to lose and you know it... you don't need to be beaten over the head with it! These three measures will usually be enough to indicate if you're heading in the right direction or not.

Stage 2: Less fat to lose (below 'dangerously high' category)

When heading into leaner territory, it's still important to lose fat, but you also want to limit the loss of lean mass or muscle tissue in the process. The law of diminishing returns is setting in, too, if you reached this point from a much heavier bodyweight. If you fall into the latter category, the rate of weight loss is now slower in absolute terms but may be similar in relative terms (something to remember).

In addition to taking your weight, photographs, and girths, you will also benefit from fortnightly caliper measurements at this stage, too. These additional measures will help you to better determine your body composition. A DEXA scan every few months or so won't hurt, either.

Now that you know where you're at and how to determine your body composition at the various stages of your lean body quest, you can begin to construct your own nutrition plan to reach your goals.

MEASURING YOUR PROGRESS

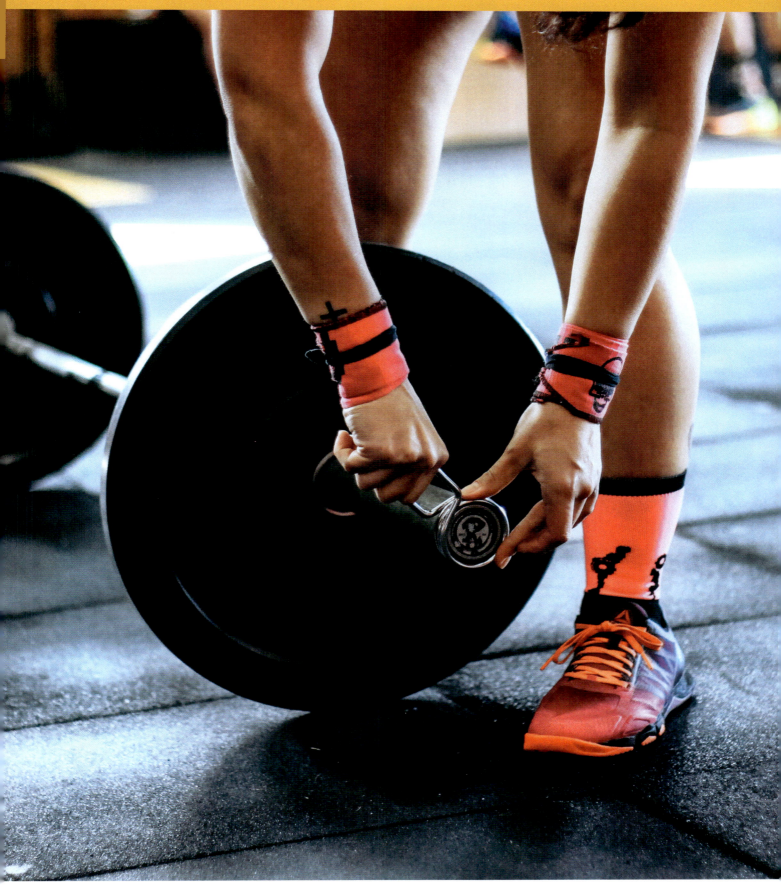

THE LEAN BODY SOLUTION   45

Designing Your Lean Body Nutrition Plan

"A GOAL WITHOUT A PLAN IS JUST A WISH".
ANTOINE DE SAINT-EXUPÉRY

Once you have established your body-composition goals, it's time to take action and start changing your own nutrition accordingly. There are two ways you can go about this:

The Principled Approach

For most people, adherence to good nutrition principles and the introduction to eating leaner, more nutritious foods (such as the ones promoted in this text) is enough to lean one down to a healthy and sustainable body fat range, without having to be too meticulous in measuring consumption. If you focus on consuming the food and recipe options we provide, you should notice a big difference in not only the way you look but also in the way you feel. For some, this approach is just what they need to not only get their body in better shape, but also to have enough variety and freedom in their diet without it 'eating away' at them mentally.

The principled approach can be especially helpful if you have struggled to maintain a lean and healthy body composition over time. Here are our seven Lean Body principles:

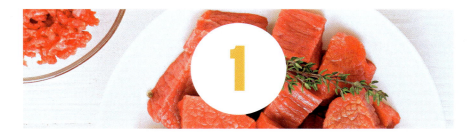

BUILD MEALS AROUND COMPLETE PROTEIN

Whether it's breakfast, dinner, dessert, or a snack on the run, including enough protein is vital for muscle repair and maintenance (amongst other important needs). Because the body doesn't store excess protein like it does with excess carbohydrates and fats, protein needs to be consumed regularly. Compared to carbohydrates and fats, protein has a higher thermic effect and generates more heat in the body when ingested. This is associated with an increased metabolic rate and energy demand from the body.

Protein also has a very positive effect on satiety (i.e. how full you feel), which is very important if you're trying to strip fat off your frame and avoid overeating. For these reasons, it's good practice to regularly include enough complete protein in your meals where all the amino acids are present for usability (plant-based eaters take note!). It can't be understated that getting enough protein is an extremely important ingredient for enhancing a person's metabolic processes and succeeding with one's lean body goals.

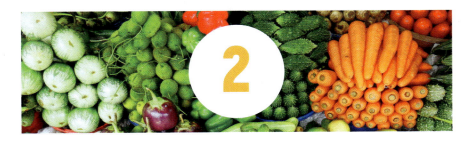

MAKE IT COLOURFUL

Including a variety of vegetables and fruit in an array of different colours will make most meals healthier and more fibrous (leaving you feeling fuller for longer). This practice also helps ensure that you are getting all the micronutrients and disease-fighting properties of a healthy diet that has enough fruits and vegetables.

Most people lack more vegetables than fruit in their diet. When most people are told to eat more vegetables, they think they have to conjure up a whole lot of new meals and snack items dedicated to just these—this is not the case.

A smart approach is to simply start adding these into meals and snacks they're already consuming. For instance, adding veggies to wraps, sandwiches, soups, stir fries, and even shakes is simple and can really bump up one's overall intake. Fruit can also be mixed in with foods like yoghurt, salads, quinoa, and oats. A lack of veggies and fruit is usually more a sign of a lack of thought than anything else.

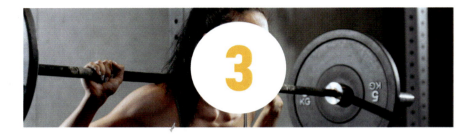

STRAIN BEFORE SUGARS AND STARCHES

More carbohydrates can be processed by the body in the presence of the hormone insulin when they are being utilised for fuel by the muscles (glycogen), rather than being stored as fat on your frame. When are insulin levels naturally elevated? During and after intense exercise. This is part of the reason why we like higher-intensity forms of exercise like resistance training when it comes to lean body goals. Hence, carbohydrates are usually best consumed around intense workout times (particularly during the few hours right before, during, and after training).

This way, you likely only consume carbohydrates that your body utilises whilst ensuring you don't needlessly inflate a spare tyre. This principle applies to sweet and sugary foods and also starchier foods like rice, pasta, bread, and other grains that are more dense in carbohydrates. Going crazy and pigging out on sugars and starches is not recommended: 0.5–1.0 g per kilogram of bodyweight per day of these types of carbs (after intense training) is a good general guideline here if your goal is to lose fat.

For the rest of the day, carbohydrates should mainly come from less starchier forms and other fibrous sources such as vegetables and to a lesser extent fruit.

DESIGNING YOUR LEAN BODY NUTRITION PLAN

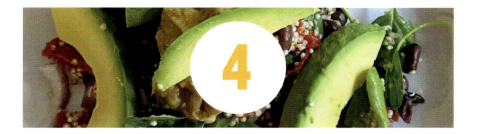

MAKE IT WHOLE

Many people talk about eating whole foods, but few realise the importance. Living off shakes and juices all the time is not only impractical, but it will often run its course quickly. A lot of the fullness we experience from food comes down to how it needs to be digested and broken down. If you're constantly missing the first parts of the digestion process and not chewing and breaking down your food, it not only has a big impact on how full you will feel, but also how long it takes the satiety signal to go from your gut to your brain. This means that it is very easy to fill up with more than required if your food is always broken down in advance.

The 'make it whole' principle also applies to processed foods. These foods are not only easier to consume in most cases, but also usually have a lot of the nutritional value lost in their processing (and commonly lack dietary fibre). To ensure you're getting the most out of your food both from a satiety and health standpoint, it's wise to make the majority of your food whole food. If you're eating something from a packet, also realise that the longer the ingredients list is, usually the further away the food is from being a proper whole food.

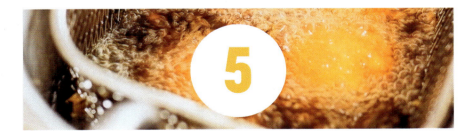

WATCH OUT FOR BAD FATS

The average western diet contains an excessive amount of fat from highly refined cooking oils, processed snack foods, fatty deli meats, and highly processed dairy products. A reduction of these

THE LEAN BODY SOLUTION

sources of fats and the inclusion of healthier fats will often do wonders for most people's body composition. It will also usually do amazing things for one's hormones and susceptibility to many health issues, too! We are not saying that low-fat is the key; we are saying that right-fat is the key.

The three categories of fats to pay attention to are saturated, monounsaturated, and polyunsaturated fats. We usually get enough of the first kind. The other two, however, usually need more direct attention and intervention. Quality monounsaturated fats can be sourced from foods like almonds, olive oil, and avocados. Quality polyunsaturated fat can be sourced from things like fish oil, walnuts, and ground flaxseeds. Getting the right fats in the right amounts usually results in improved blood and hormonal profiles, and can ultimately help people lose excess body fat.

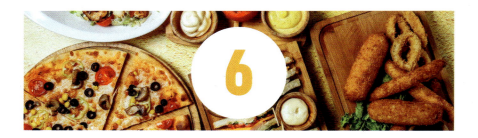

GIVE A TENTH OF ALL EARNINGS

Of all the meals you consume, you can tithe 10 per cent. This means that if your goal is to get within a healthy body composition range, a tenth of the foods/drinks you consume don't really matter that much and can come from sources not suggested in this guide. For example, if you consume four meals per day (28 per week), that means roughly three can be of similar size, but can differ from the normal make up. When for the most part, your nutrition is similar to what we put forth in this guide, your body becomes acclimated to these foods and the internal environment you're creating. So much so, that when you eat or drink a little differently from time to time, these small inputs usually have a negligible overall effect.

Not only can you keep your lean body results and health intact by observing this principle, you can also keep your sanity, too! Remember that perfection is not achievable (nor is it desirable) when it comes to nutrition. One small mistake often leads to total derailment and an all-or-nothing mindset where perfection is replaced by 'blowing' an entire diet. Context is key! This principle can also apply to undereating or overeating by ten per cent occasionally, too.

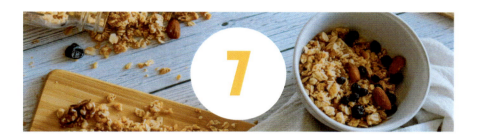

KNOW YOUR PORTIONS

Being able to properly estimate portions is an integral part of long-term lean body composition success. Although the principled approach to getting leaner doesn't require sticking to a set meals or predetermined nutrient amounts, we do encourage some form of recording initially (such as in a food diary or using a nutrition-tracking app). This way you can get to know your nutrition by inputting the foods and beverages you are consuming in their relative amounts.

Getting to know your portions and intake regularly will not only help you become more aware of what you're eating and when, but it will also help you to intuitively learn nutrient density, macronutrient composition, and the serving sizes of various foods and beverages. People who track their nutritional quantities generally have greater control of their body composition than those who don't. This is because simply examining an activity forces you to pay attention to it (yes—mindless eating is indeed true!). In other words, becoming aware of what and how much you throw down your pie hole (along with the associated triggers) makes you more self-accountable. And no, this doesn't mean zealous 'Calorie tracking'.

Knowing what you're consuming is also very important for the times you hit a plateau in your lean body pursuit. If you're aware of what and how much you are consuming, it's a lot easier to alter your intake accurately... as opposed to shooting in the dark.

If your goal is to lean down and you're consuming a surplus of certain nutrients, you are likely going to gain fat. If you're consuming the right amount of certain nutrients, however, you will likely lose fat. Even if you don't follow our example recipes per se, it is still prudent to consider the information in the coming sections to gain some perspective on your main nutrient needs for your goals. This way you can get an idea of how much of each nutrient to consume on average each day, while also avoiding being caught dumbfounded with what to do when hitting a roadblock in progress.

Tracking your nutrition and knowing your portions is imperative for adopting the 'calculative approach' in the next section and personalising your nutrition further.

How long should a person track their intake for and how do they know when it's time to stop? There is no hard and fast rule, but from our experience with coaching many clients over the years, the best time to stop is when a person reaches their desired body-composition goals and they can maintain these habitually.

If you achieve your own desired results and then start to lose course, body composition measurements and other health indicators can alert you to this. If you have fallen off track, it's likely time to start tracking your nutritional intake again.

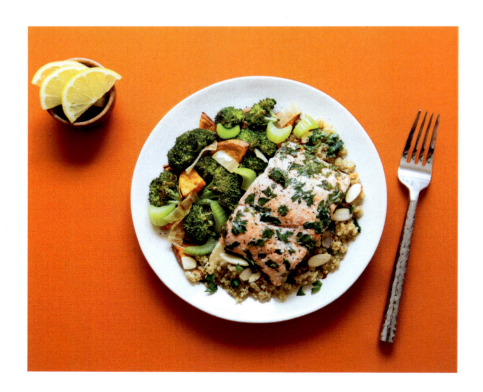

The Calculative Approach

The principled approach previously explained works great for getting most people in a leaner and healthier body composition range and staying there longer term.

This approach emphasises eating predominantly nutrient-rich, high-quality foods (like the ones we put forth in this guide) most of the time. If you focus on following these principles consistently, your satiety signalling will likely be quite good and you will intuitively learn how much to eat without having to track your intake.

However, before most people can adopt this approach and be intuitive with their eating, they first need insight regarding their nutrition. Some people also require more structure and may have very specific body-composition goals that demand further personalisation.

Depending on how far you want to go with your lean body goals (i.e. how lean you want to get) will determine how much attention you will need to give to dietary control.

Although not a longer term solution for most, there can be a time and place for structured plans to reach a leaner body composition. In fact, to have better intuition regarding foods and their various effects on the body, we recommend to all our clients that they do the calculative approach at least once for a decent amount of time (usually until they attain and can maintain a healthy body composition range without much effort).

This more personalised approach to nutrition is based around solid numbers and daily targets. In the coming sections we provide simple and practical methods we use with clients for determining nutrient requirements, along with some examples of daily eating that are constructed around these targets.

Calculating Your Lean Body Nutritional Requirements

> "CONFORMITY IS THE JAILER OF FREEDOM AND THE ENEMY OF GROWTH".
> JOHN F. KENNEDY

The Traditional Way

The common method for determining overall energy balance is usually done by factoring in a person's weight and activity level and then using a table similar to the one below to calculate the Caloric requirements to lose weight, gain weight, or maintain weight:

	Weight x Energy Factor	Bodyweight (Pounds)	Weight Loss	Weight Maintenance	Weight Gain
Activity Level	Minimal (1–2 per week)		11	13	17
	Moderate (3–4 per week)		13	15	19
	High (5–6 per week)		15	17	21

Here is an example of this method in action:

Joe, a 41-year-old man, was very active in his twenties and weighed 85 kg at 15% body fat (fair range). He has since dropped off with

CALCULATING YOUR LEAN BODY NUTRITIONAL REQUIREMENTS

his exercise and diet in his thirties and has put on 15 kg of fat. He now weighs 100 kg (220 lb) and is 27.75% body fat (dangerously high range).

Joe proceeds to track his nutritional intake and determines that his average daily energy intake comes out to be 3200 Calories (80 g fat, 160 g protein, 460 g carbs).

Joe then decides he wants to get back to where he was and lose the fat that has crept onto his frame over the last decade or so. He also decides to take up resistance training three times per week to help prevent his muscle mass withering away as he gets older. As per the energy balance table above, this would equate to an intake of 2860 calories per day as calculated below:

220 x 13 = 2860

Joe decides to cut Calories but does not change the composition of his diet—he simply decides to eat less of the same kinds of foods. Like Joe, this is the starting point for many people's fat loss goal and it's, wrongly, also the end. Many begin to start tracking Calories and try to fit whatever foods they like within these new restricted Caloric parameters. They may succeed for a number of weeks and months, however, they start to tire, burn out, and their body starts to crave the previous intake again (and oftentimes even more to avoid this situation).

They then lower their Caloric intake again in a desperate attempt to lose fat. They repeat the process only to wind up with more of the same. Then comes the rebound. The person becomes ravenous and a lot more food is then consumed than required (especially foods high in sugar and fat). All of the body fat piles back on (and often more) and this also usually replaces any lean tissue lost in the previous process.

The person then gets sick of being heavier and decides to try the process again, only to fall victim to the same innate urges—another yo-yo dieter is born.

As you can see from this illustration, energy balance does matter. However, as discussed earlier, energy balance is not the defining factor in determining body-composition change, and Calorie counting is certainly not the answer to getting both leaner and healthier longer term. This is where the concept of mass balance comes into the equation.

Macros, Micros, and Mass Balance

Nutrients can be ingested via the diet as macronutrients (e.g. carbs, fat, and protein) or micronutrients (e.g. vitamins and minerals). Nutrients can even be generated from within the body, such as when the liver creates glucose via gluconeogenesis (in the instance of a ketogenic diet).

When nutrients enter the body, they can be utilised for various functions such as energy production, tissue synthesis, and storage. Nutrients can also be discarded from the body via exhalation, faeces, urine, and sweat.

Mass balance is attained when the amount of nutrients entering the body equals the amount utilised or excreted by the body. Hence, a state of mass balance means there is no net gain or loss of nutrients over time.

Attaining a healthy body composition and good mass balance is not just about getting the balance of macronutrients right, it's also about getting the balance of micronutrients right, too. Here is an example to better illustrate this; let's consider our 41-year-old overweight man Joe again. Let's suppose Joe's diet for a long time has contained processed foods that are high in sugar and carbohydrates, and low in nutritional quality (not uncommon!).

Over the years, he has accumulated excess body fat and has also developed some nutrient deficiencies, which affect how his body functions. He then decides to gradually transition to a more nutritious diet that is rich in vegetables, quality protein, and healthy fats. In the process, his nutrient deficiencies begin to resolve and his body is better able to utilise the nutrients in his diet. His nutrient intake becomes sufficient to meet his body's essential needs, his excess body fat diminishes, and any excess nutrients are excreted. In this scenario, Joe has been effectively shifting his body towards proper mass balance.

He could further enhance this process, too, by engaging in resistance training regularly each week to help strengthen his body, enhance its systems, and encourage increased demand for bone and muscle tissue synthesis (and increased protein intake to account for the increased turnover).

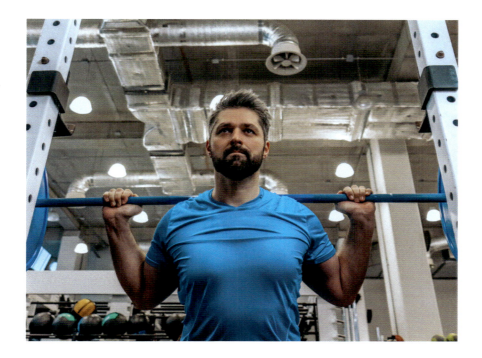

Many people in a similar predicament to Joe often don't take the appropriate countermeasures and instead mistake a steady and slow decline in metabolism for a fast one. In reality, most people are not really accounting for all of the inputs and outputs, nor are they doing their body many favours in the process.

Are there other factors that need to be accounted for when striving to achieve proper mass balance? Yes; the body's nutrient needs can vary depending on a number of factors such as age, sex, and overall health status. There are also environmental and lifestyle factors that can affect nutrient needs and metabolism, too, such as stress, activity level, and sleep (a little more on these later).

On the surface, achieving mass balance between all the macronutrient and micronutrient inputs and outputs might appear challenging (and that may be true). However, it is worth noting that a person cannot achieve perfect mass balance. What is desirable is an adequate balance of nutrients in and out of the body, and this is very attainable for most people.

There are also ways of making nutrition and mass balance easier when it comes to being leaner and healthier (which is likely the reason you picked up this text). One way we do this for our own clients is using our easy 1-2-C approach.

The 1-2-C Method

When determining a person's macronutrient requirements for their goals, the common method is to fixate on Calories and use a table such as the one in the prior 'energy balance' section. With Calories employed as the overarching factor, a bunch of multiplication, division, and subtraction are used to determine the proportion of macronutrients and fit these within the Caloric parameters.

Our approach is different and focuses on getting the key determinant of body composition change (nutrient mass) right for the person and their goals. Our method is also simple enough that any person can easily calculate and verify the numbers for themselves without much effort. As the name of this section implies, it's also a very easy way of remembering one's daily targets.

As per the 'Making Macros Matter' section, we use the following numbers for this method with our clients:

> 1 = 1 g of fat x bodyweight (kg)
> 2 = 2 g of protein x bodyweight (kg)
> C = carbs

Carbs will vary based on the type and level of activity. In the case that the client is engaging in higher-intensity exercise (such as intense resistance training), the following table is sought for the carb multiplier:

	Weight x Carb Factor	Bodyweight (Kilograms)	Weight Loss	Weight Maintenance	Weight Gain
High-Intensity Physical Activity Level	Minimal (1–2 per week)		x1.5g	x3.0g	x4.5g
	Moderate (3–4 per week)		x3.0g	x4.5g	x6.0g
	High (5–6 per week)		x4.5g	x6.0g	x7.5g

As an example, let's use Joe, the 41-year-old moderately active man, again and plug his numbers into the above table to determine his daily targets:

CALCULATING YOUR LEAN BODY NUTRITIONAL REQUIREMENTS

Fat: 100 x 1.0 g = 100 g
Protein: 100 x 2.0 g = 200 g
Carbohydrate: 100 x 3.0 g = 300 g
Total mass intake = 600 g

Interestingly, if you add up the above macronutrient numbers in Caloric values, they come out to be very similar to those that are derived from the targets in the energy balance section:

2900 vs 2860

You might now be tempted to think that overall Calories must still be the leading and guiding factor in determining body composition change. Remember, though, that mass balance and energy balance are separate balances in the body and both can go in the same or different directions. However, as you will soon see in explicit examples, it is the underlying mass balance that will dictate changes in weight and body composition (energy has no mass).

It does not end with just accounting for fat, protein, and carbs when it comes to mass balance. There are some other forms of mass that we should also factor in:

- **Fibre:** The standard minimum daily requirement for most women is 25 g of fibre per day, and 30 g for most men. Those with higher-energy requirements and larger persons (such as Joe in our example) can often consume more if required. For most people, getting an adequate amount of fibre can help promote satiety, stabilise blood sugar at lower levels, and enhance overall digestion and gut health.

  However, fibre intake can vary based on a number of factors with individual demands and tolerance levels varying from person to person. To learn more about fibre requirements, see the 'Framing Fibre' section of this text.

- **Water:** Do not overlook water, either: more than 60% of a person's body mass is water. Getting enough water is extremely important as it is involved in a multitude of metabolic processes. We have dedicated an entire section to water accordingly. See the section, 'Getting Your Water Intake Right'. Our man Joe is again used as an example, and his target came out to be 4 L per day.

CALCULATING YOUR LEAN BODY NUTRITIONAL REQUIREMENTS

- **Alcohol:** If you decide to drink, this should also not go unchecked, either. Alcohol can affect a person in numerous and profound ways (both physically and cognitively). Appetite stimulation, dehydration, and altered energy metabolism are just some of the ways alcohol can affect the body. One needs to decide whether or not consuming alcohol is worth it given their own personal situation (more on this later).

  Again, we have dedicated a section to alcohol accordingly. See the section, 'About Alcohol'.

- **Micronutrients:** It's not just macronutrients that matter when it comes to achieving mass balance. As previously mentioned, getting an adequate amount of various micronutrients is also required for a healthy and well-functioning body. There is a long list of micronutrients and going into the requirements for each would be in a magnitude beyond the scope of this text. Eating a variety of the foods from the 'Good Macronutrient Sources' section will provide many of these nutrients in good amounts.

  From time-to-time, it can be prudent to have blood tests and analysis of nutritional intake by a dietitian or qualified health professional. These measures can help determine whether a person is obtaining (and absorbing) enough essential vitamins, minerals, and other nutrients in their diet. Getting sufficient amounts of the required micronutrients is not only essential for proper metabolism and physiological function, it's also essential for staving off disease and optimising both physical and cognitive functioning.

  By now, you should be more clear on what sort of targets you can aim for with your nutrition each day in order to lean down. At this point, you may be wondering how you might put these elements together and structure your own nutrition plan. We will cover this in the coming sections along with troubleshooting methods that can be employed if you encounter stagnation with your progress.

Structuring Your Lean Body Plan

> **"ADAPTATION SEEMS TO BE, TO A SUBSTANTIAL EXTENT, A PROCESS OF REALLOCATING YOUR ATTENTION".**
> DANIEL KAHNEMAN

Meal Timing and Frequency

If you have been following along closely, you will have noticed that our general recommendation to our clients with a lean body goal is regular eating every few hours. This is due to a few reasons we have touched on earlier. The first being that protein needs regular replenishment for the growth, repair, and maintenance of lean tissue (this is especially important if you're doing higher-intensity forms of training such as strength training). Remember, that unlike excess carbs and fat, the body doesn't store excess protein as body fat. Protein tissue turnover (mass out) needs to be met with the intake of adequate amino acids from the diet (mass in).

The task of getting more protein might seem difficult, however, it becomes simple if all meals and snacks are built around complete protein (as per our guidelines in 'The Principled Approach' section). We realise that at times this approach may not be feasible due to a person's work or essential life circumstances. However, the human body is the human body and it does not contemplate and negotiate metabolic processes based on a person's schedule. Every 2–3 hours is optimal, and every 4–5 hours at a stretch is advised for most of our client's with lean body goals.

Muscle protein synthesis is not the only reason why protein should be consumed regularly. Remember that protein also has a very positive effect on satiety (i.e. how full you feel). Hence, regular consumption of protein will often result in a person eating less overall and dissuade them from overeating. If you're a person who regularly skips breakfast (and no, coffee is not breakfast), gets hungrier as the day goes on, and backloads the latter half of your day with excessive eating, then take note!

Using Joe again as an example, here is how he might structure his meals and snacks over time to reach his original targets:

- **Breakfast: Quick & Warm Protein Fruit Muesli**
  (fat: 29 g, protein: 40 g, carbs: 60 g)

- **Snack:** 2x **Coconut Rough Protein Balls**
  (fat: 10 g, protein: 20 g, carbs: 18 g)

- **Lunch: Reuben-Style Turkey Sandwich**
  (fat: 15 g, protein: 38 g, carbs: 47 g)

- **Lunch Side: Spicy Red Pepper Tomato Soup**
  (fat: 2.5 g, protein: 3 g, carbs: 20 g)

- **Post-Workout Snack: Better Choc Banana Protein Smoothie**
  (fat: 3 g, protein: 27 g, carbs: 36 g)

- **Dinner: Zesty Chicken & Black Bean Burrito**
  (fat: 7 g, protein: 25 g, carbs: 64 g)

- **Dinner Side:** 2 serves of **Sofrito**
  (fat: 14.5 g, protein: 4 g, carbs: 36 g)

- **Dessert: Choc Mint Protein Mousse** with 2x **Cocoa Black Bean Brownies** (fat: 18 g, protein: 65 g, carbs: 36 g)

The specific recipes used above can be found in the 'Lean Body Recipes' section of this text.

The structure above is about as close as one gets to hitting total daily targets:

Fat = 99 g
Protein = 222 g
Carbs = 317 g
Total mass intake = 638 g
Cals = 2849

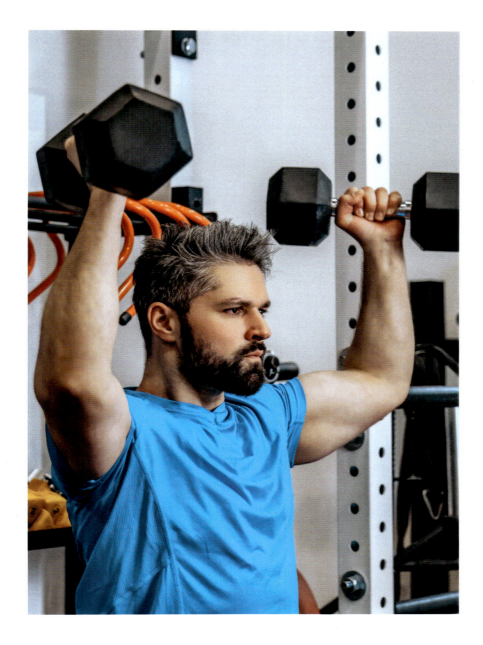

In this example, if Joe was not able to take a break and eat his morning snack at work, he could simply combine this with his breakfast. Alternatively, he could also create a structure with fewer but bigger meals for that particular day.

You may have also noticed that Joe's biggest meals of the day are astutely placed and coincide with his workout time. This way, more of the carbohydrates that he consumes will be utilised during his workout for energy and replenishing depleted muscles thereafter (instead of being stored as body fat).

Switching Things Up

If you feel the meals or recipes in the previous example may be too elaborate for someone in your situation, you need not worry. You can definitely have easier and more basic combinations of foods in your plan. The key determining factor is whether you are picking the right kind of foods and you're eating them in the right amounts. Refer to the 'Good Macronutrient Sources and Substitutions' section of this text for ideas here.

If you're getting sick of a particular meal or food, then you can simply swap it out for another food on the list or one of our Lean Body recipes that falls within your targets (i.e. macronutrient targets).

Having clients switch up their foods over time is not something we try to make them avoid; instead, we often welcome it! This way they have flexibility within parameters and can help themselves (both mentally AND physically) to a variety of good foods, while also ensuring that they get an adequate amount of nutrients from all of the food groups.

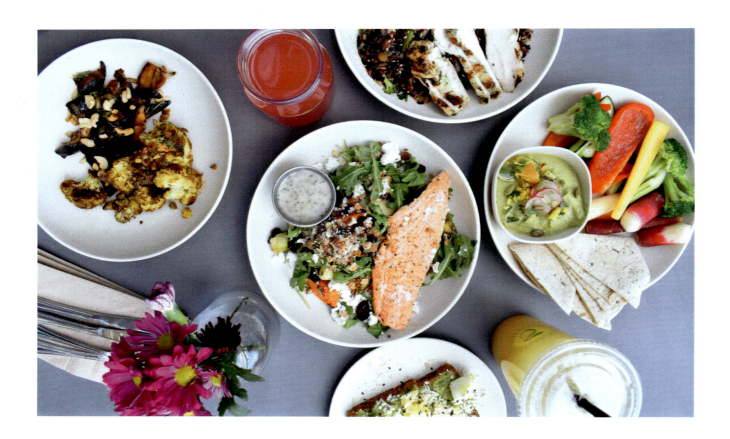

If you're doing all this and find you start to halt with your fat loss, then it's likely you are not accounting for everything you are consuming. If you're consuming other foods and beverages that are not accounted for in your plan (more on these soon), it's very likely that you will gain fat. This is why it is important in the developing stages to keep track of your intake and see what might be causing you to stall or go in the wrong direction with your body composition.

The occasional social occasion is okay as long as it's, by definition, 'occasional', and what is consumed is thought about in advance and factored into the equation. It's important to remember, too, that you have the most accuracy and influence over your nutrition if you prepare your meals yourself. Constantly relying on takeaway, dining out, or situational food options is a much harder path to losing fat than if you put yourself in charge and know exactly what you're putting in your mouth (you're also far less inclined to succumb to social pressures this way, too).

To help you get started with your lean body lifestyle, we have provided a plethora of tasty recipes in the 'Lean Body Recipes' section that you're welcome to use. We have tested these on our clients over the years and tweaked them for the best results possible. These can provide you with some practical ways you can structure your meals to fit your daily plan, as well as some easy swaps if you get bored. Again, feel free to substitute with your own options and ideas. As long as you're staying within your personal targets and your meals are congruent with the principles in this text, you will see great results with your body over time.

If you're unsure about how to structure your nutrition to get all the necessary macronutrients and micronutrients in the right amounts for you and your situation, then consider our Lean Body Program. We have dealt with a lot of clients from all walks of life who've had many unique challenges and problems to solve. Our qualified coaches and dietitians can work with you personally to help you construct a plan that is simple to follow, enjoyable to consume, and flexible enough for your lifestyle. The program is designed to support people each step of the way so that they can not only learn and advance at a faster pace, but also so they can enjoy better results longer term. Visit **theleanbodyprogram.gr8.com** for more info.

Troubleshooting Nutrition and Overcoming Stagnation

> "WE CANNOT SOLVE OUR PROBLEMS WITH THE SAME THINKING WE USED WHEN WE CREATED THEM".
>
> ALBERT EINSTEIN

It's not unusual to encounter plateaus in progress when leaning down—in fact, it is wise to expect them at some stage. It's knowing what to do in these situations that will determine whether stagnation or further advancement will be the proceeding pattern going forwards. To illustrate this best, let's use Joe again as an example.

Joe started off well with his established targets (as devised in the '1-2-C Method' section) and after a couple of months has lost 6 kg (~13 lb) of body fat and is down to a bodyweight of 94 kg (~207 lb). He is now in the fair range for his age category with a body fat percentage of around 23%. However, Joe's fat loss has plateaued over the last couple of weeks; he often now finds his energy levels are a bit depleted throughout numerous times of the day. He also is not doing enough work at a high enough intensity (relative to his body size) in the gym, and thus he's not depleting glycogen as much as he originally anticipated. Despite this, Joe desperately wants to get down to his goal weight of 85 kg and 15% body fat.

Joe is really determined and wants to waste no time with delayed progress in his weight loss. To get to his goal, Joe decides to follow conventional wisdom. He abruptly lowers his 'Calories' in an effort to lose fat again. He pays no attention to composition of his diet and decides to slash 1000 Calories equally between fat, protein, and carbohydrate.

His daily intake numbers then begin to look like this:

> **Fat:** 100 x 0.66 g = 66 g
> **Protein:** 100 x 1.3 g = 130 g
> **Carbohydrate target:** 100 x 1.96 g = 196 g
> **Total mass intake =** 392 g
> **Cals =** 1900

Although this work's initially from a weight-loss perspective, Joe begins to lose his muscle mass with the lower than required protein intake. His energy levels start to crash even further and his body ravenously starts craving lots of food (understandably). Joe's diet now becomes unsustainable and he rebounds in a big way. He starts to consume a lot more food—especially foods high in sugar and fat (see examples in 'Not All Foods Are Created Equal' section). He overcompensates, and within a short amount of time, he is consuming far above even his initial intake targets at a bodyweight of 100 kg.

After not too long, Joe has gained A LOT of body fat and is in a worse position than where he started with his goals. Not only is the physical detriment on Joe quite substantial in this scenario, but the psychological impact on him is even more profound. He begins to either doubt his ability to attain a better body composition (resolving to 'live large'), or he begins a series of similar attempts at various times in the future that all amount to the same outcome (yo-yo dieting).

Joe's story is unfortunately not uncommon. It typifies the approach of many people in a similar position and is an experience that may sound quite synonymous to that of your own. It is a clear illustration of why Calories in, Calories out is not an effective method for getting leaner and healthier longer term.

But you're now probably asking yourself what could have been done instead in this all-too-common situation? What could have Joe done to overcome his fat-loss plateau?

In short, Joe could have changed the composition of his diet. Remember, body composition change is a mass balance equation, not an energy balance equation. Losing fat mass is about creating a deficit in mass, not in energy. Remembering that carbohydrates are the macronutrient most responsible for weight gain (and also that they're not an essential nutrient), should provide some hints as to what could be done instead in this kind of situation.

With this in mind, Joe could have made one small tweak to his daily targets: he could have decreased his carbohydrate intake while increasing his fat intake as follows:

	Previous Intake	New Intake
Fat	100 g	190 g
Protein	200 g	200 g
Carbohydrate	300 g	150 g
Total Mass Intake	600 g	540 g
Energy	2900 Cals	3110 Cals

The increase in fat from 100 g to 190 g would make him feel more satiated and he would also have more energy throughout the day. This is because fat is a denser fuel source (9 Calories per gram) in contrast to carbohydrate (4 Calories per gram).

This is only one part of the outcome, though. As the energy portion from fat increases, Joe's overall mass intake decreases due to the higher-energy density of fat.

Thus, by increasing his fat intake by 90 g and reducing his carbohydrate intake by 150 g, Joe would ingest 60 g of mass less per day. That may not seem like much, but if we do some quick maths, it adds up to almost a 2 kg loss after 30 days:

60 g x 30 = 1800 g (1.8 kg or ~4 lb)

This loss in mass is assuming Joe's water intake (from both food and drink), insoluble fibre, and his vitamin and mineral intake (e.g. sodium) has not been substantially affected by the dietary interventions and everything else remains reasonably constant. It's important to note, too, that the amount of mass lost can be more or less, depending on which macronutrient Joe chooses to manipulate.

Not only will the type of macronutrient dictate how much mass is lost, it can also dictate the kind of body mass that is lost. For instance,

Joe could negatively affect his body composition and lose excessive amounts of lean mass if he were to reduce his protein intake by 150 g instead of his carbohydrate intake by the same amount.

Alternatively, if Joe achieved his mass deficit by lowering his fat intake from 100 g to 60 g while keeping his carbohydrate and protein intake the same (300 g and 200 g, respectively), he may negatively affect his hormonal system by undereating fat.

Joe's choice to lower only his carbohydrate intake by 150 g and increase fat intake by 90 g could also result in more 'mass out' in the form of fat than expected. One major reason for this is that consuming even small meals or snacks containing between 15 to 30 grams of carbohydrates is typically enough to initiate an insulin response for most people. Insulin is the body's main storage hormone and, thus, any amount of carbohydrate that spikes Joe's blood sugar and triggers an insulin response can promote fat storage.

Hence, the decision to lower carbohydrate intake by 150 g while increasing dietary fat intake by 90 g would likely result in a good amount of fat loss. In this scenario, you should also notice from the table that Joe's Calories were higher than with his previous target (3100 vs 2900). This means that Joe would be deriving more energy from his new intake and would likely not feel as hungry when eating more dietary fat and less carbohydrate as illustrated. This example again proves that body composition is a mass balance equation and not an energy balance equation (at weight stability, energy balance can be positive or negative). With this in mind, if Joe hit another plateau and was still not at an appropriate body composition, he could further reduce his carbohydrate intake and increase his fat accordingly.

How far could Joe ultimately go with his fat loss? Would he get down to 85 kg eventually? We have seen it done plenty of times before. Although it's hard to pinpoint exactly how lean Joe could eventually get, we can say with confidence that with proper adherence to the mass balance principles, Joe would be able to reach close to his genetic potential with his physique. It's worth noting, too, that not all losses in weight will be losses in fat mass. It is inevitable that some lean mass will be lost along with fat mass (especially when approaching leaner body fat ranges).

Another proviso to consider here is that Joe is now in his forties (not his twenties) and needs to put his goals in better perspective.

He is now at a typically busier and more stressful time of his life and a body fat level of 15% would also now put him in the 'very lean' (as opposed to 'fair') range for his age category. Though time is usually not on a person's side when it comes to getting in their best shape, it can and has been done plenty of times before with the right plan in place. Like Joe, most people consume far too many carbohydrates for their age and training status. They instead should be eating more quality protein and relying on fat as the predominant fuel source for getting leaner.

If you're interested in how to fuel your body on fat, we cover this in depth in our Lean Body Program, at **theleanbodyprogram.gr8.com**.

Lifestyle Factors Affecting Nutritional Requirements

We have previously covered the nutritional factors that directly influence a person's body composition and can have an impact on their overall health status. It is important to note, too, that there are some indirect lifestyle factors that can also seriously shape a person's nutrition and overall health. Here are some aspects to consider:

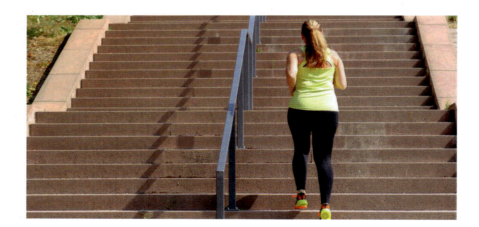

EXERCISE

Done correctly, exercise can improve metabolic health, heart, and bone health. It can also do wonders for a person's mental health and sleep. Exercise will also increase the demands on the body to provide energy and can assist with enhancing body composition change. However, an important point needs clarifying here: if a person can only maintain a healthy body composition by doing a high amount of exercise, then their diet is wrong—there is no sugar-coating this (pun intended).

Exercise has numerous health benefits, but if a person depends on it to maintain their body fat level within a healthy range, then their nutrition needs work. Trying to change the outputs without properly managing the inputs will not get anyone very far with their health or body-composition goals. You've likely heard the saying, "You can't out-train a bad diet". We will take it further and say, "You can't (nor should you try to) out-train a bad diet".

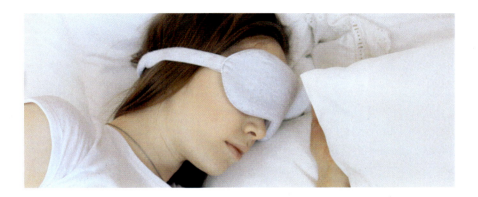

SLEEP

Sleep is a very important and often overlooked factor when it comes to a person's health and body composition. Sleep assists and allows for a host of functions; it is critical for repair and tissue turnover (this includes building muscle AND burning fat), it helps improve physical performance, it enhances immunity, and it supports better mood regulation (sounds like something you should be getting plenty of—right?!). Sleep also plays a role in regulating important hunger and metabolic hormones (such as leptin and ghrelin).

Routinely sleeping less than 6-7 hours per night can not only lead to overeating and weight gain, but it has also been linked to various lifestyle diseases such diabetes, heart disease, and cancer. If you're planning to get in shape and stay in shape, then you would be wise to prioritise sleep. The general recommendation for most adults is around 7–9 hours of sleep per night.

Proper sleep is foundational to a healthy lifestyle and a lean body. Without adequate sleep, any adjustments you make to your eating habits become less effective. Every major system, organ, and tissue in your body suffers when you lack sleep. Thus, sleep is not a luxury, but a necessity. Be sure to prioritise a healthy sleep schedule and stick to it.

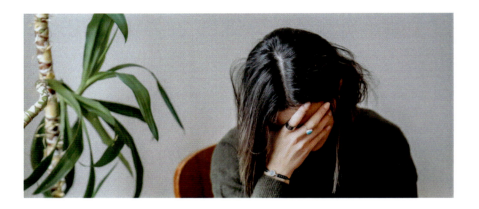

STRESS

If not properly managed, stress can have a big impact on a person's nutrition, body mass, and overall health. When someone experiences stress, their body can release a hormone called cortisol. Cortisol can increase appetite and cravings for energy-dense (high-sugar and high-fat) foods. This can lead to vast overeating and fat gain over time.

Stress can also trigger emotional eating where food is used as a way to cope with negative emotions. This can result in serious fat gain and compromised health over time (both physical and mental). Stress can not only trigger overeating—it can also trigger undereating as well. As you will soon see, eating well below one's requirements for proper mass balance is not a good thing.

Undereating Can Be as Dangerous as Overeating

If you have been diarising your nutrition and calculating some nutritional targets to lose fat, and these targets came out higher than what you have been eating on average each day, then don't go any further—contact an experienced dietitian (or send us a message so we can point you in the right direction). A state of consistent undereating can cause irreversible damage and is associated with the following over time:

- Nutrient deficiencies
- Reduced metabolism
- Muscle loss
- Bone loss

If you fall into this category and have been under eating or following strict diets for more than a few months, it's time to fix this in order to not cause any further longer-term damage. Do seriously consider reaching out and getting some help to reverse this. Doing so will likely save you a lot of heartache in the future and it's unlikely any further lowering of your nutritional intake right now will make you lose fat anyway.

With all this talk around food and nutrition, it's likely that you're hungry now. Steady yourself though and put down the fork! It would be erroneous to address the food you're consuming without also considering how you consume it.

Knowing the Difference Between Hunger and Appetite

Hunger and appetite are two different but often confused sensations relating to food. Hunger is a physiological drive that is controlled by your body's need for energy and nutrients. When you are hungry, your body may produce physical symptoms such as low energy, a growling stomach, light-headedness, and general weakness.

On the other hand, appetite is a psychological drive that is influenced by external factors such as emotions and stimulus of the senses (taste, smell, sight, etc.), as well as social situations and other cues (like reading a nutrition text!). In a nutshell, appetite is the desire to eat, whereas hunger is the need to eat.

Many people justifiably beat themselves over the head about the times they have given in to appetite.

There will be times though when you'll likely be hungry when trying to lose body fat. This should be expected from time to time when you're taking in less energy producing mass than you're excreting, and your body is breaking down tissue (preferably fat) in place.

Yes, it can be a little uncomfortable at times dealing with hunger. But, do you know what happens after 45–60 minutes of having a hunger signal? It goes away! Yep, this signal is cyclical and is governed by a hormone called ghrelin.

Sometimes, all you need to do is just have a glass of water and wait it out.

But before resorting to these kinds of measures, the rate at which you cram food down your pie hole also needs to be addressed.

It takes the satiety signal around 20 minutes to travel from your stomach to your brain to tell you that you are full. This signal is governed by another hormone in your body—leptin. Hence, if you're shovelling food down too quickly, it's easy to consume a lot more than you actually need. The lesson here is to slow down your eating. This way you will not only reduce the risk of consuming in excess and putting on fat, but you will also savour the taste of your food and enjoy it more... not to mention feel a lot less bloated in the aftermath.

There is another lesson to learn, too, when it comes to better managing hunger and appetite: food selection matters!

Not All Foods Are Created Equal

Often, the people who get hungry a lot whilst trying to lose fat, do not do themselves any favours with their food selections. These people are usually overly focused on 'Calories' rather than the nutrient quality of their food. As you should now know, not all foods are created equal and many foods have the tendency to stimulate appetite and fat gain, while others have the opposite effect.

When eating predominantly higher-quality foods with lots of good nutrients (like unprocessed meats, vegetables, nuts, etc.), a person's hunger signals usually closely match their intake and energy needs. On the other hand, when consuming primarily lower-quality, processed foods (like fast foods, soft drinks,

TROUBLESHOOTING NUTRITION AND OVERCOMING STAGNATION

candy, biscuits, etc.), these offer very few nutrients and often negate the body's ability to regulate a person's intake and energy requirements via appetite cues.

As mentioned in the previous section, ghrelin is the main hunger and appetite-stimulating hormone. It and can be stimulated by the following kinds of foods:

- Low-protein or low-fibre meals
- High-sugar and high-carbohydrate foods
- Highly palatable, pleasurable, and brain-rewarding foods
- Combinations of the above

Revisiting our example from earlier in this text on Calories, eating 70 g of sugar is not the same as eating 70 g of lean protein (even though the 'Calories' are the same). Hence, the quality of a food and how your body metabolises that food has a BIG impact on whether or not you will be leaner and healthier longer term. With this in mind, here some specific foods to watch out for that meet the criteria of the four points above in standard quantities:

- **Refined flour and grains:** white bread, white rice, and white pasta. Most flatbreads, wraps, and tortillas
- **Breakfast cereals:** corn flakes, puffed rice, flavoured and quick oatmeal, refined wheat cereal
- **Baked goods:** cakes, cookies, pastries, muffins, donuts, and croissants
- **Processed snack foods:** crackers, potato chips, biscuits, oat, and granola bars, etc.
- **Fast foods:** burgers, fries, chicken nuggets, pizza, hot dogs, fried chicken, etc.
- **Sweets and desserts:** lollies, chocolates, puddings, ice cream, and sweetened yoghurts
- **Sugary beverages:** soft drinks, energy drinks, fruit juices, sweetened teas, sports drinks, flavoured milks and coffee drinks, flavoured waters, sweetened smoothies, sweet and sugary alcoholic drinks/mixes
- **Condiments, sauces, and spreads:** ketchup, barbecue sauce, sweet chilli sauce, honey mustard, tartar sauce, aioli, ranch dressing, sweet and sour sauces; sweet and creamy salad dressings, mayonnaises; chocolate spreads, cream cheese spreads, jams, and sweetened nut butter spreads
- **Deli meats and cheeses:** marbled or fatty cuts of ham, roast beef, and various cured sausages such as bologna, salami,

pepperoni; cured or smoked meats such as pastrami and corned beef; processed cheese slices and cheese spreads; full-fat cheddar, Swiss, brie, blue cheese, and some cream cheeses

Now we are not saying you should outlaw these foods. What we are saying is that regular consumption of these kinds of foods is not conducive to reaching one's leaner body composition and health goals in the longer term. With our clients, we recommend that they consume no more than 10% of their overall intake from these kinds of foods (remember this rule from the 'Principled Approach' section).

Besides, there are a lot of better ways of preparing many of these kinds of foods in ways that incorporate much better nutrients and whilst still maintaining their flavour. Many examples are provided in the 'Lean Body Recipes' part of this text. We also provide principles and methods you can utilise if you choose to create your own great-tasting food.

But before we go there, let's look at the smaller and often underestimated elements of nutrition that often add up to sizable differences.

Five Fatty Foods That Add Up Quickly

Sometimes there is a significant difference in the macronutrient density of seemingly similar foods. These differences can catch you off guard if you're not aware and take significant chunks out of your daily allowances.

Fat is one particular macronutrient that most people fail to account for properly in their daily nutrition. There is nothing wrong with fat—you need it as part of a lean and healthy diet. However, it can be very easy to over consume fat, particularly if carbohydrate intake is higher, and fat requirements are minimal (~1 gram per kilogram of bodyweight). In this case, fat has a smaller daily allowance per gram (as opposed to that of carbs and protein) and keeping fat intake in check is vital for optimising one's body composition and health.

Here are five fatty foods that can add up quickly and balloon your fat intake if you're not careful:

TROUBLESHOOTING NUTRITION AND OVERCOMING STAGNATION

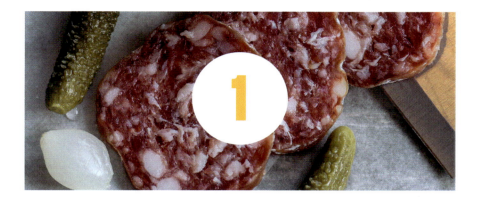

FATTY RED MEATS

There is a big difference between having 200 grams of beef ribs instead of 200 grams of beef tenderloin. Having 200 grams of the latter compared to the former, means you consume an extra 45 grams of fat. Cured meats also usually contain a relatively large amount of fat per portion and can easily add up.

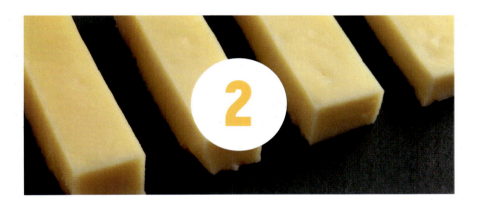

DAIRY

Full-fat milks and cheeses contain a lot more fat than their lower fat alternatives. Often you will feel just as satisfied both in terms of quantity and taste on the alternatives. Dairy is easy to over consume so be sure to make your selections from this food group wisely. Choosing low-fat milk, Greek yoghurt, cottage cheese, and other cheese varieties can make a big difference if you're struggling to control your overall fat intake.

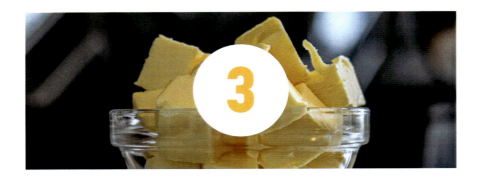

OILS AND BUTTERS

Using tablespoons of butters and cooking oils to coat pans and trays adds a lot more fat to meals than using cooking sprays. Cooking in non-stick pans and skillets can also help you significantly reduce fat from the cooking process. Common spreads like peanut, almond, and dairy butters quickly add up, too, and should be properly portioned out and accounted for.

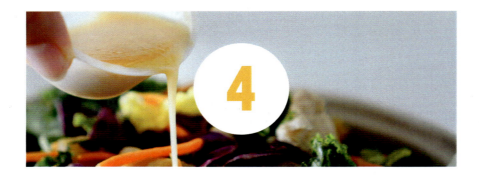

DRESSINGS

Pouring an oily dressing all over the top of your salad is a good way to add a lot of often unwarranted fat to a meal. A leaner alternative is to coat the salad bowl lightly, then put the salad in and toss it to flavour the whole salad. If you're going over the top with standard salad dressings, an even better idea is to use salad dressing sprays. You can find these in some stores or you can buy an empty bottle and pump your own.

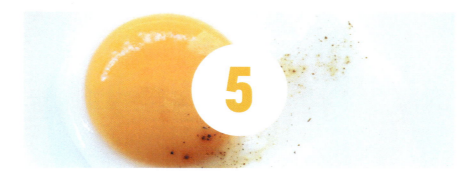

EGGS

Using fewer whole eggs and substituting these with more egg whites will drastically cut fat (the yolks) in a meal. Not to mention bump up the protein intake. Having one too many whole eggs in a meal can easily blow out a daily fat target if not properly accounted for.

These five foods can definitely add up and go under one's radar if not careful. Let's now look at another important but often overlooked aspect of nutrition: fibre.

Framing Fibre

> **"A SHOE THAT FITS ONE PERSON PINCHES ANOTHER; THERE IS NO RECIPE FOR LIVING THAT SUITS ALL CASES".**
> CARL JUNG

Fibre is essentially all the "non-digestible" carbohydrates that we obtain from primarily plant-based foods in the diet. Higher-fibre foods tend to be less carbohydrate-dense and less processed compared to low-fibre foods.

Foods rich in fibre include legumes, beans, nuts, seeds, oats, fruits, vegetables, and unprocessed wholegrain foods (e.g. breads, cereals, and pastas with the word 'whole' as the first ingredient).

There are two different types of dietary fibre (soluble fibre and insoluble fibre) and each have distinct characteristics:

Soluble fibre: This type of fibre dissolves in water and forms a gel-like substance in the digestive tract. It is found in foods such as oats, legumes, and various fruits and vegetables (e.g. apples, oranges, berries, carrots, broccoli, sweet potato). Soluble fibre can act as a prebiotic and cultivate gut bacteria.

Insoluble fibre: This type of fibre does not dissolve in water and remains relatively intact as it passes through the digestive system. It is found in foods such as whole grains, nuts, seeds, and many vegetables. Insoluble fibre can add bulk to the stool and speed up the transit time of food going through various parts of the digestive tract to promote more regular bowel movements.

In terms of weight management, fibre increases satiety by adding volume to meals without contributing much nutrient mass. It also

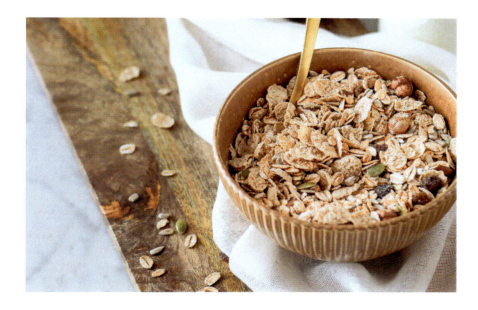

slows down the digestion and absorption of fats and carbohydrates to help promote lower and more sustainable blood-sugar levels.

Fibre also influences gut motility, which is the movement and contractions of the muscles in the gastrointestinal tract that propel food and waste material through the digestive system. This process ensures the proper digestion and absorption of nutrients, as well as the elimination of waste products.

The recommended daily intake of dietary fibre varies depending on the age, sex, activity level, and overall health status of the person. The standard minimum daily requirement of fibre for women is 25 g per day, and 30 g per day for men. Those with higher energy requirements and larger persons can in most cases consume more if required.

The Purported Benefits of Fibre

- **Easier excretion and elimination:** the presence of fibre can add bulk to stools and stimulate the muscles of the intestines to promote proper peristalsis (the wave-like muscle contractions that propel stool through the digestive tract). Thus, dietary fibre can play a role in promoting regular bowel movements to help reduce the time that waste spends in the colon and help prevent constipation. Fibre can also bind to certain toxins such as potential carcinogens in the digestive tract and facilitate their elimination from the body.

- ✓ **Cultivate gut microbiome:** The gut microbiome is involved in various functions such as digestion, nutrient metabolism, immune system regulation, and protection against pathogens. It helps break down certain dietary components that the human body cannot digest on its own. It also produces various vitamins and helps maintain the integrity of the intestinal barrier. Fibre can serve as a source of nutrition for beneficial gut bacteria. As the bacteria ferment fibre in the large intestine, they produce short-chain fatty acids (SCFAs), which provide nourishment to the colon cells and support a healthy gut environment.

With these purported benefits, many assume that everyone should get a certain amount of fibre each day in their diet. However, there are also some purported drawbacks of fibre too depending on the situation and the person.

The Purported Adverse Effects of Fibre

- ✗ **Digestive discomfort:** Some people may experience bloating, gas, abdominal cramps, and other gastrointestinal distress when consuming high-fibre foods. This can be especially more pronounced if there is a sudden increase in fibre intake without allowing the body to adjust gradually.

- ✗ **Nutrient absorption:** High-fibre foods (particularly those containing insoluble fibre) can bind to certain minerals like calcium, iron, and zinc, reducing their absorption. However, this is usually not a concern if the diet is varied and includes a range of nutrient-rich foods.

- ✗ **Personal tolerance:** Fibre needs can vary from person to person. Some people may have specific medical conditions or gastrointestinal disorders that require them to limit their fibre intake or avoid certain types of fibre. For instance, inflammatory bowel disease (IBD) patients may have an atypical gut microbiome that may not contain sufficient quantities of bacteria that normally ferment fibre that enters the colon. This can eventually cause irritation and inflammation.

In fact, people with the lowest bacterial diversity usually become more inflamed after consuming fibre. If those with higher levels of inflammation had some 'bad bacteria' already present in their gut (or alternatively, not enough of the 'healthy bacteria'), it's possible that eating more fibre is just adding more fuel to the fire.

Ketogenic diets are a common resort for many people suffering from various gut and digestive system disorders. As these diets are high in fat, they tend to restrict many carbohydrates (including fibrous ones) that trigger inflammation in affected persons. Reducing the intake of fermentable carbohydrates such as certain fibres and sugars can help alleviate symptoms associated with various gut motility and gastrointestinal conditions.

Those on ketogenic diets can produce SCFAs to nourish the colon from other non-fibre sources such as ketones and certain amino acids. It should be noted, though, that this production is relatively small compared to what can be achieved through the fermentation of dietary fibre. With that said, the specific amount of short-chain fatty acids (SCFAs) that the body needs for optimal function is not well established. SCFAs—including acetate, propionate, and butyrate—play important roles in various physiological processes such as energy provision to colon cells, gut health, and influencing metabolic and immune functions.

While there is no recommended daily intake for SCFAs like there is for other nutrients, it is understood that having an adequate supply of SCFAs is beneficial for overall health. The exact amount of SCFAs needed may vary from person to person and this is influenced by factors such as diet composition, gut microbiota composition, and overall health status.

The frequency of bowel movements can also vary from person to person and what is considered 'regular' can differ among individuals. Generally, a range of three bowel movements per day to three bowel movements per week is considered normal. However, what is more important than the frequency alone is the regularity and consistency of bowel movements for each individual.

For most people, having consistent bowel movements is an indication of a healthy digestive system. Bowel movements should be relatively easy to pass and should not cause pain or discomfort. Faecal matter should also have a formed shape and not be overly watery or hard.

Right vs Wrong, or Matter of Context?

Fibre tolerance tends to be dependent on the person. Most people can tolerate fibre in the generally recommended amounts and this nutrient is usually considered to be helpful for digestion and overall gut health.

General fibre requirements are not solely based on the premise of increasing SCFA production. Fibre can also support lower and more stable blood sugar levels and enhance feelings of fullness.

However, mindlessly consuming fibre with the thought that it will make you healthier may not be the best idea (especially in the form of highly refined fibre supplements or fibre-fortified foods). Fibre can be helpful for most people but it is not a magic bullet for digestion, gut health, or any other health condition.

There are also no hard health outcomes relating to singular factors of nutrition— rather it is a combination of factors that contribute to one's overall health.

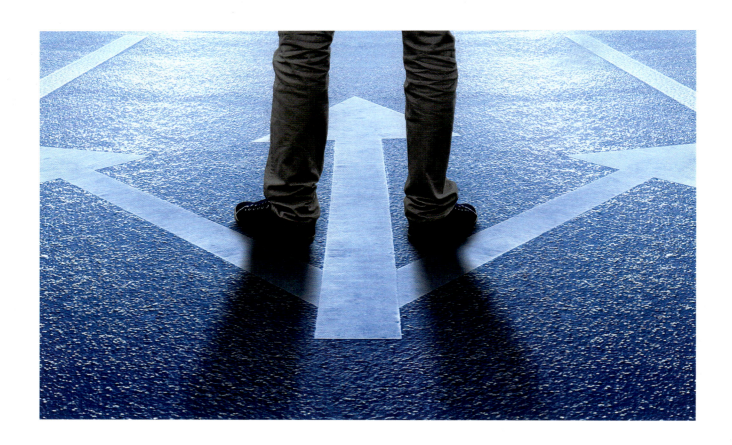

Fibre is just one of many factors that can influence gut health and motility. Others include intake and nutrient composition, physical activity, hydration, stress levels, and certain medical conditions.

Dietary fibre can potentially have harmful effects, but context is very important. The main cause of these effects appears to come from the absence of healthy gut bacteria and not necessarily from the fibre itself.

Although not an essential nutrient, fibre can play a role in most people's diet in assisting with nutrient digestion and excretion. It can also be helpful in stabilising blood sugar levels and enhancing satiety when carbohydrates are present in the diet.

General fibre requirements are thus not universal and can differ from person to person based on the person's sex, age, goals, activity levels, and overall health status.

When carbohydrates are in the diet, consuming more fibrous foods (if well tolerated) can be helpful if a person is looking to avoid overeating and putting on excess body fat. However, if you're consuming fibre, but you're having issues with the effects it may have on your gut or digestive system, it would be prudent to consult a qualified health professional in this area.

Becoming leaner and healthier doesn't stop with fibre or the foods you eat, either. It would be a great disservice to only talk about what you eat and neglect what you drink. Yes, we are talking about not only those beverages you have daily, but also those ones you may be having late at night (the alcoholic variety).

In the coming sections, we will look at not only which fluids are best to consume when aiming for a lean body, but also how to determine how much fluid a person may require on a daily basis.

Choosing Leaner Beverages

"THE ACCUMULATION OF SMALL OFFENCES CAN POISON EVEN THE PUREST OF RELATIONSHIPS".
ANONYMOUS

Changing drink choices can be one of the easiest ways to get leaner with less effort. Many drinks such as store bought beverages are unsuspectingly loaded with sugar (some can deliver over 100 g of sugar in a single serving!).

Nevertheless, there are still drink options that are low in sugar (and artificial sweeteners) that are sweet enough and quench your thirst - you just need to pay attention to them. In the following section, we'll outline which drinks will be satisfying and can be consumed regularly if you're looking to be leaner and healthier. We will also highlight the ones that should be consumed sparingly or even avoided. We have broken these drinks down by popular categories:

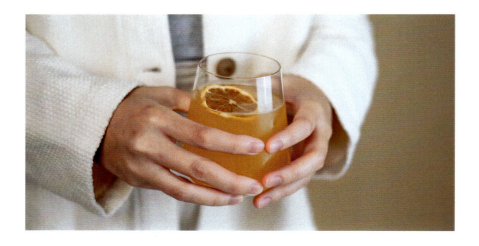

Common Drink Choices to Look Out For

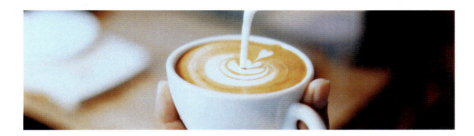

COFFEE

This common morning wake-up drink seems mandatory for many people in order to start their day. However, one needs to be careful they are consuming predominantly coffee and not a sugar bomb that leads to a midday energy crash. If you like the taste of coffee and you can learn to love the simple options like black coffee or espresso, these will keep your blood sugar (and body fat) a lot lower.

Sometimes this means buying a higher-quality coffee so that it has better natural flavour and can be enjoyed more. If switching to a simpler cup of coffee just doesn't work for you, then coffee plus skim milk and/or a natural sweetener is a good next best. Don't forget about iced coffee and blended coffee for hot days, too. Again, the same rules apply.

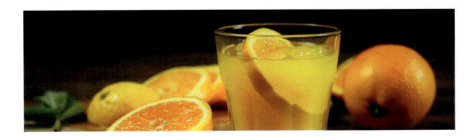

FRUIT JUICE

Now when we say fruit here, we don't just mean the bottled kind you find at the store and served at breakfast time; we also mean the commercial ones you can have blended up and put into a big Slurpee cup. While juice does come from fruit, it contains little of the health benefits that eating whole fruits does. This is because fruit juice removes the fibre and the nutrients. The typical varieties you find on the shelf at the grocery store are also often processed through cooking to be shelf stable. The end result is sweet beverages that are packed with sugar.

If you feel the need for having something sweet and fruity, you're far better off having… fruit! If you want something in liquid form, blending fruits at home to make a smoothie is the next best option. We have outlined the best ways to do this in the '4 Steps to Making Nutritious Shakes and Smoothies' section of this text. This section along with examples in the 'Lean Body Recipes' segment will give you some great ideas for making your own delicious and nutritious smoothies.

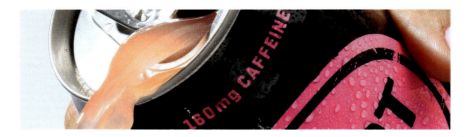

ENERGY DRINKS

Energy drinks are heavily advertised in the culture of action and extreme sports. With this also comes a proclivity for the marketed drinks to contain dangerous levels of caffeine, stimulants, and other chemicals that are harmful to the body in high doses. Energy drinks can also be very addictive and often become a crutch for the user in a lot of cases. Instead of being called 'energy drinks', they should be called "temporary-energy drinks".

This is because as soon as the sugar, caffeine, and other stimulants wear off, you're left with long-lasting fatigue that's far worse than any temporary energy-high was good. This unfortunate effect doesn't mean that there are no options to improve energy, though. Thankfully, some natural remedies can create enhanced alertness, without wrecking your body. Simply drinking tea or coffee is usually enough to wake most people up. Adding peppermint oil or ginseng to a beverage is an easy way to perk up, too. Beetroot juice is also a very good alternative that is far more nutritious and rarely causes energy crashes.

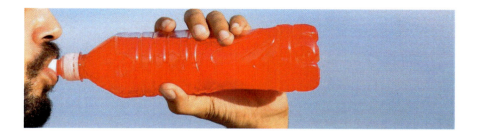

SPORTS DRINKS

If you're an endurance athlete or you work out intensely for more than two hours each day, you may need a sports drink to replace glycogen and electrolytes lost during training. But for the average person trying to lose fat, sports drinks aren't necessary, and they're adding a heap of sugar to the diet. If you like to drink these for the flavour, try adding some EAAs (essential amino acids) to water or opt for some of the aforementioned naturally flavoured alternatives instead.

For an easy electrolyte-infused beverage, a great alternative is unsweetened coconut water. These contain ample amounts of the two main electrolytes (sodium and potassium) without all the sugar and artificial sweeteners found in sports drinks.

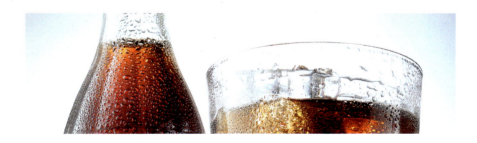

SODA

Sugary sodas and soft drinks are a major contributor to fat gain for a large number of people. They are so addictive and easy to drink that many don't even realise a single can of soda has the equivalent sugar of a bowl of ice cream. Artificially sweetened sodas can also contribute to fat gain inadvertently for some people by spiking blood sugar and causing their body to crave real sugar.

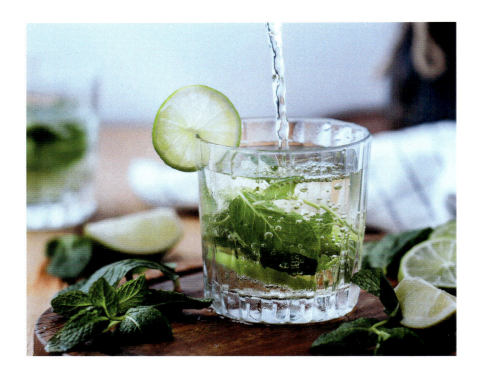

We are not the biggest fan of consuming lots of artificial sweeteners like aspartame and sucralose (usually 951 and 955 abbreviations on labels). There are also no significant health differences between dark sodas and light sodas as some like to claim. If you feel the need to have a sweet soda, naturally sweetened mineral waters are a far better option in our view. There are some homemade options for these as well. Mineral and sparkling water with added fruits such as lemons and limes are a great alternative. These contain more micronutrients than simple zero-calories sodas that have very little nutritional value.

Kombucha may be a decent option to help someone switch off of sugary sodas, as these are less sweet and naturally carbonated. However, despite many manufacturers' claims, these still contain a decent amount of sugar and are processed in a similar way in the body as a sugary soft drink is.

If you are trying to kick a soda habit, all these of these alternatives will not be as sweet to your taste buds if they are familiar to super sweet beverages. With a little time, though, your taste will adjust, your preferences will begin to change, and any previous cravings will be overshadowed by improved energy levels and feelings of well-being.

Are 'Diet' and 'Zero-Sugar' Beverages Okay?

Many people believe that a 'diet' beverage means a healthy one. However, this is far from the truth. While these drinks may not contain any sugar, they are sweetened with chemicals that can inadvertently cause fat gain and potentially have negative effects on your health if consumed regularly. In many scientific reviews of people drinking diet or regular soda, researchers find that there tends to be no difference in weight between these groups over time. Meaning that those drinking the 'diet' or 'zero-sugar' sodas often go on to gain just as much fat as those drinking full sugar sodas.

Why is this? There's a couple reasons driving fat gain with diet sodas. The first is that these beverages are super-sweetened with chemicals like aspartame which is 200 times sweeter than regular sugar. In drinking these ultra-sweet beverages, the brain often doesn't know the difference as to whether what's being consumed is sugar or not. In response, the release of insulin in the body can be signalled in a similar manner to what occurs when consuming items rich in sugar. This will often lead a person to consume sugar elsewhere in their diet to satisfy the cravings and, as a result, gain body fat. Furthermore, diet drinks have been shown in many cases to negatively alter gut microbiomes by increasing the abundance of certain bacteria that are associated with metabolic disorders like obesity and type 2 diabetes. At the same time, these drinks also decrease the amount of bacteria required for good gut health.

Although more research is needed in this area, we tend to err on the side of caution by not recommending regular consumption of 'diet' or "zero sugar' artificially sweetened beverages. This is especially in consideration of the inadvertent fat gain they can cause and the potential risk to one's health they may pose longer term.

Getting Your Water Intake Right

> **"THOUSANDS HAVE LIVED WITHOUT LOVE, NOT ONE WITHOUT WATER".**
> W. H. AUDEN

If there is one critical element we forget about when it comes to our nutrition and health goals, it's water. We're often surrounded by water but often we forget its importance. Water comprises more than 60% of your makeup and is involved in thousands of processes in your body!

Hence, you will miss out on a BIG part of the health, body composition, and performance results you could be getting if you don't get your water intake right.

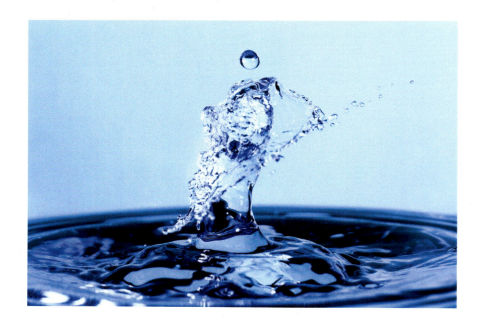

GETTING YOUR WATER INTAKE RIGHT

The problem is, we're often advised to "drink more water", yet few of us really know how much is required for our body size. We are also often unaware of what factors drain our body water and what other quantities of water come into the body (apart from drinking the straight stuff).

How do you get the required amount of water for your Lean Body goals? Follow these general guidelines:

3 Simple Steps for Staying Hydrated

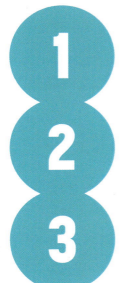

1. For bodily functions, 30 mL of water per kilogram (2.2. pounds) of bodyweight each day is a good general intake recommendation.

2. Did you have any other fluids today? tea, coffee, shakes, etc? If so, subtract these.

3. Did you exercise today and/or have exposure to heat? If so, take your weight before training/heat exposure and subtract your weight afterwards from this amount—whatever total weight you lost (in L/kg needs to be multiplied by 1.25 and consumed).

To see this in practice, let's use our example of Joe the 100 kg (220 lb) 41-year-old moderately active man from earlier.

1. 30 mL multiplied by 100 (weight in kg) = 3000 mL (3 L)

2. He had 180 mL of almond milk in his post workout snack: 3 L – 0.18 L = 2.82 L

3. Joe also trained and lost 1 L/kg of body water: 1 L x 1.25 = 1.25 L + 2.82 L. Therefore, on a day like this, Joe needs to drink roughly 4 L of water.

THE LEAN BODY SOLUTION

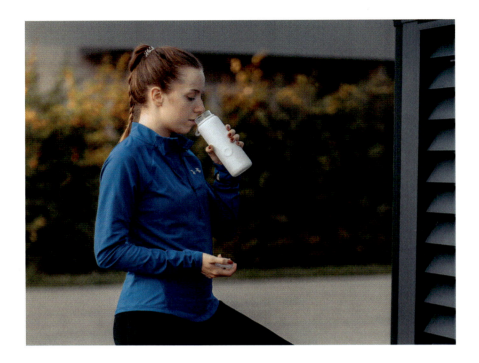

Dehydration Signs to Look For

Consider the following combination of factors regularly to assess whether you are dehydrated:

Thirst: This is the body's natural mechanism to signal the need for fluid intake. If you're feeling thirsty, it's often a sign that you may need to drink more fluids.

Urine colour and frequency: Monitoring the colour of your urine can provide some insight into your hydration status. Pale yellow or clear urine generally indicates adequate hydration, while darker urine can suggest dehydration. Also, if you're urinating regularly throughout the day, it's a positive sign of hydration.

Physical signs and symptoms: Dryness of the mouth, fatigue, dizziness, cramping, headaches, and decreased urine output can all be signs of dehydration. Feeling energetic, alert, and having good overall well-being can indicate proper hydration.

Body weight: Monitoring your body weight can give you an idea of whether you're adequately hydrated or not. A sudden drop in weight can indicate fluid loss, while a consistent weight suggests proper hydration.

Other Factors Affecting Hydration

Personal hydration needs can vary based on factors such as age, type, and level of activity, the climate, and overall health status.

Caffeinated substances are often blamed for dehydration, but often these become less diuretic over time as the body adjusts to regular intake.

Alcoholic substances, on the other hand, can predictably cause dehydration regularly. If you choose to drink, you should be prepared to drink more water (more on this soon).

It's not just the climate to consider either when it comes to dehydration. Hot environments and workplaces can increase fluid loss and often catch people off guard.

It's also important to consider electrolytes that may have been lost along with larger amounts of fluid and replenishing these at the earliest possible time.

Again, it's important to monitor the dehydration signs and symptoms from the previous section and take regular proactive measures to stay hydrated. Prioritising hydration is not only essential for your health and your performance, it also does wonders for satiety and preventing overeating.

Understanding Alcohol

"SOMETIMES THE GREATEST GAIN IS TO LOSE WHAT IS WEIGHING YOU DOWN".
ANONYMOUS

Before talking about alcohol, it's best to define what alcohol is exactly. The alcohol that you find in beverages such as wine, beer, and spirits is actually 'ethanol' or 'ethyl alcohol'. And it is the only type of alcohol that you can drink without causing serious damage to your body (at least in the short term).

In Australia (where one of the authors resides), one standard drink contains 10 g of pure alcohol. As this is the standard drink size in many countries, it will be referred to in this book. Just be mindful that this amount is different in some countries. For instance, in the United States, one standard drink contains 14 g of alcohol.

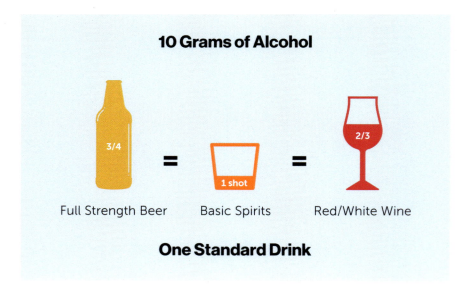

Not only can standard drink amounts differ from country to country, drinking guidelines can, too. In Australia, for instance, to minimise harm, the current public health guidelines recommend healthy men and women drink no more than 10 standard drinks in a week and no more than four standard drinks on any one day. In Ireland, the guidelines currently recommend up to 17 drinks per week for men and no more than 11 per week for women, with two alcohol-free days per week. In countries such as Belgium, there are different recommendations based on gender, with no more than 21 standard drinks for men and 14 for women consumed each week.

These differing guidelines may seem confusing; however, regardless of the differing amounts, anything over the recommended amounts is considered heavy drinking in most countries. And as different as the guidelines are between countries, there is one consistent growing trend in most countries, and that is the recommended limits on alcohol consumption are getting lower over time.

And you may be wondering at this point, what is the safe amount of alcohol you can get away with before it affects not only your health but also your body composition? We will get to this, but first, it's worth clarifying why the recommended amounts of alcohol for women are lower than that of men in many regions. Yes, this is due to some more obvious biological differences (which will be covered shortly), but it's also due some not so obvious differences that a lot of the research is now pointing towards.

Even in countries like Australia where the recommended standard drink amount is the same for both genders, the research and accompanying guidelines also suggest that women need to be particularly careful regarding how much they drink. Why? At the same higher levels of consumption, women are not only more vulnerable to arising health issues than men, but they're also vulnerable to developing more total health issues than men.

Apart from pregnancy complications (whether trying to conceive or during the pregnancy itself) and hormonal issues (e.g., accelerated menopause, disrupted normal menstrual cycle) specific to females, some of the conditions women are more likely to develop than men—with the same degree of alcohol consumption—include liver damage, brain function abnormalities, heart problems, infertility, mental health disorders, and various cancers.

UNDERSTANDING ALCOHOL

As for the more obvious biological reasons as to why a woman's body generally cannot tolerate the same amount of alcohol at any given time than that of a man, there are a few. First, alcohol (or ethanol) by nature is both water and fat-soluble. This means it can pass through all the cells and tissues of your body, including the blood-brain barrier. Because ethanol is soluble in water, it moves into water spaces throughout the body, such as your bloodstream, extracellular spaces, and intracellular spaces. However, it does not accumulate in your adipose tissue (or fat) because it prefers to reside in water. Just in case you think alcohol is converted into body fat, it isn't. However, this doesn't mean it cannot increase fat gain in other ways (more on this soon).

In essence, alcohol is restricted to a finite water volume in the body. This water volume is called total body water (or TBW for short) and it differs between men and women. Generally speaking, a higher percentage of a woman's body mass is fat compared to that of a man's. On average, the TBW in women is 55% of their body mass, whereas it is 68% in men. Because women have a lower percentage of body water and a higher percentage of body fat than men, women will tend to have a higher blood alcohol content (BAC) compared to men if they drink the same amount of alcohol. Thus, the higher BAC in females puts them at greater risk of impairment compared to males, for example, since more alcohol reaches the brain and at a faster rate.

It's not just differences in TBW that also allows men to be able to drink more before becoming impaired (and possibly even overdosing). The main underlying factor as to why women can generally tolerate less alcohol than men is due to women possessing lower levels of an enzyme called alcohol dehydrogenase (ADH). This enzyme is involved in breaking down alcohol in both the stomach and the liver. Men have highly active forms of ADH in their liver and their stomach, with its presence in the stomach alone reducing the absorption of alcohol by 30%. By contrast, females have almost no ADH in their stomach and the ADH in their liver is also far less active than that of males.

Of course, there are other factors that can influence how alcohol is processed and how it affects your body, such as bodyweight, hydration status, and overall health status.

Hydration level is one factor that can be easily and quickly varied. Alcohol is a diuretic and sends you to the bathroom more frequently.

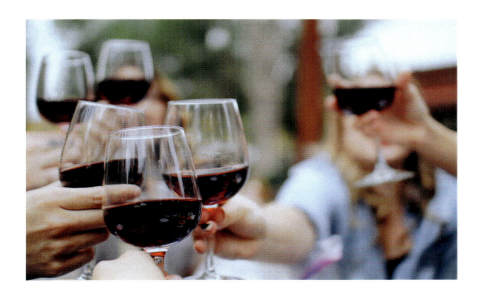

This is because when you consume alcohol, it suppresses the release of the antidiuretic hormone vasopressin, which controls how much water the kidneys reabsorb and retain. This reduces fluid retention and increases urination. This water loss through increased urination can lead to dehydration.

However, you don't only excrete more fluid when you drink alcohol, you also excrete more electrolytes (such as sodium, potassium, and magnesium) which are essential for body and brain functions. This is often why many people feel a lot better after having electrolyte drinks the day of a hangover.

Thus, the common advice to drink more water when consuming alcohol will allow your body to better process the alcohol and reduce potential damage, but it's also wise to replace the lost electrolytes, too.

However, it's not just your total body water and hydration status that alcohol has effects on. Alcohol has more broader implications for a person's overall health and body composition.

Alcohol's Effects on Health and Body Composition

Ethanol is a dense fuel source. When you consume alcohol, it is metabolised by the liver and converted into acetate, a substance that can be used as an immediate source of energy by the body.

However, alcohol is not only a fuel source, it's also a toxic molecule. Thus, the body doesn't have a storage place for alcohol like it does with carbohydrates and fat. Again, just because alcohol itself doesn't store well as body fat, that does not mean it cannot augment fat gain (particularly when consumed in higher quantities).

Unlike other energy-providing mass that you consume such as protein and fat, alcohol lacks any essential nutrients your body needs.

Revisiting the concept of available energy versus effective energy from earlier, alcohol contains a lot of readily available energy, but the effectiveness of this energy as a fuel source for the body is low due to its negative impacts on nutrient absorption and overall function.

The energy derived from alcohol is often not used for beneficial bodily functions but instead goes towards metabolising the alcohol itself and dealing with its toxic effects.

When alcohol is consumed, the body prioritises metabolising it over other nutrients. This causes a reduction in the use of other energy substrates (such as dietary fat and carbohydrates) and begins to store these as body fat until the alcohol is excreted from the body. This is especially true for dietary fat, which can be reduced to around 25% less oxidation in the presence of high amounts of alcohol in the bloodstream.

Alcohol can not only disrupt fat metabolism and make you fatter, taken consistently at too high a dose, alcohol can also impair protein synthesis along with anabolic signalling—meaning that you will struggle to both gain and retain muscle mass.

These are some more reasons why it's erroneous to think in terms of Calories in and Calories out when it comes to what we consume—especially with regard to alcohol. Calories can give us an idea of the energy content of a substance, but they do not provide us with any clarity on how much energy is derivable from it for the human body.

Although we, the authors, do not condone drinking in general, there are some practical precautions that will be covered later if you do decide to drink. Having an occasional drink or a big night on the booze every now and then won't do too much damage compared to if you're having a couple of drinks most nights or heavily drinking every weekend. The latter can prove disastrous for one's health and can cause long-term detrimental effects on both your body and your brain.

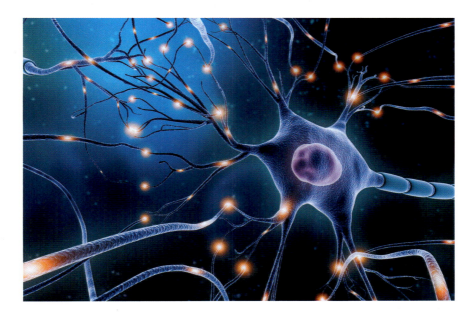

And why can't your body handle much alcohol at any one time? This comes down to how alcohol is metabolised and how your body deals with this toxin. When processed by the liver, most of the ethanol in your body is metabolised into acetaldehyde, and then into acetate by enzymes like alcohol dehydrogenase (ADH) and aldehyde dehydrogenase (ALDH).

Acetaldehyde is very toxic to the mitochondria and your cells. To mitigate these effects, the liver converts it to acetate so that your body can deal with it and break it down further to water and carbon dioxide for easy elimination. However, your body cannot do the conversion of acetaldehyde to acetate quick enough when you're drinking a lot, so the acetaldehyde builds up and wreaks havoc in your body while your liver struggles to process it all. It's acetaldehyde that is the major contributor to bodily symptoms associated with intoxication such as facial flushing, nausea, and even vomiting. Acetaldehyde is also a known carcinogen and can be a contributing factor in the development of alcohol intolerance—a condition where the body lacks the proper enzymes to break down the toxins in alcohol.

It's not acetaldehyde, though, that causes you to feel drunk but rather ethanol's effects on the brain. When ethanol crosses the blood-brain barrier, it affects the central nervous system by acting as a depressant and slowing your brain activity down—this is what often leads to the signs of intoxication such as impaired coordination, slurred speech, and altered judgment. One experiment to measure the effects of alcohol on the body is to use vital sign measures (e.g., a heart rate monitor); it's shocking how much distress someone's body is in even after just a couple of drinks.

To make matters worse, high alcohol consumption can increase the body's production of the stress hormone cortisol. Over long periods of time, this can lead to increased lean tissue breakdown and muscle loss.

Furthermore, alcohol can affect blood sugar levels, leading to fluctuations and drops in glucose. These fluctuations negatively impact how insulin functions and how much food your body craves (which is usually more than required).

It doesn't stop there, either. Just one serving of alcohol in the evening can significantly decrease growth hormone secretion during sleep. Growth hormone (somatotropin) plays a crucial role in the metabolism of your muscles, bones, and brain, as well as in blood-sugar maintenance.

If you're a man, you especially need to worry. Excessive drinking decreases testosterone and severely compromises building muscle mass over time. Heavier drinking is also known to increase estrogen levels, which can result in some very feminising effects (can you say "gynecomastia"?).

Adding more insult to injury, alcohol can also cause damage to the organs involved in digesting, absorbing, and processing nutrients—leading to nutrient deficiencies in those who drink often.

Excessive alcohol consumption has also been found to increase production of the main hunger and appetite hormone ghrelin, making your body crave more food. Alcohol can also affect neurotransmitters in your brain such as neuropeptide Y and serotonin, which are involved in regulating hunger and appetite. The likelihood of increased food cravings and a desire to eat more when consuming alcohol are further heightened by the stimulation of these neurotransmitters. Alcohol can also lower inhibitions and impact your brain's reward system by triggering the release of dopamine, a neurotransmitter that's associated with pleasure and satisfaction. This can lead to decreased self-control and increased desire for pleasurable foods. Hence, overeating and making unhealthy food choices are usually the result.

And if you're using alcohol to wind down and get to sleep, be aware of how alcohol affects the quality of your rest. While alcohol can induce feelings of relaxation and sleepiness, it can also disrupt your sleep cycle, thus decreasing your sleep quality. It does this in a few different ways. Apart from the obvious ones like having to get up to go to the bathroom frequently during the night because alcohol is a diuretic, alcohol also suppresses melatonin production and interferes with your circadian rhythm. Also, as alcohol starts to metabolise more, the sedative effect wears off and can cause a rebound and waking-up effect. This prevents you from getting both the deep sleep and rapid eye movement (REM) sleep you need because the alcohol in your system keeps you in lighter stages of sleep. This is why you might still feel tired after a full night's sleep if you've been drinking.

Consuming alcohol regularly and excessively can also trigger inflammation across the entire body, including in the gut, liver, the face, the joints, and the brain. Higher alcohol consumption has also been linked to high blood pressure, increased triglycerides, heart disease, stroke, DNA damage, and various cancers.

As you can see, the argument against alcohol is a weighty one indeed. Alcohol isn't essential for good mental or physical well-being in any way, and there's no reason to think that pouring poison down your piehole improves your life in any way. If you're someone who drinks but struggles to cut back, it's no surprise: alcohol is currently among the most misused addictive substances on the planet. In the United Kingdom, almost 60% of adults 18 years and over reported drinking in the past week. In the United States, two-thirds of the adult population drank excessively in the previous year. About 13% of American adults also meet the criteria for alcohol use disorder (or AUD).

Given the addictive nature of alcohol, it's easy to see how one or two planned drinks can easily turn into seven or eight!

And what should you do if you fall into the trap and drink heavily every now and then? What can you do mitigate the negative effects (at least in the short term)?

Below are some tips to reduce the damage from alcohol and help safeguard your body composition:

7 Practical Tips If You Decide to Drink

From a body composition standpoint, if you're active and not trying to get super lean, following the health guidelines for alcohol consumption mentioned earlier won't greatly affect your body composition.

However, if you're trying to get really lean, it's probably not a wise idea to consume alcohol given the fact it can stimulate your appetite when you're likely already eating less than usual.

If you're not trying to get shredded and you decide to drink heavily (again, not advised), here are seven tips to safeguard your body composition—and to some extent—your health:

1. If you decide to drink, be sure to not do so on an empty stomach: food does prevent the rapid absorption of alcohol into the bloodstream. Eating a meal with a mixture of protein, fat, and complex carbs before drinking appears to be better than having the equivalent meal made up of just one macronutrient. Having just sugars and simple carbohydrates is the worst tactic, as these are quickly absorbed by the body so they won't be much help in slowing down the absorption of alcohol in the digestive tract.

2. When drinking, remember to account for the alcohol content, along with any carbohydrates present in the drinks. If consuming distilled spirits, they're best combined with low/no-sugar mixers (e.g., vodka with soda water).

3. When having beer or cider, remember that 'low carb' and 'light' are not the same thing. Consider varieties that are both low carb and lower alcohol by volume (ABV): that is, an ABV of 4–5% or less. Remember that stouts and darker ales tend to be higher in carbs and have a higher ABV than other beers.

4. When consuming wine, consider lower ABV (around 10–12%) and lighter versions of red and white wine. Brut varieties are generally the lowest when it comes to sparkling wines. Sweet, aromatized, and fortified types of wines are all high in sugar, and it's wise not to overconsume these.

5. If you find yourself drinking heavily, remember that eating more protein and less fat usually results in less fat gain after drinking (all else being equal).

6 Drinking plenty of water before, during, and after higher amounts of alcohol consumption, along with replenishing electrolytes, can really help to mitigate alcohol's adverse effects.

7 If you have succumbed to a big night on the drink and you're feeling various hunger and appetite effects, consuming more protein will not only help the body store less fat, but it can also help curtail some of the negative effects alcohol has on muscle growth and repair.

Again, most of these tips are safeguards from doing more damage than one should if excess alcohol is consumed. They are not in any way put forward to promote the consumption of alcohol. Excessive alcohol consumption can have negative effects on your body composition and health regardless of how you adjust your diet to compensate for the excess. If in doubt, it's always wiser to abstain from alcohol. By nature, it's an addictive substance and designed to get people hooked. This is why we, the authors, do not recommend alcohol to anyone in any amount if they're looking to take charge of their body and their health.

Now that you know the best kinds of foods and beverages to focus on for leaner body composition and good health, it's time to look at how you can practically put these together and incorporate them into your own daily nutrition. But before you do this, though, first ensure you have proper tools in place.

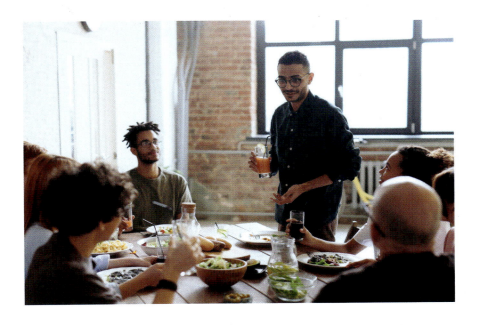

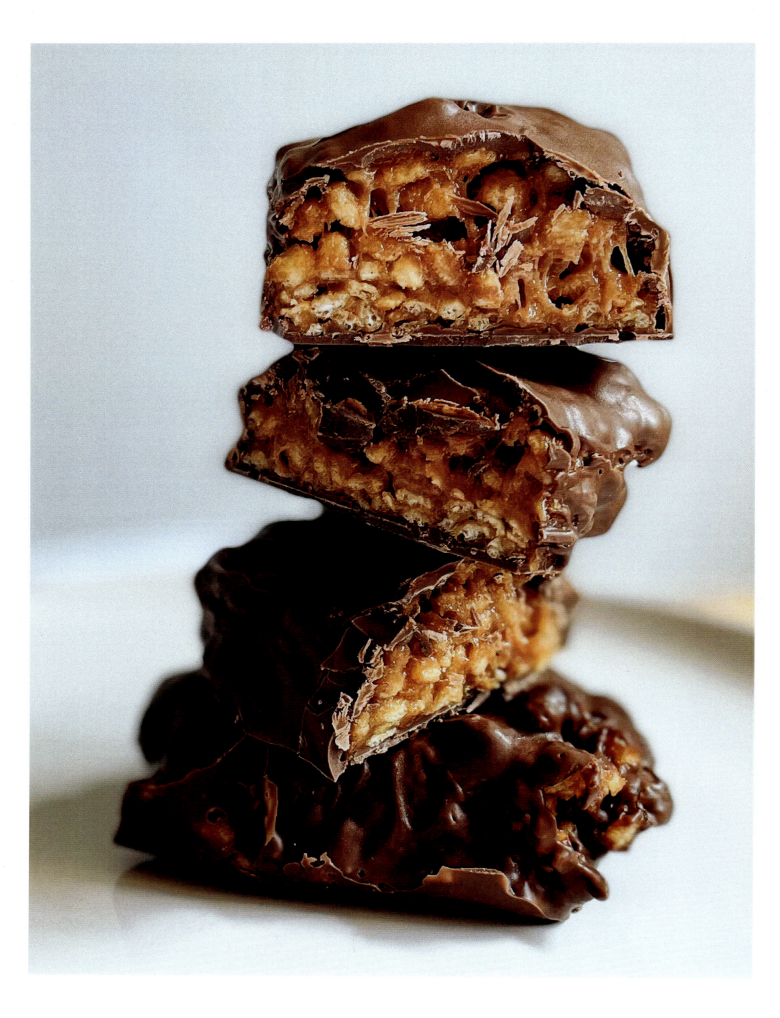

THE LEAN BODY KITCHEN

Kitchen Equipment Essentials

> **"EFFICIENCY IS DOING THINGS RIGHT;
> EFFECTIVENESS IS DOING THE RIGHT THINGS WITH THE RIGHT TOOLS".**
> PETER DRUCKER

Just as a carpenter needs both materials and tools to build a house, you will likewise need both materials (food) and tools (kitchen equipment) to construct your meals and nutrition plan. If you don't have the equipment, you can't prepare it. The more input you have with the preparation process, the more of a handle you will have on your results.

People wonder why they struggle to eat lean and clean—when we look at their kitchen, we are often not surprised. Constructing a nutrition plan without kitchen equipment is like trying to become a pilot without an aircraft to fly. If you're committed to your lean body goals, you will invest in the equipment required to enable you to achieve those goals. Get some skin in the game! Ensure your kitchen is equipped with the following from day one, or it's very unlikely you will be able to do… well anything:

- **Blender:** Vitamix, Blendtec, Ninja, or Nutribullet brands
- **Standard oven:** Ensure bake, broil/grill, and stove-top cooking options.
- **Knives and cutting surfaces:** Three standard knife sizes are recommended: small paring knife (10 cm), medium utility knife (14 cm), and a large chef knife (23 cm).
- **Pots and pans:** Non-stick cooking material is best to avoid relying on large amounts of oil when cooking—especially when it comes to frying.

KITCHEN EQUIPMENT ESSENTIALS

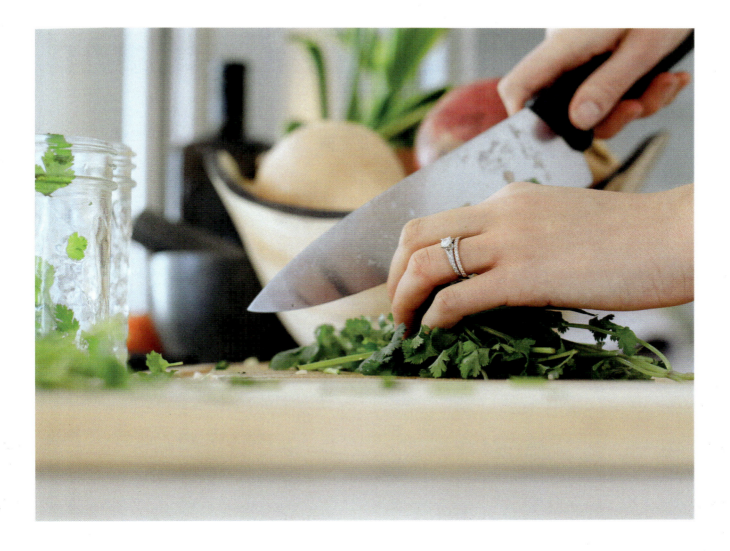

- **Measuring cups:** Cups divided into ¼, ⅓, ½ and 1 cup measurement are standard.
- **Measuring spoons:** A set of ¼ tsp, ½ tsp, 1 tsp. and 1 tbsp measurements is recommended.
- **Baking pans:** Choose non-stick material in a variety of sizes.
- **Grater:** The best options will have small and larger size holes for grating.
- **Mixing bowls:** Small, medium, and large bowls will allow for more ease when preparing recipes.
- **Kitchen utensils:** It will help with cooking to have at least tongs, a spatula, and a vegetable peeler.
- **Grill (standard or portable/benchtop):** Propane or charcoal are acceptable.

Preparing, Packing, and Storing Your Meals

> **"PREPARING YOUR OWN FOOD IS A REVOLUTIONARY ACT OF RECLAIMING YOUR HEALTH AND INDEPENDENCE, EMPOWERING YOU TO TAKE CHARGE OF WHAT YOU PUT INTO YOUR BODY".**
>
> JAMIE OLIVER

Part of having a great diet is the essential need to be able to prepare, store, and pack your meals. The healthiest possible meal is useless if you find you don't have time to prepare it frequently, or if you can't take it with you on the go. The best way to fail with your body composition and health goals is to try and cook each meal when you're already hungry and likely don't have the energy. The old adage of 'failing to plan is planning to fail' definitely has merit here.

With the right tools, though, you should be able to conveniently make and store big batches of meals, as well as eat them conveniently before they expire. And if you're really pressed for time, we give you some advice for sourcing your own pre-prepared meals in advance. We do believe that everyone can and should prepare at least some of what they eat each week. Apply the tips below to ensure you can keep up with your lean eating plan by preparing, storing, and packing your meals in the best way possible.

PREPARING, PACKING, AND STORING YOUR MEALS

Step 1: Preparing

- When preparing all meals, make sure to keep cutting surfaces clean and sanitised. Never use already dirty knives or dirty cutting surfaces—clean all dishes as soon as possible after they're used. This keeps equipment in its best shape and keeps your food safe.

- Make sure to avoid any cross-contamination by using different equipment for meat and dairy, produce, and bread. When these pairs of food mix, they can create unhealthy bacteria on surfaces. Separate equipment for raw and cooked should also be a given.

Step 2: Packing

- Some tips when purchasing storage containers are to choose glass over plastic (zero chance of toxic chemicals in glass) when possible and make sure that the containers are dishwasher safe.

- Containers do wear down over time. Old storage containers that look foggy or permanently are disfigured should be thrown out and replaced.

- When packing prepared foods in containers, always store them into ready-to-eat serving sizes. This saves time by making them ready to grab and go out the door whenever needed.

Step 3: Storing

- After food is cooked and prepared, never leave it out. Refrigerate all cooked foods and freeze foods that need to be stored for longer than a few days (see table below for guidelines). Nearly all foods and beverages can be frozen.

- Different types of foods will vary with storage times. Raw and unpackaged items that are not sealed/air-locked will generally last a few days when refrigerated, while most packaged items should be consumed within one to two weeks. This is especially true for meat and dairy—never exceed two weeks of storage.

THE LEAN BODY SOLUTION

- When removing foods from storage to eat, always thoroughly smell them before heating up or consuming them. Never eat anything that smells questionable. Throw out food if it smells or looks like it's gone bad in any way. Never try to reheat bad food. Below is a table that can be used as a guideline for the shelf life of common meats:

Type of Meat	Raw, Unpackaged Shelf Life	Cooked Shelf Life
ground beef	2 days in fridge 4 months frozen	4 days in fridge 3 months frozen
steaks and cuts of beef	3 days in fridge 10 months frozen	5 days in fridge 3 months frozen
poultry	2 days in fridge 9 months frozen	4 days in fridge 4 months frozen
fish (lean varieties) e.g. halibut	2 days in fridge 6 months frozen	4 days in fridge 6 months frozen
fish (fatty varieties) e.g. salmon	2 days in fridge 3 months frozen	4 days in fridge 6 months frozen
prawns, shrimp, scallops, crab, other seafood	2 days in fridge 6 months frozen	4 days in fridge 3 months frozen

Outsourcing

We realise that for some, meal preparation is not always feasible with a very busy lifestyle. This is not an excuse to opt for take-out, though. There are smarter ways to source your meals than picking up your phone and looking for the nearest cuisine that jumps out at you. One such way is to hire a personal chef for a few hours each week to do the above three steps for you. Chefs are pros and will often bring all the required food and kitchen equipment to cook, pack, store, and label your meals, as well as clean up after each bout of meal prep. This option is also more affordable and easier than most think—especially when compared to eating take out regularly.

PREPARING, PACKING, AND STORING YOUR MEALS

The next best option if you're time poor is to use a food-preparation service. There are many companies that can deliver lean and healthy meals to your door that are congruent with your goals. Most of these companies also have nutritional information available for each meal, so you can build these into your lean body diet, too. Often you can order as little or as many of these meals as you like—i.e. your whole week of eating doesn't have to be something sourced from a packet if you don't need it to be. One of the authors actually used these services for some of his meals for a little while as he was finalising this guide.

Of course, we would prefer that when you can, you learn to build the skills and prepare your own lean and tasty meals. There is a lot of subliminal learning that happens in this process and you also build life skills that you will inevitably need. When push comes to shove, though, we would prefer that you can pivot rather than fall over with your lean body goals and outsource if required.

Now that you have your kitchen ready with the proper tools in place it's time to start making some nutritious and tasty food!

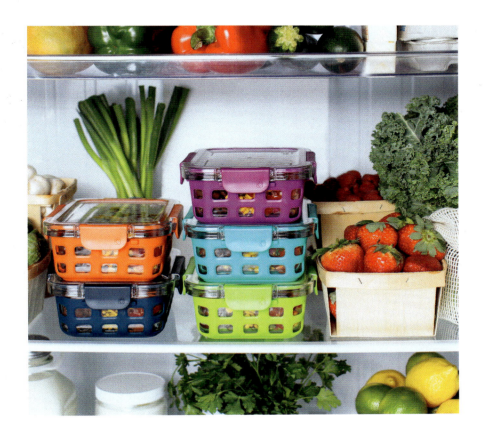

THE LEAN BODY SOLUTION 113

Principles for Making Your Own Lean Body Recipes

"GIVE A MAN A FISH AND YOU WILL FEED HIM FOR A DAY. TEACH A MAN TO FISH AND YOU WILL FEED HIM FOR A LIFETIME".
PROVERB

It's one thing to follow a recipe book and cook up its contents, it's another to eat these meals every day for the rest of your life. Don't get us wrong; there is a large variety of great recipes in this text. However, we know that there is a plethora of cuisines and dishes out there... and we're also mindful that your tastes will vary over time. For this reason, we want you to know how to tweak other recipes in your favour—or even create your own lean body recipes!

Knowing how to do this is easier than you think. It will also feed you well for a lifetime!

The following section will show you exactly how to tweak your nutrition in a proficient manner without destroying your results. Whether you want a smoothie, a salad, a sandwich, or a snack, we will teach you the lean body way for any occasion. In fact, these are the exact same principles we used to create all of the Lean Body Recipes within this guide.

In this section, we have laid out these food preparation principles with simple visuals that you can easily refer to.

4 Steps to Making Nutritious Shakes and Smoothies

"WILL IT BLEND?"
TOM DICKSON

Shakes and smoothies are a great way to quickly add protein and other nutrients to your diet. However, few people realise that they can put A LOT more taste and nutritional value into these concoctions.

Use the below tips when making shakes and smoothies to add more nutrients, boost your health and performance, and improve your recovery from workouts.

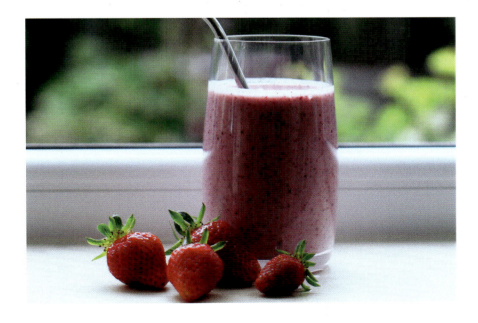

4 Steps to Making Nutritious Shakes & Smoothies

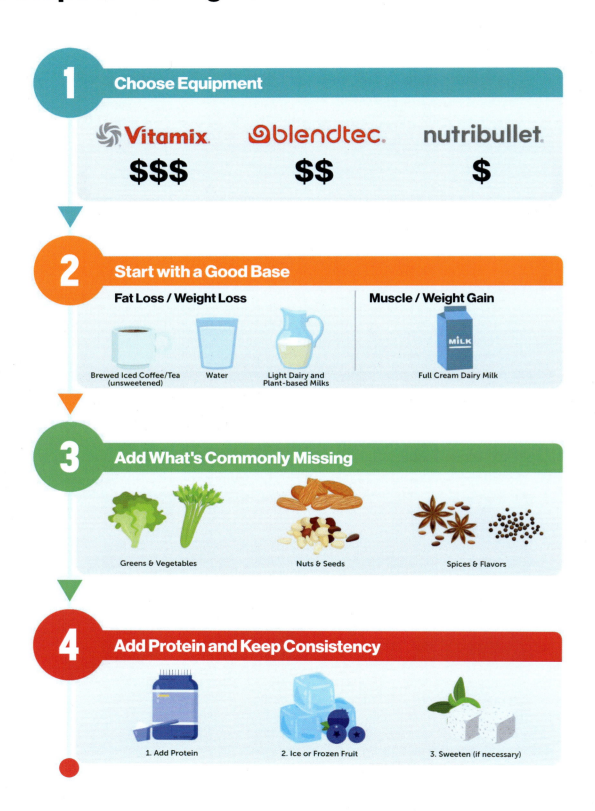

Ingredient Options

Nuts & Seeds

- Ground flaxseeds
- Chia seeds
- Hemp seeds
- Nut butters - almond, peanut, cashew
- Tahini
- Pumpkin seeds (ground or chopped)
- Nuts - cashews, almonds, walnuts, pecans, Brazil nuts, pistachios

Protein

- Animal-based protein powder - whey, casein, egg
- Greek yoghurt
- Cottage cheese
- Plant-based protein powder - pea, soy, rice, hemp
- Silken tofu

Base Liquids

- Water
- Brewed Tea
- Unsweetened Almond, Oat, Soy, or Coconut
- Milk
- Dairy Milk
- Brewed iced tea/coffee (unsweetened)
- Coconut water
- Kefir

Spices & Flavours

- Cinnamon
- Ginger
- Turmeric
- Nutmeg
- Cardamom
- Cloves
- Black pepper
- Cayenne pepper
- Vanilla extract
- Cacao powder/nibs
- Maca powder
- Peppermint extract
- Lemon or lime juice

Sweeteners

- Stevia
- Agave nectar
- Erythritol
- Monk fruit
- Xylitol
- Yacon Syrup

Fruits

- Apple
- Mango
- Berries
- Avocado
- Lemon Slices
- Peach
- Pineapple
- Cherries
- Bananas
- Papaya
- Pears
- Oranges
- Grapefruit
- Kiwi fruit
- Pomegranate

Vegetables

- Cucumber
- Kale
- Spinach
- Collard Greens
- Rocket Leaves
- Cooked Pumpkin
- Cooked Sweet Potato
- Beetroot
- Concentrated Greens Powder
- Carrots
- Celery
- Zucchini
- Fennel
- Swiss chard/Silverbeet
- Watercress
- Broccoli
- Cauliflower

4 STEPS TO MAKING NUTRITIOUS SHAKES & SMOOTHIES

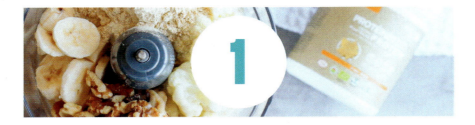

STEP 1: CHOOSE EQUIPMENT

With smoothies, you may be churning up a barrage of ingredients. To do this well and not get a 'chunky' smoothie that will require chewing, you will need good hardware to get the job done.

The esteemed **Vitamix** blenders are currently the best option on the market by far. They also come with the highest price tag. **Blendtec** blenders are a nice alternative with a slightly lower price. For even more affordable options, look into **Ninjas** or **Nutribullet** blenders. The latter options can often get the job done, but just require longer blending periods for everything to get completely liquidised. For more information on deciding on which blender is right for you, visit **performancerevolution.com.au/will-it-blend-a-review-of-popular-blenders** to read our comparative guide to top blenders on the market today.

STEP 2: START WITH A GOOD BASE

Making a base with the proper liquid is essential if you are to achieve lean body goals. Cow's milk can be a great option if you're looking to build muscle and put on weight, but this should be limited if you're trying to lose weight and burn body fat (especially high-fat whole milk varieties). If you have to have milk and your goal is to lean down, opt for a low-fat dairy milk.

When making smoothies or shakes as part of a fat-loss plan, water is the obvious answer when it comes to the leanest base ingredient. Home-brewed teas can also be a great substitute for higher-fat and higher-sugar base liquids. If you're looking for a creamier texture, non-sweetened versions of soy, almond, or coconut milk offer a great way to enhance the flavour, too. These alternatives can thicken your drink and provide a creamy taste without all the carbohydrates and fat of their fully sweetened counterparts. These lighter, creamy base liquids also mix well with protein powders, too.

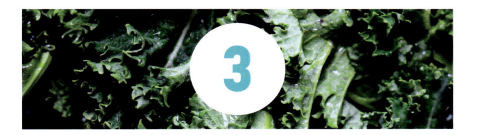

STEP 3: ADD WHAT'S COMMONLY MISSING

To maximise the benefits of your smoothies and shakes, you should examine which nutritious foods are commonly missing from your diet and look to add these in where possible. Most people don't get enough quality leafy greens or antioxidants in their diet. With smoothies, it's easy to add these foods while not really affecting the overall flavour. To fill some of the common nutritional gaps, you could try the following:

- Toss in up to 1 cup of greens (e.g. rocket, spinach, or kale). Also note that freezing greens first will help reduce any bitterness they may have in your smoothie.

- For more fibre and healthy fats, add 1–2 tbsp of ground flaxseed or chia seeds.

- To pump up antioxidants, add a teaspoon of cinnamon or ginger. Stronger-tasting spices like turmeric, cloves, and allspice should be added in ¼ to ½ teaspoon amounts.

Refer to the 'Ingredient Options' table above to give you some more ideas on how to add what's commonly missing from most shakes and smoothies. Remember too not to be too liberal with nuts and nut butters. These are very tasty but also very dense in fat, so definitely measure out your servings and don't just heap these ingredients in. For example, 1 tbsp of nut butter or a 1/4 cup of nuts is a good limit for most. These amounts will give you a good amount of flavour and texture without blowing out your daily fat intake.

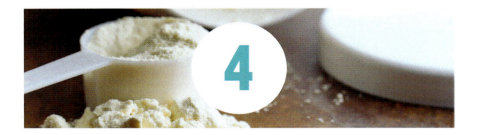

STEP 4: ADD PROTEIN AND KEEP CONSISTENCY

When it comes to smoothies, there can be some bad ingredient combinations that result in either a thick and undrinkable sludge, or a thin and almost watery liquid. The ideal consistency should be something in the middle of this range. To achieve this, add the ingredients as per the previous two steps, and then finish by adding in protein powder along with half cups of ice until the desired consistency is reached.

Lastly, you can sweeten a smoothie by adding fruits such as mangos, bananas, apples, blueberries, kiwi, or papaya. When these kinds of fruit are cut into chunks and frozen, they will enhance the texture and sweetness of your shakes and smoothies.

Some protein powders will be flavoured and sweetened already (preferably naturally). However, if you're not adding protein powders, or you're chasing a bit more sweetness (without resorting to sugary sweeteners like honey), then you can add some natural sweeteners such as stevia, monk fruit, xylitol, and erythritol.

Here are some example recipes that follow the steps we have just outlined:

> **FOR NUTRITIOUS SHAKES AND SMOOTHIES EXAMPLES, SEE THE SECTION 'POST-WORKOUT SHAKES AND SNACKS'**

5 Steps to Making Tasty, Clean, and Lean Sandwiches

"SANDWICHES ARE LIKE LOVE; THEY COME IN MANY VARIETIES, BUT EACH ONE IS SPECIAL IN ITS OWN WAY".

ANONYMOUS

Sandwiches are a common and convenient option, especially for busy working professionals who need a quick meal to power them through the workday. They can provide a delicious source of nutrition, but only IF they're made right. Sandwiches are also the perfect pairing with a variety of foods too (soups, salads, fruits, etc.). To make a high-quality combo of sandwich and pairing, follow these easy steps below:

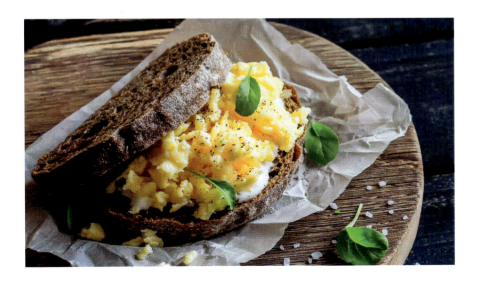

5 STEPS TO MAKING TASTY, CLEAN, AND LEAN SANDWICHES

Sandwich Making Guide

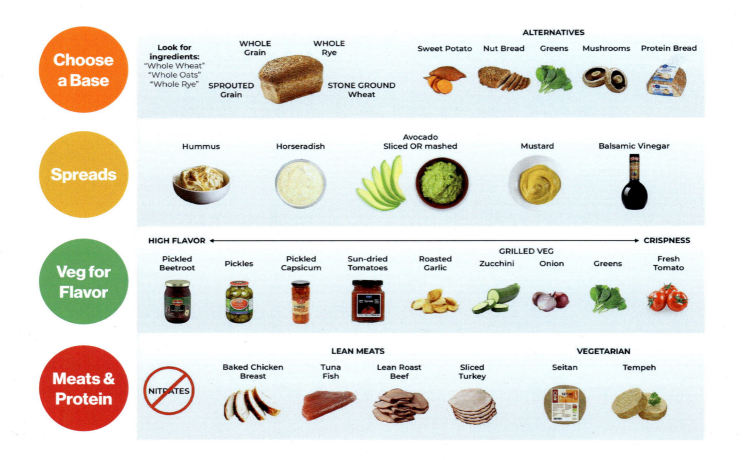

Perfect Sides for Sandwiches

Fruit	Salad	Soup
• Pears • Mango • Kiwi • Apples • Berries • Banana • Melon	• Spinach Salad • Kale Salad • Rocket • Collard Greens • Cabbage	• Tomato • Mushroom • Chicken • Barley • Split Pea • Lentil • Chili

THE LEAN BODY SOLUTION

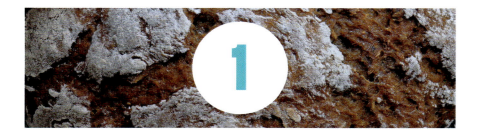

STEP 1: CHOOSE BREADS WISELY

There's now dozens of loaves available in the average grocery store. Unfortunately, few pass the test of supporting a healthy and lean body. Luckily there are a few key ways to find a good choice.

First, stay away from any bread that lists "enriched white flour" as an ingredient. You want whole ingredients that are as unprocessed as possible. Whole wheat, whole rye, stone ground wheat, oat flour, and sprouted breads are some healthier alternatives. If you're struggling to get enough protein, then high-protein breads can definitely help—some of these have up to 25 g of protein per serve (two slices). While you're skimming the nutrition label, it's also smart to check for added sugars or sweeteners and to steer clear from any breads that have 4 g of sugar or more per slice.

Alternatively, you can also find breads made from nut flours, which have less carbohydrate in exchange for a higher fat content. These are a good option for people who wish to avoid grains, but still want to include sandwiches in their diet. Then finally, a person can always substitute bread completely for large romaine lettuce leaves, portobello mushroom caps, or even slices of roasted sweet potatoes. These may not all fit the large amount of ingredients typical sandwiches would, but still work well and provide a lot of extra nutritional value of their own.

FOR TASTY, CLEAN, AND LEAN SANDWICH EXAMPLES, SEE THE SECTION 'LUNCH AND DINNER'

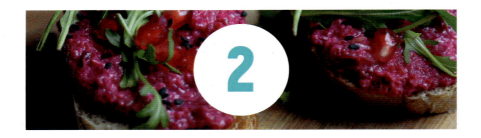

STEP 2: USE SPREADS THAT DON'T BREAK A NUTRITIOUS SANDWICH

Covering a sandwich with regular mayo or cheese certainly makes it tasty, but certainly not healthier. Instead, use one of our recommendations above (like avocado) for a healthier source of fat. This can be added as strips in place of cheese or mashed and spread instead of mayo. Don't forget about also utilising mustard, horseradish, balsamic vinegar, or hummus. All of these add bold flavours whilst contributing very little to your waistline.

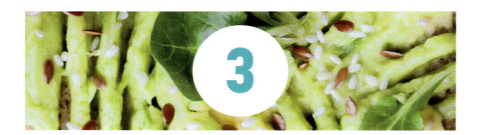

STEP 3: INTEGRATE VEGGIES FOR FLAVOUR

Many people forget that vegetables can provide TONS of flavour. Pickled vegetables like pickled beets, cucumber, and capsicum can add a lot of REAL flavour to your sandwich. To plan ahead, try grilling a bunch of veggies like red onion, mushrooms, or zucchini. Doing this will bring out more intense flavours and change good-tasting veggies into GREAT-tasting veggies.

If you don't have time to grill veggies ahead of time, buy store-bought sun dried tomatoes or roasted garlic—these can add a tasty savouriness to any sandwich. Lastly, don't forget to add greens for body and crispness. Rocket, spinach, kale, and collard greens have the highest nutritional content and make great additions.

5 STEPS TO MAKING TASTY, CLEAN, AND LEAN SANDWICHES

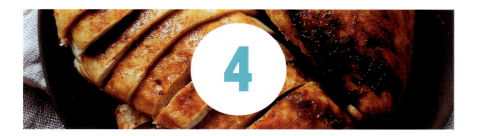

STEP 4: BE SURE TO ADD MEAT OR ANOTHER PROTEIN

With sandwiches, people often opt for the common store-bought deli meat. However, most meats can be highly processed, overly salted, and contain harmful preservatives. Be sure to find meats without added nitrates or salts. Good options include baked or roasted chicken breast, and roast beef.

If you're looking for a meat-free option, there are still plenty of high-protein additions. Avoid straight tofu, which will not have much flavour by itself. However, tempeh or seasoned seitan will provide lots of flavour. When choosing packaged mock meats, make sure the ingredient list is short and doesn't contain oil or salt as one of the first few ingredients.

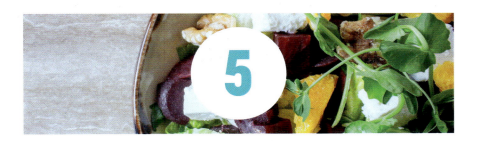

STEP 5: FINISH WITH A PERFECT COMBO

Sandwiches sometimes can't contain all we need, which is okay, because they make great additions to other nutritious foods. Ideally, a sandwich combined with a vegetable soup or simple salad makes a perfect nutrition combo.

For the more busy working professional, a sandwich lunch paired with a simple piece of fruit is also a great quick option to complete a great meal. Consider your sides when making sandwiches so you can make up for any nutrients that may be missing.

THE LEAN BODY SOLUTION

4 Simple Steps to Super Soups and Stews

"WANT SOME SOUP?"
DIN DJARIN (THE MANDALORIAN)

Due to their hunger-satisfying properties and because they're often packed with good ingredients, soups and stews have long been recognized as a leaner and healthy dish. Unfortunately, many store bought and ready-made varieties of soups and stews can be high in added sugar, salt, and preservatives, while being low in nutrients like protein and vitamins.

Making delicious and nutritious soups of your own is easy, though—you just need to know how with a simple method. Soups and stews offer a great way to make lean and tasty meals in big batches, while also being a great accompaniment and side, too.

Here is a simple four-step method for making lean, tasty, and appetising soups, and stews.

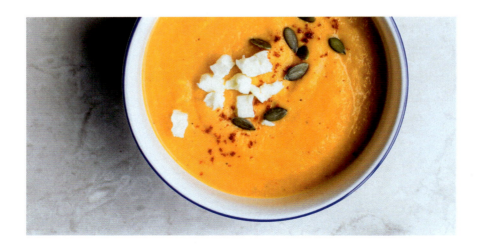

Simple Steps for Soups and Stews

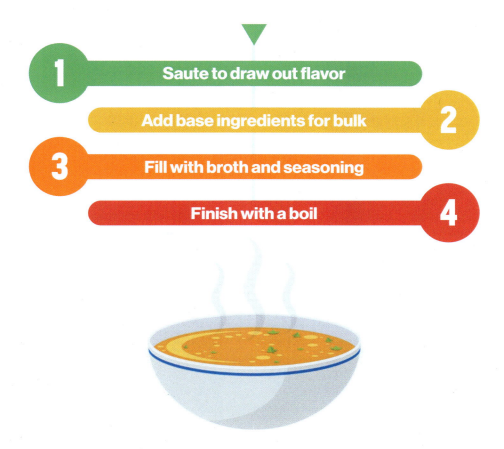

1. Saute to draw out flavor
2. Add base ingredients for bulk
3. Fill with broth and seasoning
4. Finish with a boil

Ingredient Options

Veggies to Saute	Base Ingredients	Broths & Liquids	Spices & Seasonings
• Diced Onions • Green Onions/Chives • Minced Garlic • Diced Carrots • Diced Celery • Diced Capsicum • Mushrooms	• Quinoa • Beans (black, kidney, etc.) • Barley • Lentils • Brown Rice • Wild Rice • Split Peas	• Water • Butternut Squash Puree • Chicken Broth • Tomato Puree • Vegetable Broth • Beetroot Puree • Sweet Potato Puree	• Savoury Spices: Cumin, Coriander, Paprika • Italian Spices: Basil, Oregano, Thyme, Parsley • Garlic & Onion Powder • Woody Spices: Cinnamon, Allspice, Cloves, Nutmeg • To taste: Salt, Black Pepper

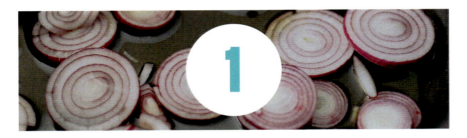

STEP 1: SAUTÉ TO DRAW OUT FLAVOUR

When starting a soup, the most common first step is to sauté some common ingredients to draw out the beginning flavours of your dish. Most often this involves dicing a combination of vegetables: carrots, celery, onion, and garlic are some popular ones that come to mind. Once this is done, these can be added to a pan and cooked over medium heat.

Many recipes call for adding large amounts of oil and butter at this stage, however, a better (and less messy) technique is to just use non-stick cookware: this will ensure you don't overdo it with fat. If you do this right, you will only require a small amount of oil (e.g. ½ tbsp) along with a small amount of broth (e.g. ¼ cup).

This provides a good way to draw out the flavour while still softening the vegetables. In applying this, be sure to sauté your mixture of vegetables and liquid for 3–5 minutes. If your recipe contains meat, this is a good time to add meat in strips or diced cuts and continue cooking until your meat is well done. If you've added onion, they will have turned slightly translucent by this stage, too, signalling you're ready for the next step.

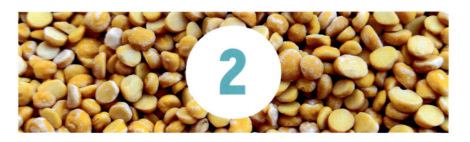

STEP 2: ADD BASE INGREDIENTS FOR BULK

Now you're ready to set the tone of your soup or stew. Most base ingredients for soups often include a grain, a bean, or some type of root vegetable. You can decide on a soup with cooked brown rice, legumes, or sweet potato, for instance. Some soups and stews make a base out of a vegetable like butternut squash, tomato, beets, or pumpkin.

In addition to the base ingredients, you can add in other secondary chopped vegetables here for flavour combinations and additional nutrition value. Secondary ingredients are added in lower amounts than the bulk so that soups don't have competing flavours. Common additions include chopped broccoli, mushrooms, okra, capsicum, green beans, scallions, corn, turnip, and zucchini.

The goal here is to bolster your base ingredients with a well-suited combination. The exact choice of ingredients is up to you and our recipes can give you a lot of guidance and mouth-watering ideas. Feel free to experiment, too! Once you've added base ingredients along with secondary ones, it's time to move on to Step 3.

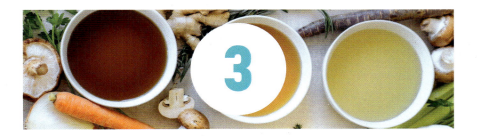

STEP 3: FILL WITH BROTH AND SEASONING

Next, you're going to fill up the soup with a light broth and add seasonings to intensify flavour. Look for lighter liquids like veggie or chicken broth, low-sugar tomato sauce, or light coconut-cream broth. A useful trick here is to open a ready-to-eat can of your favourite soup and add this as a broth. When recipes have a lot of ingredients and seasoning, adding water often works fine, too. Choosing a large amount of broth (3–4 cups) will result in a lighter more liquid-like soup, whereas adding just a small amount (1–2 cups) will create a chunkier-like stew.

After deciding on broth type and amounts, the next step is to add seasonings. Again, our sample recipes can add a lot of guidance and ideas here. Common soup seasonings can be quite varied based on the flavour of the soup you're searching for. Consider adding any of the following seasonings and spices: cumin, coriander, chilli powder, bay leaves, onion powder, garlic powder, turmeric, cinnamon, tamari, ginger, cayenne pepper, coriander, parsley, basil, oregano, thyme, red pepper flakes, fennel, paprika, mustard powder, or nutritional yeast.

After adding these and mixing well, taste your soup to see where the flavour is sitting. If it's too strong in flavour, add broth to dilute it. If too weak, add more seasoning. When just right, add a pinch of salt and pepper to your liking and move on to the next step.

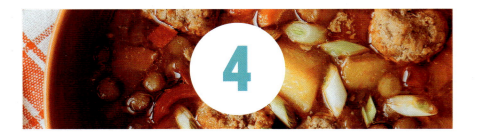

STEP 4: FINISH WITH A BOIL

Lastly, you'll want to bring your soup mixture to a boil by turning your heat to high. Similar to how steeping tea draws flavour out, your boil provides the final heat to absorb all the flavour from your ingredients. Boils can be as short as five minutes or as long as 20 minutes, depending on the ending flavour you're going for. In general, the longer the boil, the deeper and more pronounced flavours of your soup are going to be.

Make sure to stir the mixture every few minutes and watch to make sure it's not boiling out of your pan or burning. The thicker soups are the ones that will require more frequent stirring to prevent any burning or sticking of ingredients to the bottom of the pan. Once your boil is done, let your soup cool and enjoy your final product.

10 Tips to Lean and Delicious Salads from Start to Finish

"LET FOOD BE THY MEDICINE AND MEDICINE BE THY FOOD".

HIPPOCRATES

Salads are great to have because they provide more nutrients than practically any other dish! They also help include vegetables, healthy fats, and protein sources that are often missing from the diet. Because they're so nutritious, it's hard to get enough energy to feel full from eating salads. So when making salads, make them big!

Vegetables contain a lot of nutrient density and fibre, whilst also being very low in effective energy. Hence, BIG salads are often a great way to get leaner and stave off hunger at the same time.

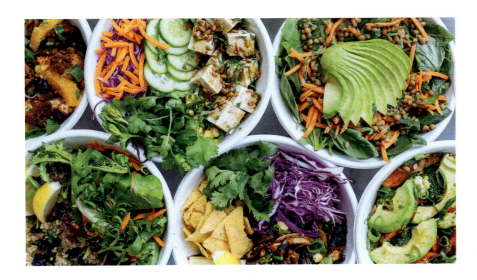

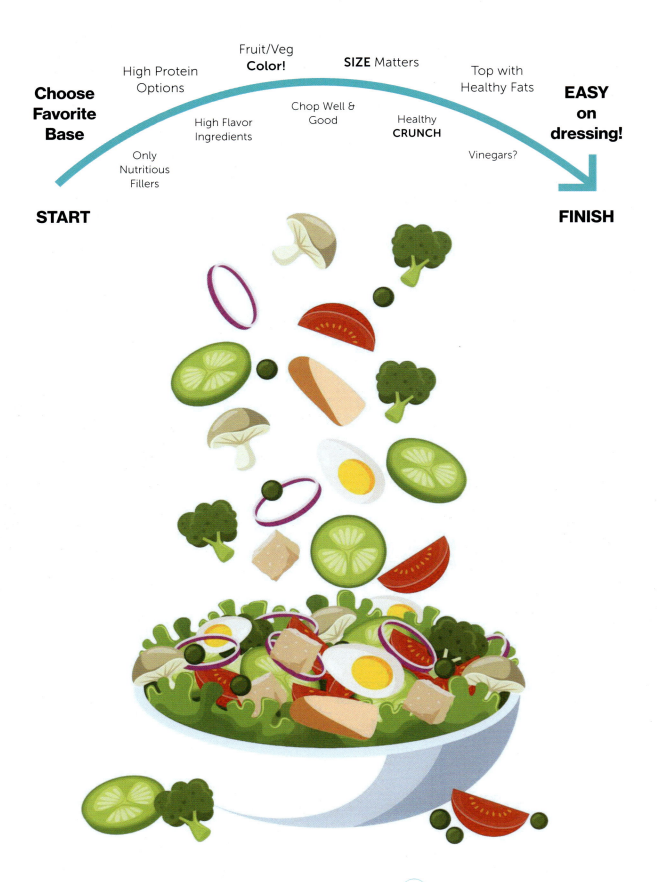

10 TIPS TO LEAN AND DELICIOUS SALADS

Ingredient Options

Veggies & Fruits

- Greens: Spinach, Romaine, Rocket, Kale
- Crunchy: Carrots, Celery, Capsicum, Cucumber
- Cruciferous: Broccoli, Cabbage, Shredded Brussels Sprouts
- Flavour: Beetroot, Swede, Snow Peas
- Fruits: Strawberries, Apple, Dried Cranberries, Pears, Grapes, Mango

Ingredients for Bulk

- Grains: Quinoa, Brown Rice, Barley
- Cooked Legumes: chickpeas, kidney beans, black beans, edamame etc.
- Cooked Lentils
- Mushroom
- Tomato
- Boiled Egg

High Flavour Ingredients

- Roasted Garlic
- Onion, Chives or Scallions
- Sunflower or Sesame Seeds
- Fresh Parsley or Coriander
- Roasted Walnuts or Sliced Almonds
- Minced Jalapeno
- Minced Ginger

Dressings

- Vinegars: Red Wine, Balsamic, Rice, Apple Cider
- Tahini
- Lemon or Lime Juice
- Avocado: Cubed, Sliced or Mashed
- Olive Oil (use small amounts)
- Orange Juice
- Miso Paste

Meats and Protein

- Grilled Chicken & Turkey
- Roast Beef & Steak
- Fish & Seafood: Tuna, Salmon, Shrimp, Crab, Lobster, etc
- Tofu (vegetarian)
- Tempeh (vegetarian)
- Seitan (vegetarian)

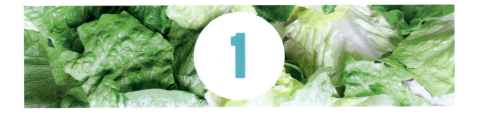

STEP 1: CHOOSE YOUR FAVOURITE BASE

Everyone likes a different kind of green. Some prefer just green lettuce, while others like spinach or the crunch of cabbage. Choose the base that you prefer the most, or do a mixture of multiple kinds. The vegetables with deep colours like kale or red cabbage will provide the most nutrients, but if those aren't your favourite, mix them with a lighter leafy base like romaine lettuce or rocket leaves. Combining can suit your taste preference while also pumping up the nutrition.

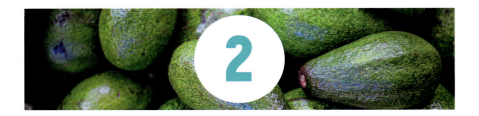

STEP 2: INCLUDE ONLY NUTRITIOUS FILLERS

It's important to leave out low-nutrition fillers that often creep into many store-bought salads and ruin them. Foods like mayonnaise, white breads, cheeses, etc. are to be left out if you're looking to get leaner and healthier. In their place, add foods like cooked pumpkin, couscous, avocado, cooked legumes, and lentils. Doing so will keep salads packed with vitamins and minerals, while still keeping them nutritious and lean enough.

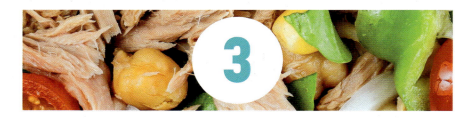

STEP 3: SELECT HIGH-PROTEIN OPTIONS

Salads have traditionally been thought of as the dieter's food, but there's no reason why a salad can't also be high in protein, lean, and filling at the same time. Some great protein sources that can really add some bulk and flavour include grilled chicken and turkey, roast beef and steak, salmon, and tuna (cut fillet or canned), cooked prawns/shrimp, crab, and lobster. High-protein vegetarian options include chopped tofu, seitan, and tempeh.

10 TIPS TO LEAN AND DELICIOUS SALADS

STEP 4: ADD HIGH-FLAVOUR INGREDIENTS

If you just always expect a salad to taste like vegetables or vegetables with dressing, you're missing out. Salads can and should contain high-flavour ingredients like olives, artichoke hearts, sun dried tomatoes or pickled items like beets and onions. These will give you the desire to keep making salads over and over again.

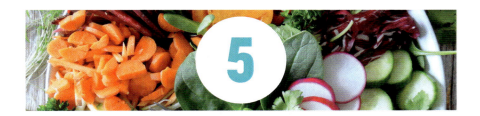

STEP 5: GET COLOURFUL WITH YOUR VEGGIES

A beautiful-looking salad isn't just more pleasing to the eyes, it's also a sign of health-promoting compounds in our foods. Having a wide variety of vegetables is healthier than having the same produce day after day. So when making your salads, try to fill the rainbow by adding as many colours as you can. Some great examples are red capsicum, orange carrots, yellow corn, white cauliflower, purple cabbage, and green broccoli.

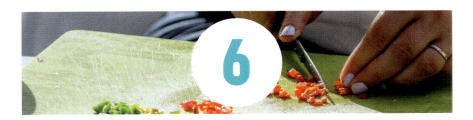

STEP 6: CHOP WELL AND GOOD

When making a salad and adding ingredients, taking some extra time to carefully chop items really pays off. You don't want to have to cut up every bite because pieces of vegetables are too big to fit in your mouth, but you also don't want to have things so small that it's hard to get them with your fork. The best balance comes from following this rule: chop all items to a small enough size that they're able to fit completely in your mouth in one bite. With practice, you'll find what size each vegetable or fruit works best for yourself.

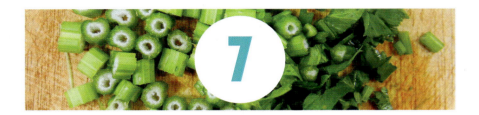

STEP 7: GIVE IT A HEALTHY CRUNCH

Texture is important with salad, too. Nothing is more unappetizing than a soggy salad that has no crunch to it. It's actually the chewing texture that helps us eat slowly and tells our body that we're getting full, too. So with the softer bases of spinach, lettuce, or rocket leaves, make sure to add crisp vegetables like celery, carrots, and capsicum. These all add a nice variety of mouth feel and will make a salad more filling and satisfying.

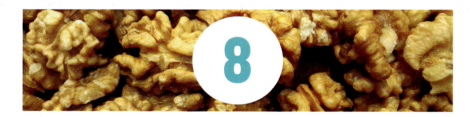

STEP 8: TOP WITH HEALTHY FATS

Since salads often contain a lot of vegetables, one will want to remember to add some healthy fats. This is because vegetables are rich in fat-soluble nutrients, so having a small amount of fat is needed to absorb these beneficial compounds. Try adding a handful of healthy nuts like almonds or walnuts, or sprinkle some ground flaxseeds or pumpkin seeds into the mix. Healthy oils like olive oil and flaxseed oil can also be added with the bonus of providing added flavour and enhanced texture.

10 TIPS TO LEAN AND DELICIOUS SALADS

STEP 9: DON'T FORGET ABOUT VINEGARS

Flavoured vinegars are growing in popularity and these tasty dressings often provide little to no sugar! This makes them great for salads. Look for balsamic, apple cider, red wine, or aged vinegars. These will provide high flavour while keeping the salad lean.

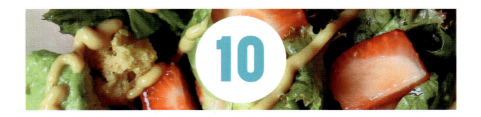

STEP 10: GO EASY ON THE DRESSING!

The number one way the average person turns a salad unhealthy is by adding high-fat or high-sugar dressings. When choosing dressings, look for ones that are more oil-based and less cream-based as these will naturally be leaner. Also pay close attention to your portion size. More than 1.5 tablespoons of dressing should never be needed on a serving of salad. A little bit of dressing goes a long way and the key is to ensure it is mixed well. Some people like spray oils because they easily coat the salad without providing excess oil. Another technique is to use a fork to stir ingredients or put a lid on a salad with dressing and shake it vigorously to coat each item with flavour.

FOR LEAN AND DELICIOUS SALAD EXAMPLES, SEE THE SECTION 'LUNCH AND DINNER'

Super Sides for Complete Meals

"YOU COMPLETE ME"
TOM CRUISE (JERRY MAGUIRE)

Sometimes to hit our nutritional needs and target amounts, it is necessary to have sides with our main meals. Sides are normal and shouldn't be considered as cheating if they are within one's requirements and for hitting their nutrition targets. A lot of people tend to be a bit lost when it comes to choosing the best sides and pairings with their meals. The lists below can help solve this problem.

Fruits *(can be combined with a sandwich)*

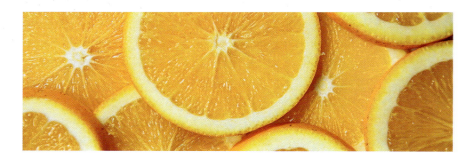

- mango slices
- cherries
- orange slices
- grapes
- pear slices
- kiwi fruit
- apple slices
- berry varieties
- melon slices/chunks
- pineapple slices/chunks

THE LEAN BODY SOLUTION

SUPER SIDES FOR COMPLETE MEALS

Soups *(can be combined with a sandwich or salad)*

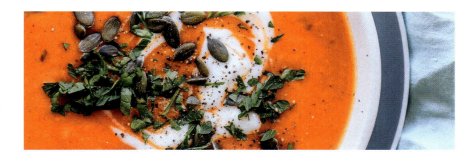

- tomato
- barley
- butternut squash
- chicken
- black bean
- mushroom
- split plea
- lentil
- chilli

Salads *(can be combined with sandwiches or soups)*

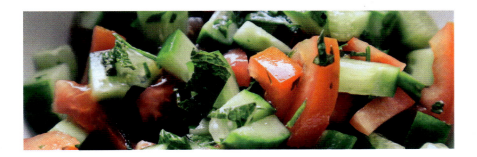

- kale salad
- Niçoise salad
- coleslaw salad
- rocket salad
- Caesar salad
- spinach salad
- tabouleh salad
- quinoa salad
- romaine salad
- Israeli salad
- Mediterranean salad
- grilled vegetable salad

FOR EXAMPLE SUPER SIDE RECIPES SEE THE 'SIDES' RECIPE SECTION

Leaner Snack Alternatives and Ideas

"LIFE IS ALL ABOUT MAKING CHOICES, FINDING THE RIGHT ONES, AND EMBRACING BETTER ALTERNATIVES ALONG THE WAY".
OPRAH WINFREY

Snacking can be an effective way to control daily hunger and satiety while providing sustained energy. However, not all snacks are lean or healthy. Many common snacks that people choose to eat can be filled with extra sugars, excessive salt, and unhealthy oils. So finding lean snacks with minimal processing should be the goal when planning out what to eat between meals.

Thankfully, many unhealthy snacks can be easily swapped with healthier alternatives that are just as enjoyable and still convenient. Here are some common swaps that a person can consider:

- Homemade veggie chips in place of high-fat potato chips
- Protein cookies instead of sugary biscuits
- Protein bars and balls instead of candy bars and lollies
- Mixed raw or roasted nuts instead of sugar-coated and salted peanuts
- Greek yoghurt with fruit instead of sugary flavoured yoghurts
- Protein ice cream instead of ice cream
- Homemade protein muffins instead of cakes and muffins
- Brown rice cakes instead of white-flour crackers.

FOR LEANER SNACK RECIPES EXAMPLES, SEE THE SECTION 'SNACKS AND DIPS'

A Brief Word on Supplements

"DON'T SWEAT THE SMALL STUFF".
RICHARD CARLSON

There is a reason we used the word 'brief' in the title and chose to keep this section small. Supplements have a very small place in your overall lean body plan—period. In fact, we would rather you get all your nutrients from whole foods.

There is a very tiny window where supplements may be applicable. For instance, a protein powder if you're travelling or looking to top up a shake or smoothie with a bit of extra protein. Some fish oil if you're not getting enough essential fatty acids from your diet. And maybe some caffeine if it helps you kick through your workouts harder on longer days. But that's about it!

Supplements are as the word implies; to 'supplement' your diet— not be a replacement. Think of supplements like the cherry on a sundae. Most people put the cart way in front of the horse and rely on pills and potions way too much.

Supplements are not a be-all-end-all replacement for quality nutrition (despite what many weight loss and supplement companies market to you!). Most supplements on the weight-loss market are a complete waste of money and, worse yet, a waste of your attention. Most have hyped up claims and don't even do a fraction of that they purport to. They simply distract you and get you into a 'quick fix' and 'magic pill' mindset.

And that's where we will leave supplements for that very reason. Focus on your diet and lean down with real food... Real food like what you're about to see in the next section.

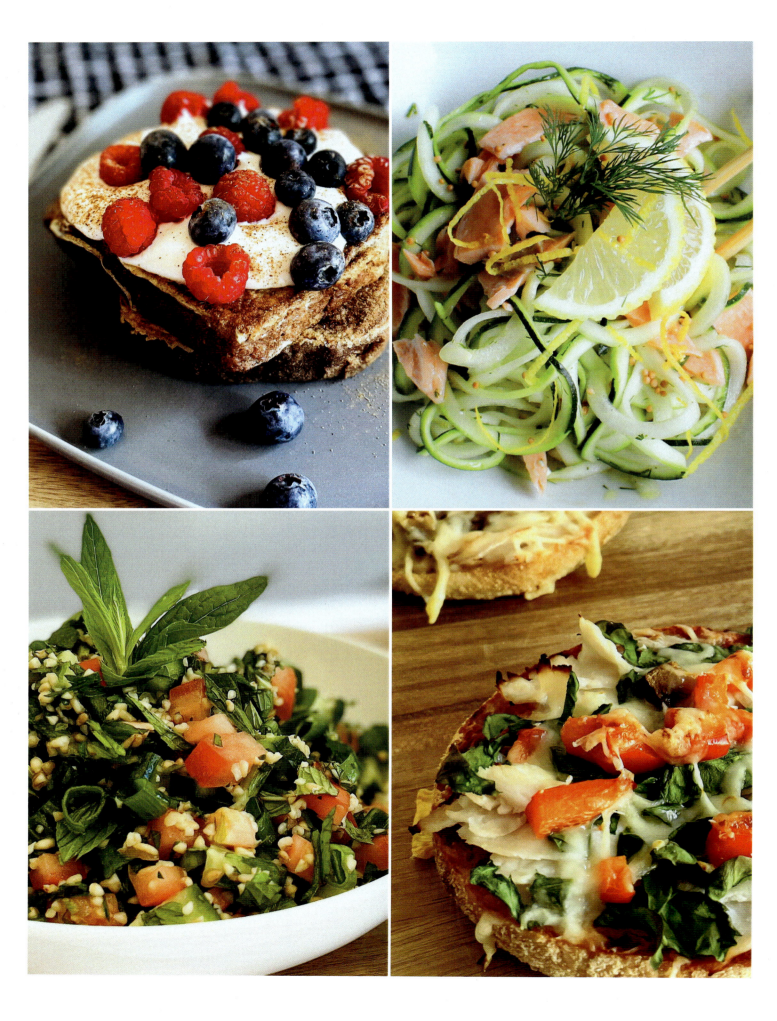

THE LEAN BODY RECIPES

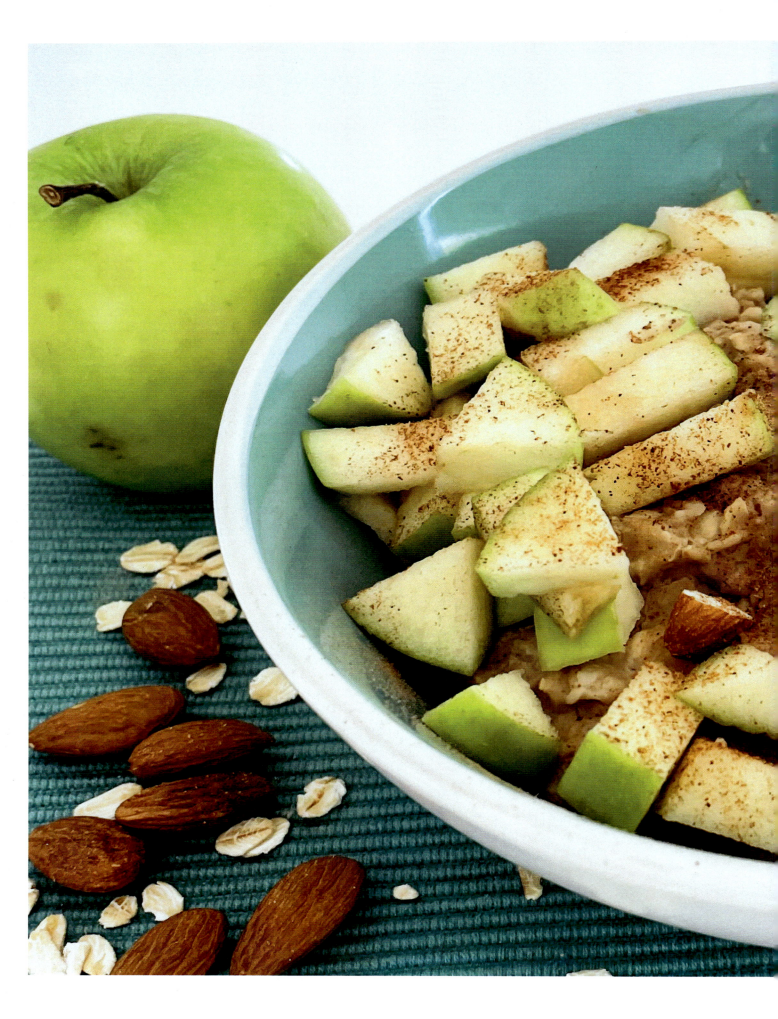

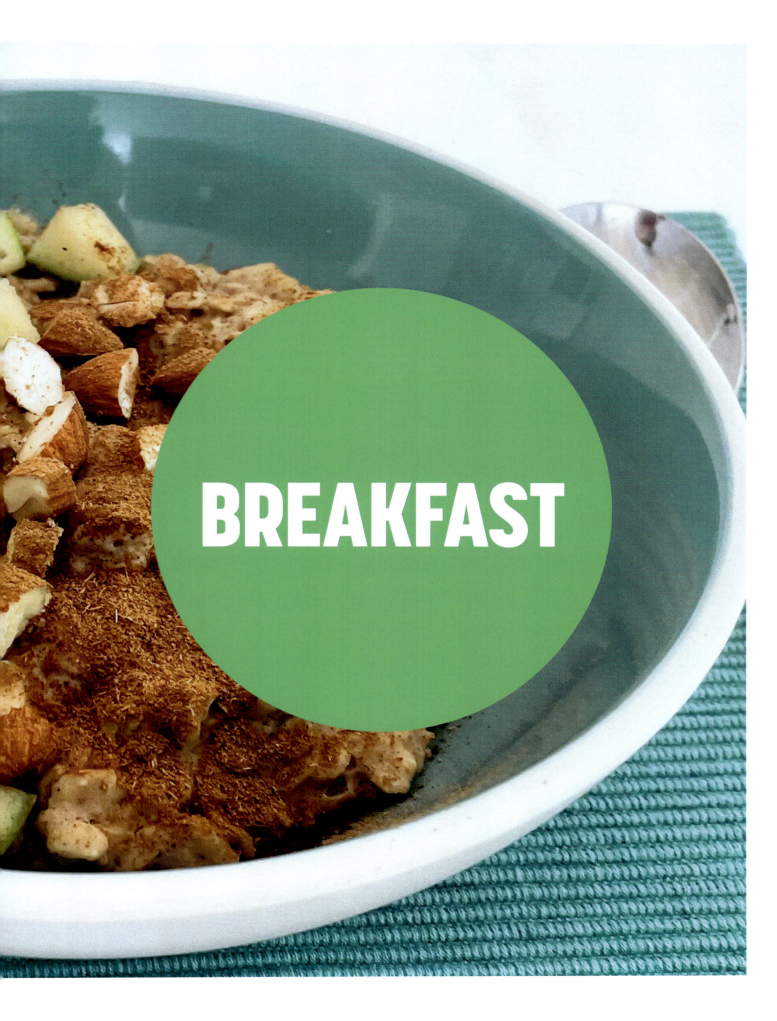

BREAKFAST

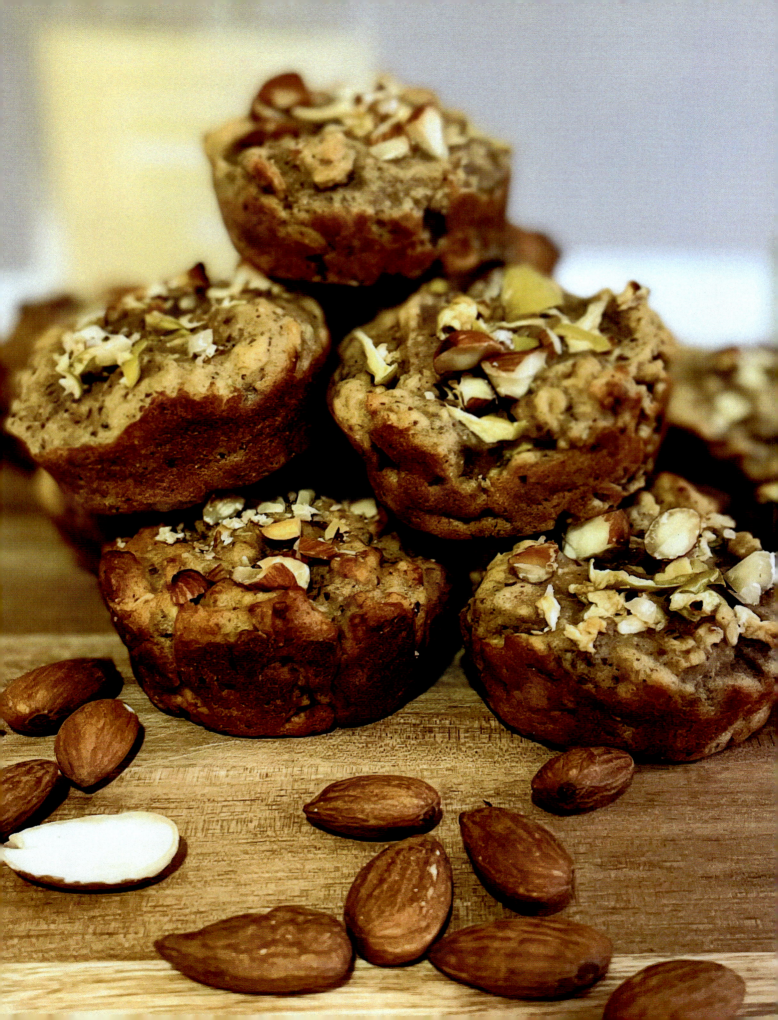

BREAKFAST

Breakfast Protein Muffins (V)

SERVINGS: 12 MUFFINS

MACRO BREAKDOWN (per muffin)

FAT: 7G

PROTEIN: 14G

CARBS: 17G

RECIPE HIGHLIGHTS

These muffins are protein packed, deliver essential omega-3s, and have a good dose of iron and magnesium. The muffins can be stored frozen and simply reheated in a microwave. Busy mornings and quick breakfast options just got easier.

INGREDIENTS

- 2 tbsp ground flaxseed + 4½ tbsp hot water
- ¼ cup olive oil
- 1 banana
- ¼ cup sugar-free maple syrup (naturally sweetened)
- 3 scoops vanilla protein powder
- ½ tsp salt
- 1½ tsp baking soda
- 1 tsp cinnamon
- ⅔ cup oats
- ½ cup Greek yoghurt
- ¼ cup chopped almonds
- 1½ cups spelt flour
- ½ cup minced apple (optional)

METHOD

1. Preheat oven to 190 °C.
2. Prepare the flaxseed by mixing it with the hot water in a small bowl. Set aside to thicken.
3. In a separate bowl, mash ½ of the ripe banana, add olive oil, then add these to the flaxseed mixture.
4. Add maple syrup, yoghurt, salt, baking soda, and cinnamon to the flaxseed mixture until all ingredients are well incorporated.
5. Add the protein powder, oats, and flour to the mixture to form the batter. If the batter is too thick, try adding a small amount of milk to thin it out. Note: batter consistency will vary with protein powders.
6. Put the mixture into 12 muffin tins and top with minced apple and chopped almonds. Bake for around 30 minutes, or until a toothpick comes out clean. Let the muffins cool for at least 10 minutes after baking.

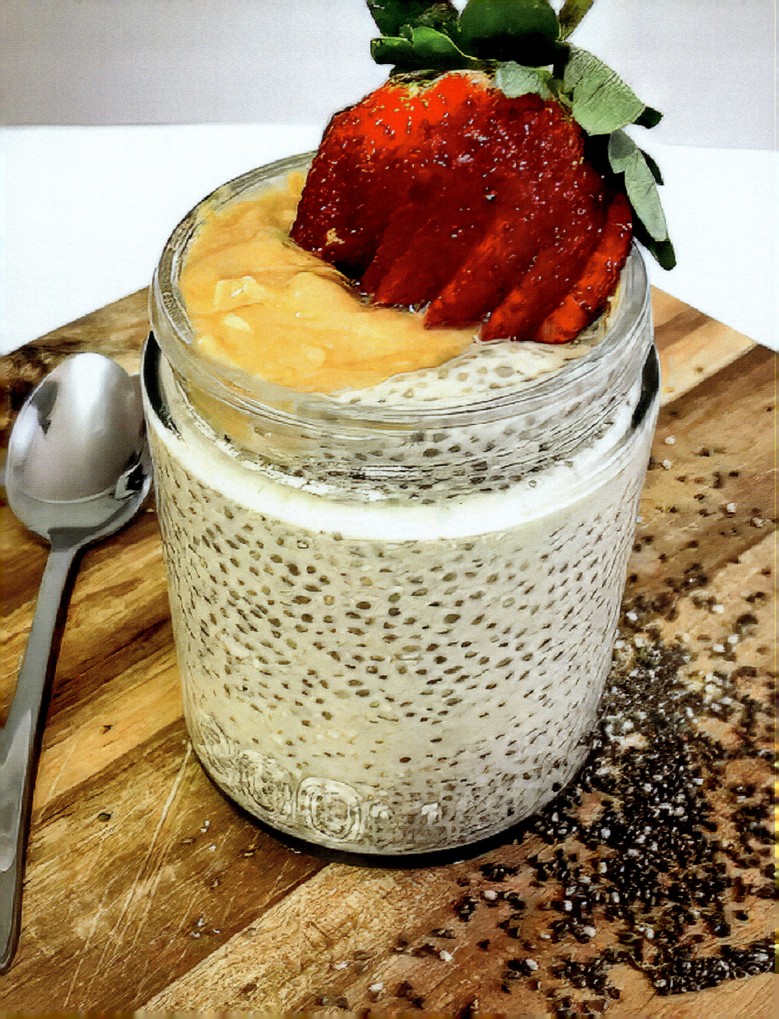

BREAKFAST

Overnight Vanilla Chia Cup (V)

SERVINGS: 1

MACRO BREAKDOWN (per serve)

FAT: 17G

PROTEIN: 32G

CARBS: 19G

RECIPE HIGHLIGHTS

This breakfast option is low in sugar and high in protein! It's also packed with calcium and omega-3s. These overnight breakfast cups are another great breakfast option for when you're on the run or rushed in the morning.

INGREDIENTS

- ¼ cup chia seeds
- 1 cup almond milk
- 1 scoop vanilla protein powder
- ½ tbsp stevia powder
- ½ cup fruit of choice topping
- 1 tsp pure vanilla extract (optional)

METHOD

1. Simply mix all ingredients except the fruit together until the protein powder is well mixed (add slightly more almond milk if needed).
2. Place mixture in a sealable glass or plastic container, and place in the refrigerator overnight.
3. In the morning, chop up your favourite fruit and top the mixture with it. The consistency should be like thick yoghurt with natural sweetness.

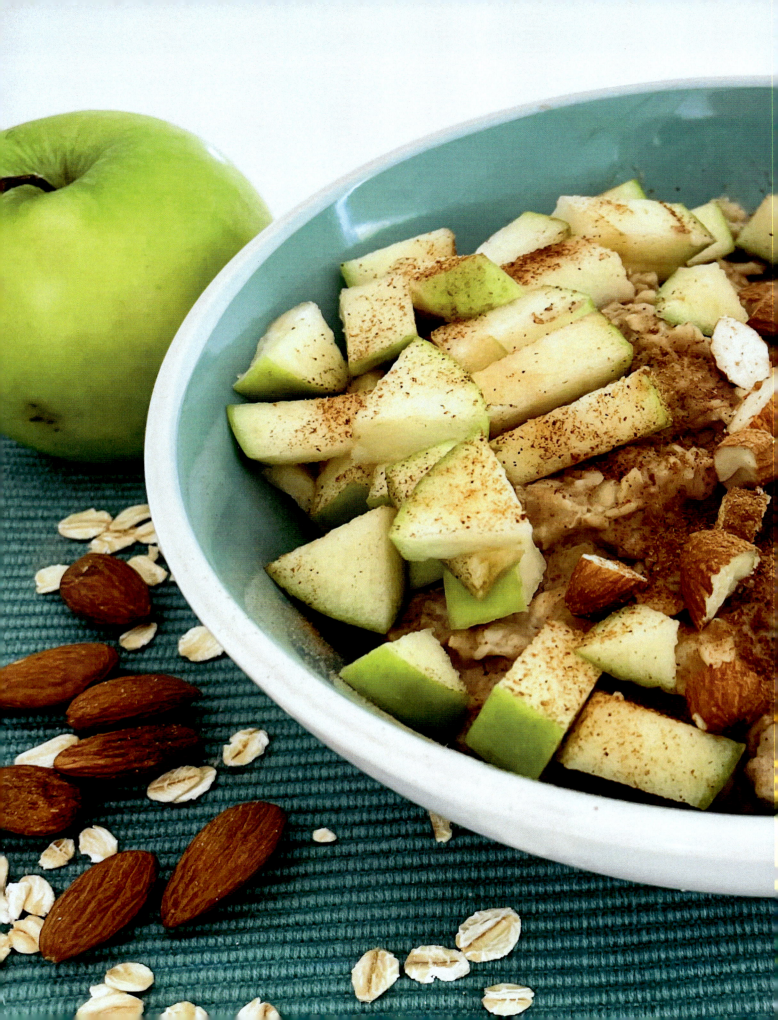

BREAKFAST

Quick & Warm High-Protein Muesli (V)

SERVINGS: 1

MACRO BREAKDOWN (per serve)

FAT: 29G

PROTEIN: 40G

CARBS: 60G

RECIPE HIGHLIGHTS

This big breakfast is perfect for those who frequently train at higher intensities and require more carbs and a higher intake of nutrients.

INGREDIENTS

- 2 cups unsweetened almond milk
- ½ cup rolled oats
- 1 scoop protein powder
- 1 tsp vanilla extract
- 1 tsp cinnamon
- ½ cup berries or chopped apple
- 2 tbsp nuts of choice

METHOD

This is a fairly quick breakfast for those fast mornings that can be either cooked on the stove top or in the microwave.

1. For pan cooking, mix oats and almond milk into a medium-sized pan, and then cook over medium heat while stirring constantly. Add whey protein and cinnamon.

2. Add 1 tsp of pure vanilla extract and cook for 2–3 minutes until the oats are breaking up. (If cooking in the microwave, microwave on high for 2 minutes.)

3. Lastly, top with berries and nuts of choice. The result is a vanilla and cinnamon protein-packed cereal that's easy and delicious!

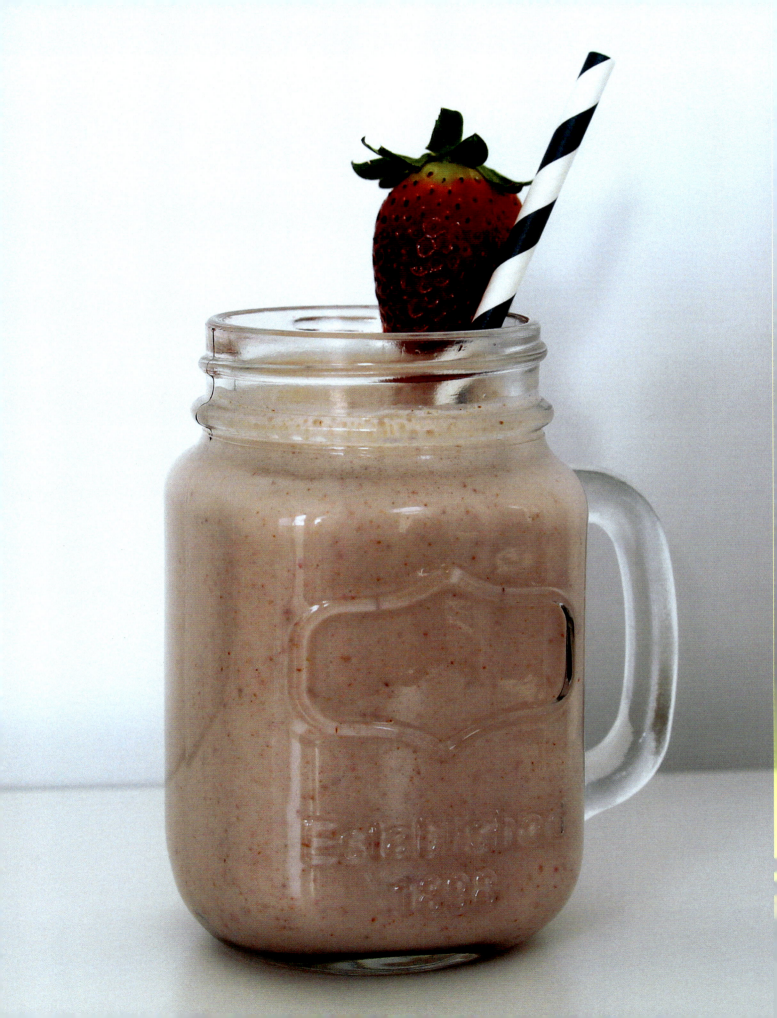

Strawberry Breakfast Smoothie (V)

SERVINGS: 1

RECIPE HIGHLIGHTS

This recipe delivers lots of protein, a heap of healthy fat, and a huge dose of vitamin C—all in one delicious creamy shake!

MACRO BREAKDOWN (per serve)

FAT: 18G

PROTEIN: 45G

CARBS: 13G

INGREDIENTS

- *2 cups unsweetened almond milk*
- *½ cup frozen strawberries*
- *2 tbsp almond butter*
- *2 tbsp avocado*
- *½ cup non-fat Greek yoghurt*
- *1 scoop whey protein isolate*
- *½ tsp vanilla extract*

METHOD

For this high-protein, creamy breakfast smoothie, you're just going to want to add almond milk first followed by the berries, almond butter, and avocado. Then top with protein sources and a touch of vanilla.

Depending on the power of your blender, you may need to keep blending on high for up to 1 minute until you end up with a smooth consistency. If it gets stuck while blending, just add a couple spoonfuls of some extra almond milk to thin it out.

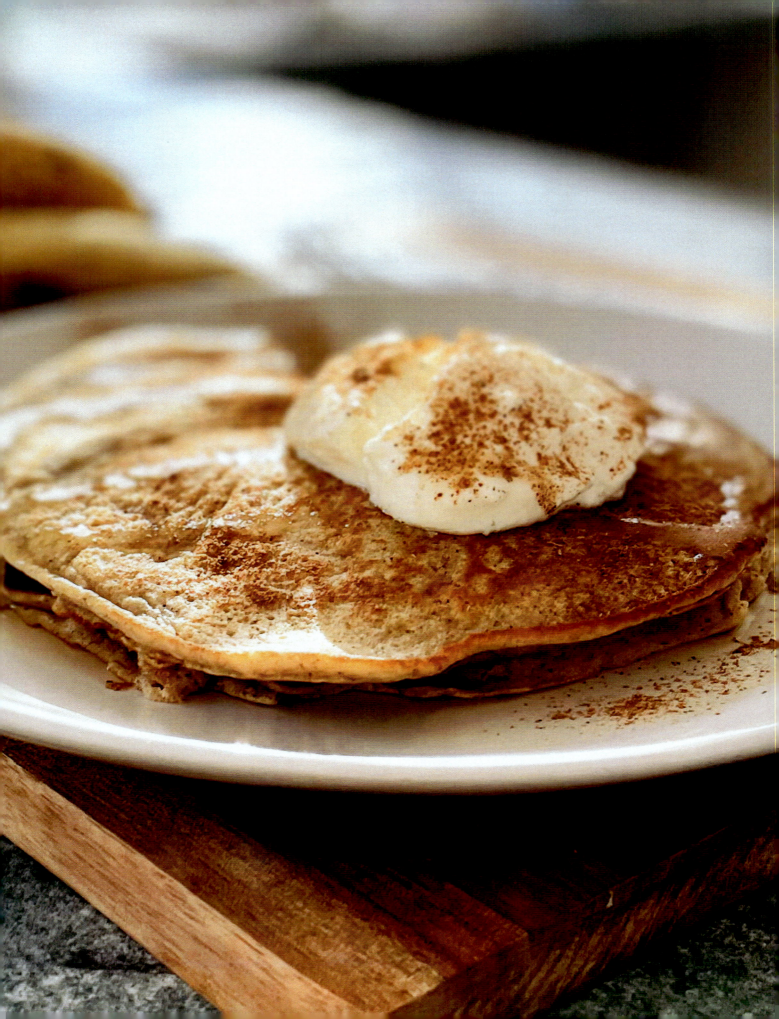

BREAKFAST

Banana-Protein Pancakes (V)

SERVINGS: 1 (2 PANCAKES)

MACRO BREAKDOWN (2 pancakes)

FAT: 16G

PROTEIN: 45G

CARBS: 26G

RECIPE HIGHLIGHTS

These pancakes will keep a person full for several hours after breakfast time. They are protein-packed and provide far less sugar than traditional butter and syrup pancakes.

INGREDIENTS

- *1 small banana*
- *30 g WPI powder*
- *1/8 tsp baking powder*
- *2 egg whites*
- *1 egg*
- *1 tsp cinnamon*
- *1 tsp vanilla bean paste*
- *Coconut oil (to cook)*
- *Low-fat Greek yoghurt (to serve)*

METHOD

1. Mash the banana in a bowl. Stir in the protein powder and the baking powder until well combined.
2. Add the egg whites, whole egg, cinnamon, and vanilla bean paste and mix using a whisk until well combined.
3. Heat a large non-stick frying pan over medium-high heat. Add a teaspoon of coconut oil and smear over the frying pan to cook the pancakes in.
4. Pour half the mixture into the frying pan to create a small pancake and cook for a few minutes until you see small bubbles appear on the surface.
5. Flip over and cook on the other side for another minute until golden brown. Repeat with the other half of the mixture to make the two pancakes.
6. Serve with a scoop of Greek yoghurt.

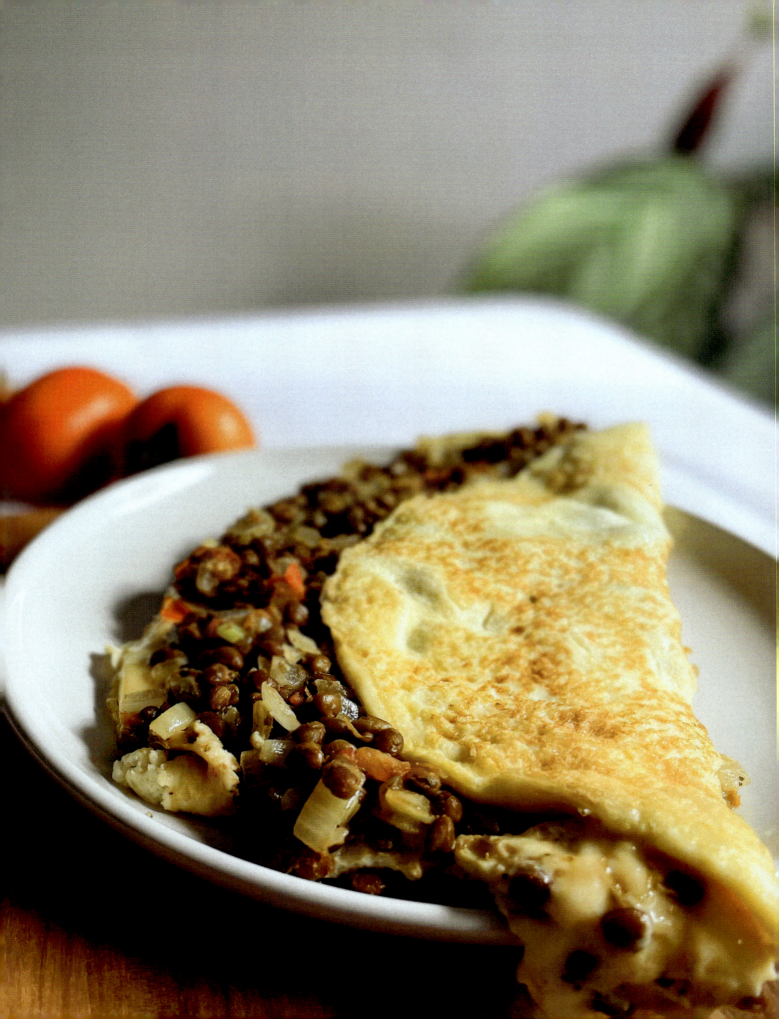

BREAKFAST

Curried Lentil Omelette (V)

SERVINGS: 1

RECIPE HIGHLIGHTS

The use of lentils increases the fibre and fullness of the omelette, while also increasing the vitamin content. This omelette is also high in protein and big on spicy flavour!

MACRO BREAKDOWN (per serve)

FAT: 10G

PROTEIN: 33G

CARBS: 26G

INGREDIENTS

- 1 teaspoon vegetable oil
- ½ small onion, finely chopped
- ½ teaspoon mild curry paste
- ½ medium tomato, seeded and chopped
- ½ cup cooked lentils, drained and rinsed
- 1 teaspoon chopped coriander
- 1 pinch of salt
- ¼ teaspoon pepper
- 1 egg
- 3–4 egg whites

METHOD

1. In a skillet, heat oil over medium heat. Sauté onion 3–5 minutes. Stir in curry paste and tomato and sauté for 2 minutes.
2. Add drained lentils and cook (stirring often) for 5 minutes or until tomatoes are soft. Stir in coriander, salt, and pepper. Set aside.
3. Whisk the egg and whites with a dash of milk and pinch of salt.
4. Heat a separate pan on medium heat and spray with oil. Pour in egg mixture until omelette forms.
5. Add lentil mixture to one side of omelette and fold then serve.

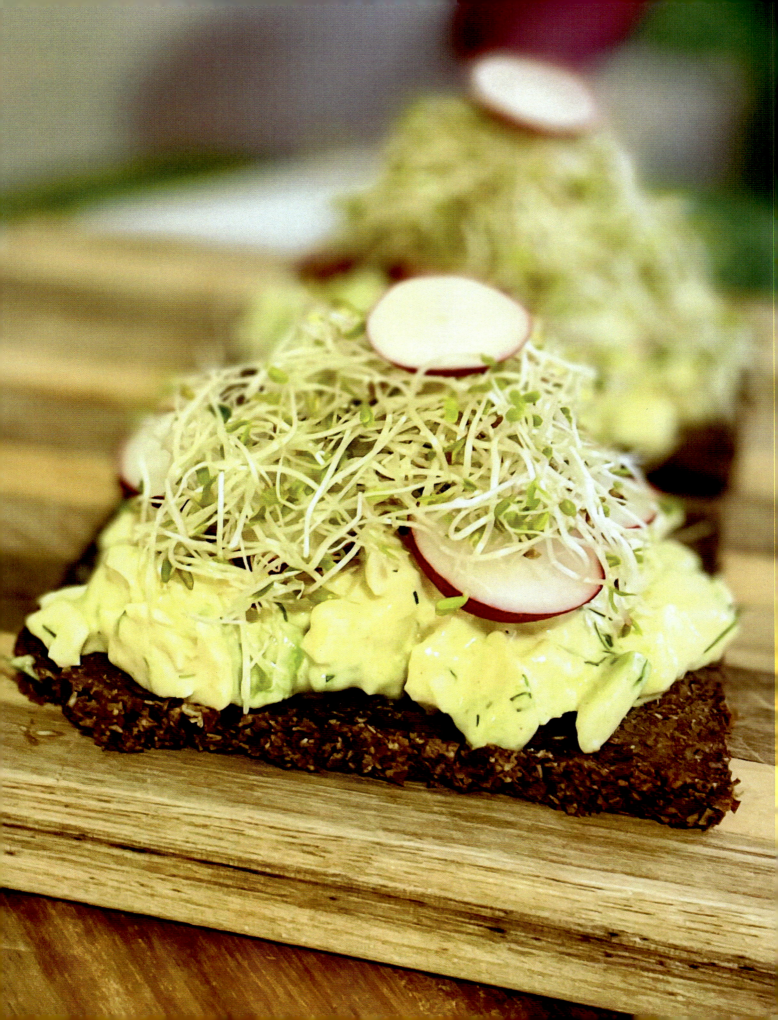

BREAKFAST

Avocado and Egg White Tartines (V)

SERVINGS: 1

MACRO BREAKDOWN (per serve)

FAT: 26G

PROTEIN: 30G

CARBS: 57G

RECIPE HIGHLIGHTS

Unlike other breads, pumpernickel comes from a whole grain (rye), which happens to have more vitamins, fibre, and overall nutrients than plain wheat varieties. This larger breakfast is great if you require more carbs and protein than the average person.

INGREDIENTS

- 1 cup egg whites
- 2 tablespoon light/low-fat mayonnaise
- 2 tablespoon Dijon mustard
- 1 tablespoon lemon juice
- ½ teaspoon finely grated lemon zest
- 1 small avocado, finely chopped
- 2 tablespoon fresh dill, finely chopped
- 4 thin slices of pumpernickel bread
- 3 radishes, thinly sliced
- ½ cup alfalfa sprouts
- Freshly ground black pepper, to taste

METHOD

1. Lightly coat a glass or ceramic pie plate with non-stick cooking spray. Pour in egg whites and microwave on high for 4–5 mins (or until egg whites are set). Cool completely then finely chop.

2. Toss the egg whites with the mayonnaise, Dijon mustard, lemon juice, and lemon zest. Stir in the avocado and dill. Chill for 30 mins. in fridge. Mixture can be stored in the fridge for up to 24 hours in an airtight container.

3. Toast the bread, then spread an even layer of egg salad onto each piece.

4. Garnish with radish, cucumber, and sprouts. Season with pepper to taste.

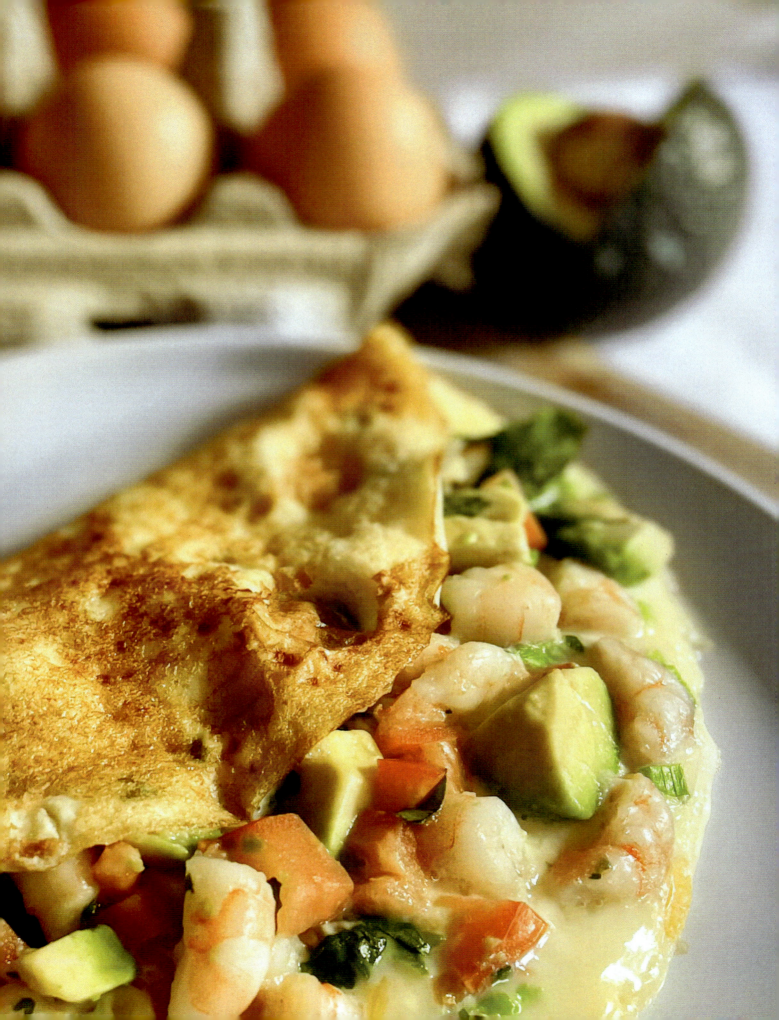

BREAKFAST

Prawn and Avocado Omelette

SERVINGS: 1

RECIPE HIGHLIGHTS

This omelette offers a good balance of fats and significantly more protein than the average omelette. It's also very low in carbs while offering a rich savoury taste. If you love avocado and prawns, you will love this combo!

MACRO BREAKDOWN (per serve)

FAT: 17G

PROTEIN: 30G

CARBS: 4G

INGREDIENTS

- ⅓ cup small or chopped cooked prawns
- ½ small tomato, diced
- ¼ avocado, diced
- Coriander, chopped (to taste)
- 1 egg
- ½ cup egg whites
- 1 tablespoon low-fat milk
- 2 tablespoon chives, finely chopped
- 1 tablespoon grated parmesan or low-fat cheddar cheese
- Olive oil cooking spray

METHOD

1. For the filling, combine small or chopped cooked prawns, avocado, tomato, and chopped coriander to taste. Set aside.
2. Beat half cup of egg whites, one egg, one tablespoon of low-fat milk. Add chives to the mixture and pour into an 8-in (20-cm) frying pan sprayed with olive oil cooking spray. Make sure the mixture covers the base and cook until almost set but still creamy.
3. Scatter the filling over one half of the omelette and the grated parmesan (or low-fat cheddar cheese) over the other half.
4. Cook for 2–3 minutes or until golden, then fold unfilled half over the filling. Slide out onto a serving plate.

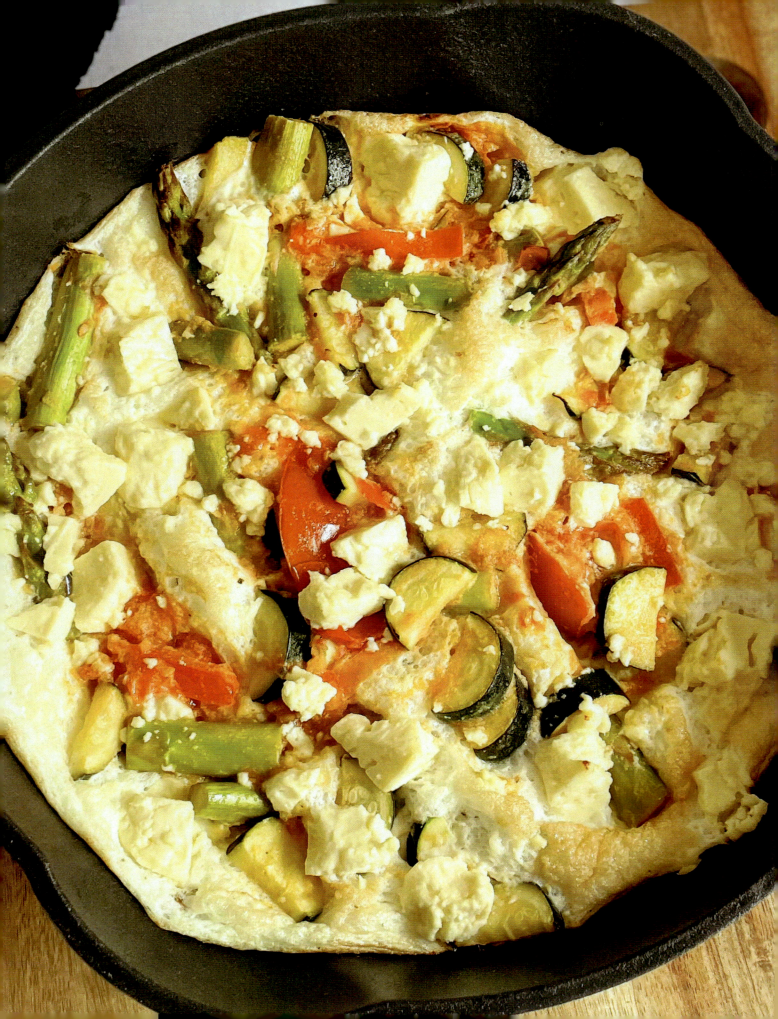

BREAKFAST

Grilled Veggie Omelette (V)

SERVINGS: 2

RECIPE HIGHLIGHTS

This very lean breakfast is low in carbs and packed with grilled vegetables to bring out savoury flavours! This omelette also has a good amount of protein and doesn't go overboard with the cheese.

MACRO BREAKDOWN (per serve)

FAT: 16G

PROTEIN: 21G

CARBS: 4.5G

INGREDIENTS

- ¾ cup chopped and grilled zucchini and tomatoes
- 5 spears of grilled asparagus
- 1 tbsp butter
- ½ small onion, chopped
- 1 cup egg whites
- 2 tbsp grated parmesan cheese
- 1½ tbsp thinly sliced fresh basil
- ¼ tsp salt
- ½ tsp pepper
- 1 tbsp basil and garlic dressing
- ¼ cup low-fat feta

METHOD

1. Grill zucchini, tomatoes, and asparagus to desire and set aside.
2. Preheat oven to 200 °C. Melt butter in a non-stick skillet set on medium heat. Add onion and cook for 3 minutes, stirring occasionally.
3. In a large mixing bowl, beat egg whites until soft peaks form. Add parmesan cheese, basil, salt, and pepper.
4. Increase heat to medium-high, spread onion mixture in pan. Add and smooth the egg mixture over the onions, cooking for 1 minute.
5. Toss grilled vegetables with basil and garlic dressing, then arrange over half of the omelette. Arrange the feta over the other half of the omelette.
6. Bake for 5 to 6 minutes or until golden: the centre should be slightly soft. Fold feta side over vegetable side and serve.

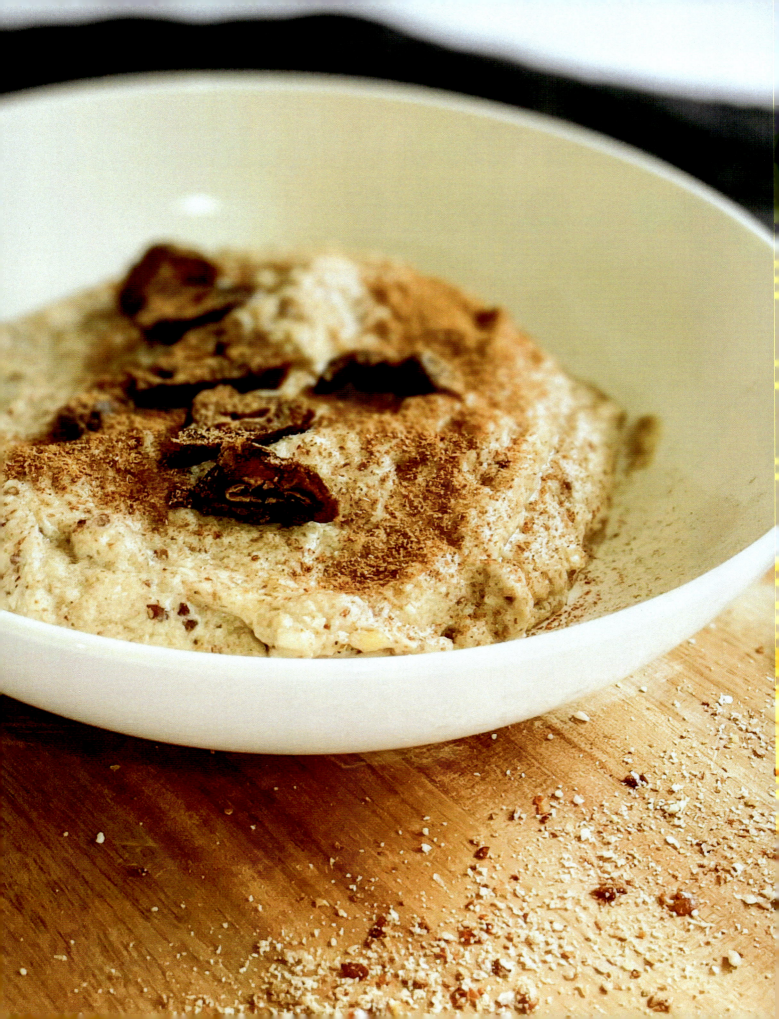

BREAKFAST

Sweet and Creamy No-Oats Porridge (V)

SERVINGS: 1

RECIPE HIGHLIGHTS

Whether you're an oats fan or not, you will love this quick, tasty recipe that can be frozen and microwaved if required. This recipe is perfect as a pre-workout breakfast if you're doing higher-intensity training in the morning.

MACRO BREAKDOWN (per serve)

FAT: 11G

PROTEIN: 18G

CARBS: 40G

INGREDIENTS

- ⅔ cup unsweetened almond milk
- 1 egg, whisked
- 2 egg whites, whisked
- 1 small banana, mashed
- 2 tablespoons LSA meal
- 1 teaspoon cinnamon
- 1 teaspoon vanilla bean paste
- 1 medjool date, chopped up into small pieces

METHOD

1. Place almond milk in a small saucepan and heat over medium heat, stirring frequently.
2. When the almond milk is warm, add the whisked egg and egg whites to the almond milk and whisk together. Continue to whisk over medium heat until the milk mixture starts to thicken (about 5 minutes).
3. Add the mashed banana, LSA meal, cinnamon, and vanilla bean paste. Whisk to combine. The mixture should start to thicken and resemble a thick porridge consistency.
4. Pour into a bowl and top with the medjool date.

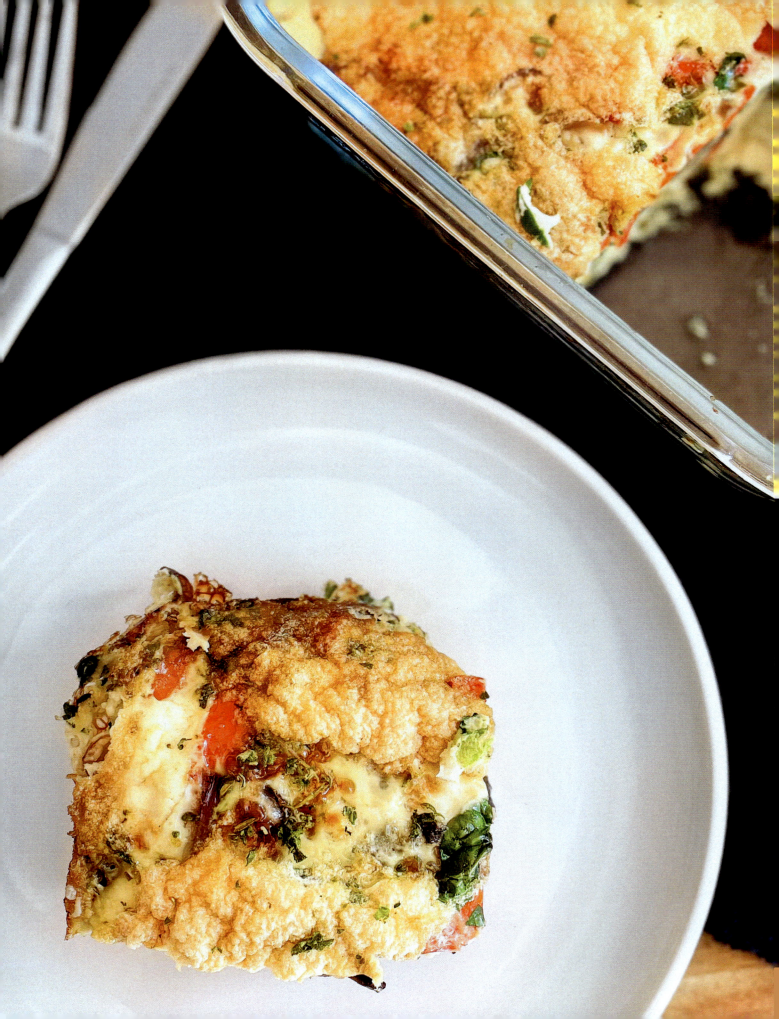

BREAKFAST

Roasted Veggie Frittata (V)

SERVINGS: 3

MACRO BREAKDOWN (per serve)

FAT: 11G

PROTEIN: 33G

CARBS: 10G

RECIPE HIGHLIGHTS

The vegetables in this breakfast dish are packed with B-vitamins to help promote energy and focus. This lower-carb and higher-protein frittata has a very flavoursome taste and can be easily stored in the fridge for when you need to quickly heat up a nutritious breakfast.

INGREDIENTS

- *2 tsp extra-virgin olive oil*
- *1 cup fresh mushrooms, sliced*
- *3 cups egg whites, beaten*
- *50 g goat cheese*
- *½ cup baby spinach, chopped*
- *1 cup red capsicum, cut into strips*
- *1 cup thin red onion wedges*
- *2 tbsp fresh oregano, snipped*
- *¼ tsp black pepper*
- *¼ tsp sea salt*
- *Olive oil cooking spray*

METHOD

1. Preheat oven to 200 °C. Lightly grease a 13x9x2-inch baking dish with cooking spray.

2. Toss olive oil, onion, capsicum, mushrooms, salt, and pepper in a large bowl until well combined. Spoon the mixture evenly into the baking dish and roast for 20 minutes (or until the vegetables are tender). Reduce the temperature to 160 °C.

3. Toss roasted vegetables with the spinach and spread the mixture into the baking dish. Sprinkle with pieces of goat cheese and pour the egg whites on top. Bake for 30 minutes (or until a toothpick inserted into the centre comes out clean).

4. Remove from oven and let stand for at least 10 minutes before serving.

5. Sprinkle with oregano to serve.

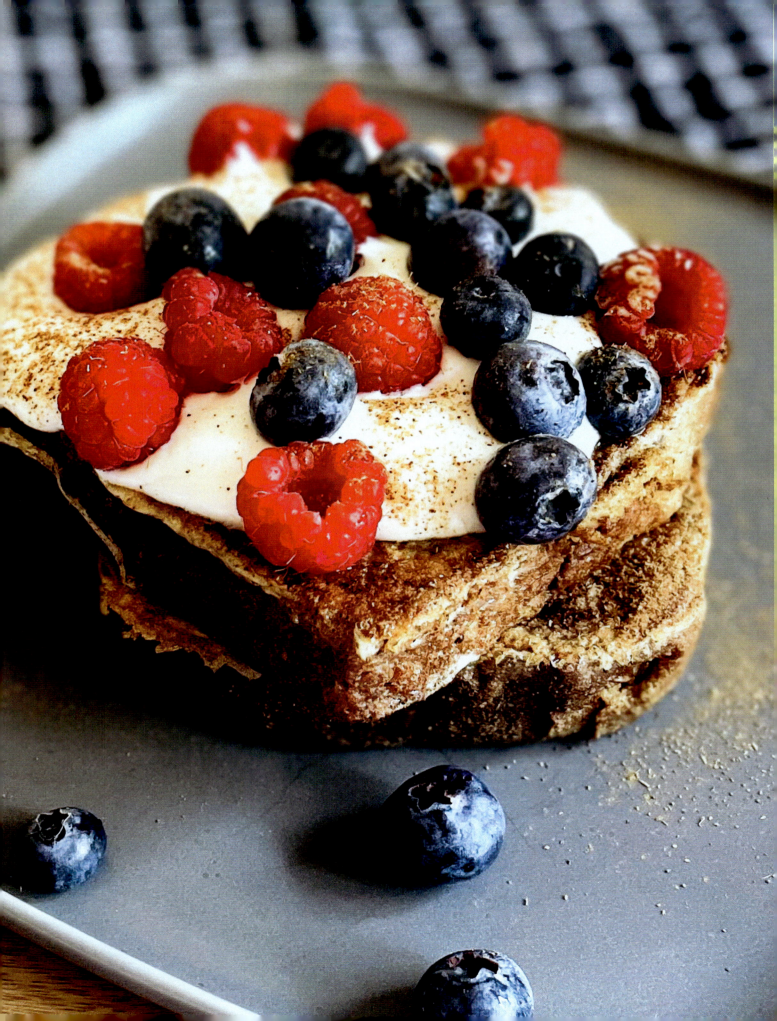

BREAKFAST

French Toast Sweet Sandwich Stack (V)

SERVINGS: 1

RECIPE HIGHLIGHTS

Most French toasts lack protein—this one does not! This sweet stack is ideally consumed as a pre-workout breakfast for those doing higher-intensity training in the morning. For a lower carb option, swap the fruit bread for high-protein or seed bread.

MACRO BREAKDOWN (per serve)

FAT: 7G

PROTEIN: 30G

CARBS: 64G

INGREDIENTS

- 2 slices of fruit bread
- 1 egg
- 2 egg whites (~70 g)
- ½ tsp cinnamon
- ½ tsp ground cloves
- ¼ cup low-fat, high-protein yoghurt
- 1 tbsp sugar-free maple syrup (naturally sweetened)
- ½ cup mixed berries
- Extra cinnamon, to serve

METHOD

1. Whisk together egg, egg white, cinnamon and cloves in a bowl.
2. Preheat a non-stick pan over medium-high heat.
3. Submerge fruit bread into egg mixture until fully covered and soak through.
4. Add to the pan and cook for 1–2 mins each side, or until egg is cooked through.
5. Meanwhile, combine yoghurt and syrup in a bowl, and mix well.
6. Remove French toast from pan and stack on top of each other on a plate. Top with yoghurt mixture and berries. Dust with extra cinnamon and serve immediately.

THE LEAN BODY SOLUTION

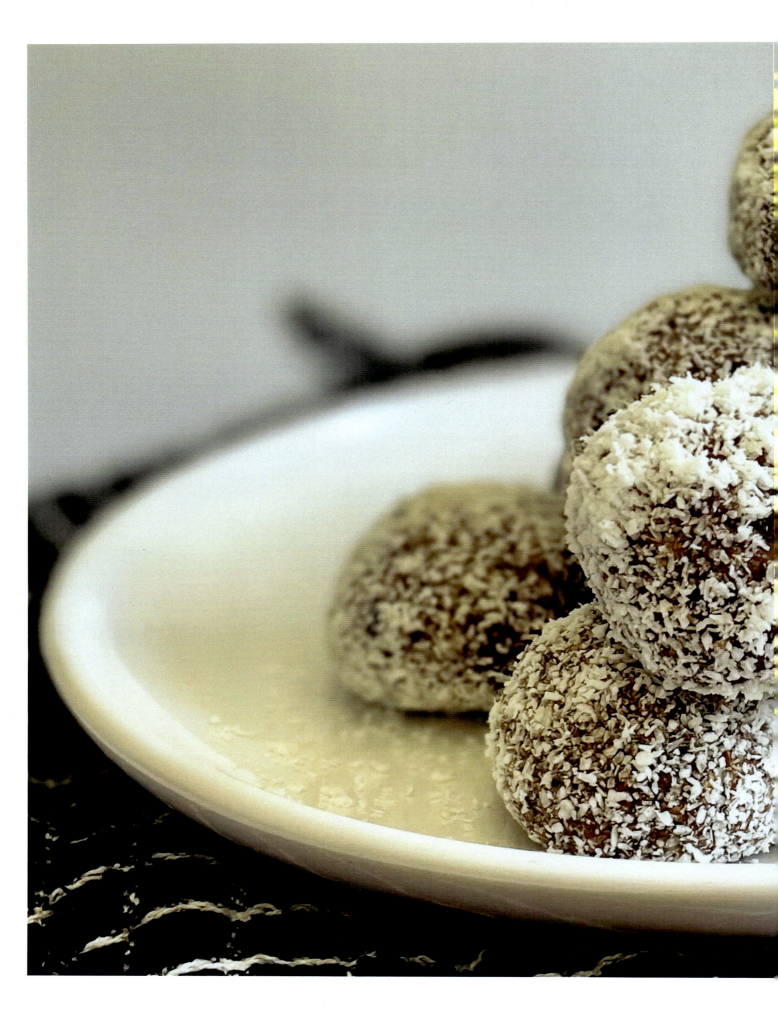

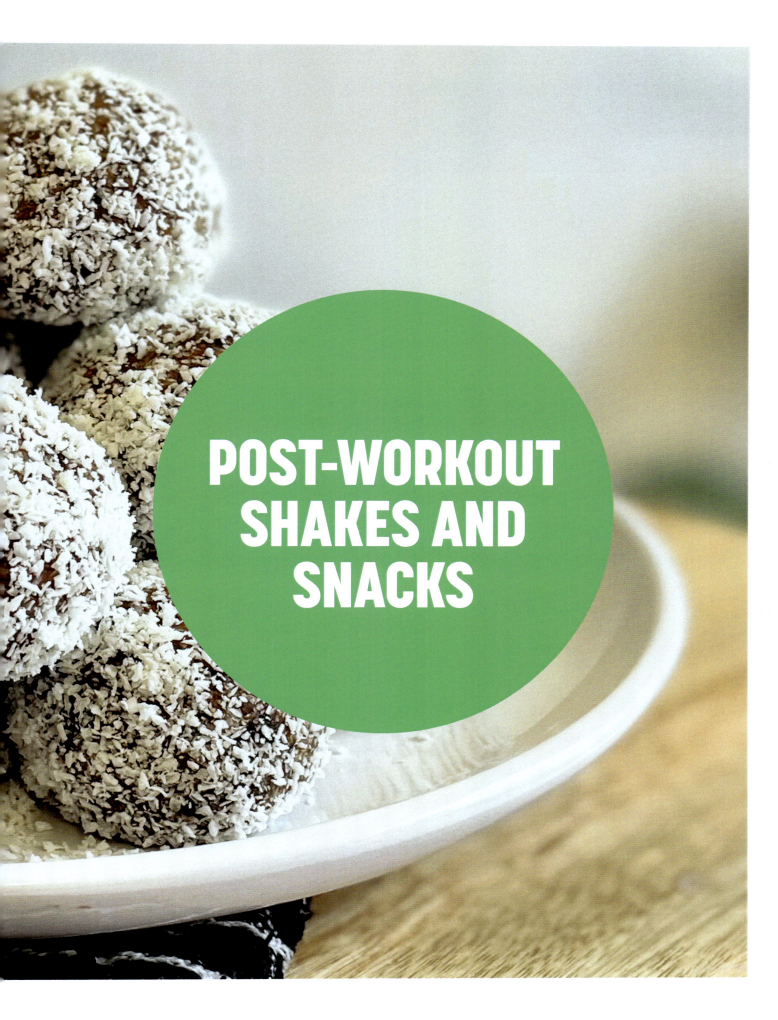

POST-WORKOUT SHAKES AND SNACKS

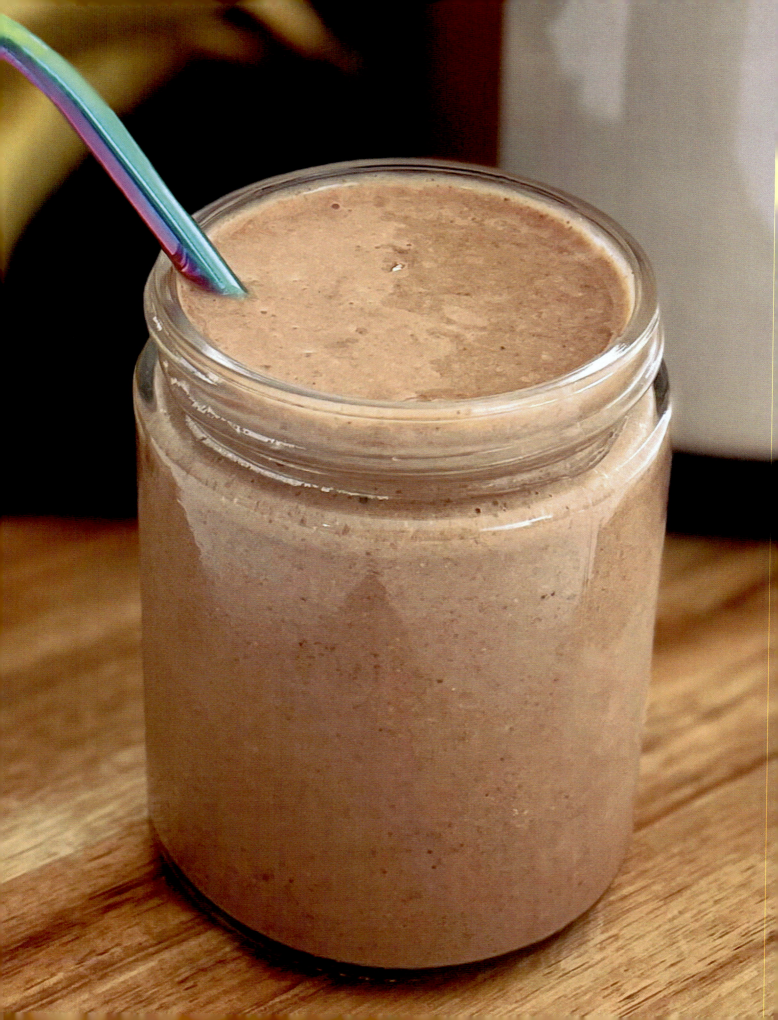

POST-WORKOUT SHAKES AND SNACKS

Better Choc Banana Protein Smoothie (V)

SERVINGS: 1

MACRO BREAKDOWN (per serve)

RECIPE HIGHLIGHTS

This delicious shake provides a quick source of carbohydrates and protein to repair muscles that have been depleted and broken down during intense workouts. The flaxseed and cacao powder add texture and promote energy long after training has finished.

FAT: 3G

PROTEIN: 27G

CARBS: 36G

INGREDIENTS

- 1 small frozen banana (cut into chunks)
- 30 g whey protein powder (plain or chocolate)
- 1 tsp. flaxseeds/linseeds
- 1 tsp cacao powder
- 1 tsp. cinnamon
- ¾ cup almond milk

METHOD

Place all ingredients in a blender and process until smooth and creamy. Serve and drink immediately.

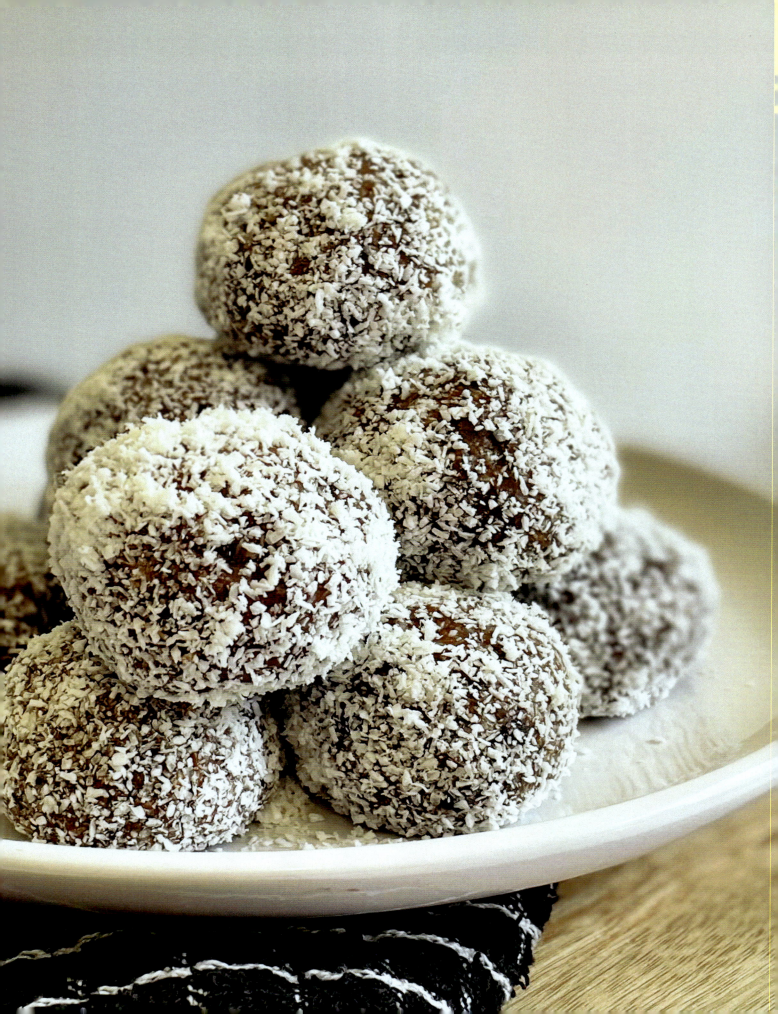

POST-WORKOUT SHAKES AND SNACKS

Coconut Rough Protein Balls (V)

SERVINGS: 8 BALLS

MACRO BREAKDOWN (per ball)

FAT: 5G

PROTEIN: 10G

CARBS: 9G

RECIPE HIGHLIGHTS

These delicious and gooey protein balls only take 5 minutes to make! Each contains 10 g of protein and they are far more nutritious and viable than overpriced store bought alternatives.

INGREDIENTS

- ½ cup pitted dates
- ¼ cup desiccated coconut
- 3 scoops chocolate whey protein powder (~90 g)
- 1 tbsp peanut butter
- 1 tbsp powdered peanut butter
- ¼ cup unsweetened almond milk
- 1 tbsp coconut oil
- ½ tsp vanilla essence
- Extra ¼ cup desiccated coconut

METHOD

1. Blend the dates in a food processor until chopped finely.
2. Add all other ingredients (except for the extra coconut) and process until well combined.
3. Place the extra coconut in a flat bowl.
4. Evenly divide the mixture into 8 portions, and roll each into a ball. Roll each ball in the extra coconut and place on a baking paper-lined tray.
5. Balls can be consumed immediately, or placed in the refrigerator for 1–2 hours to become more firm.

THE LEAN BODY SOLUTION

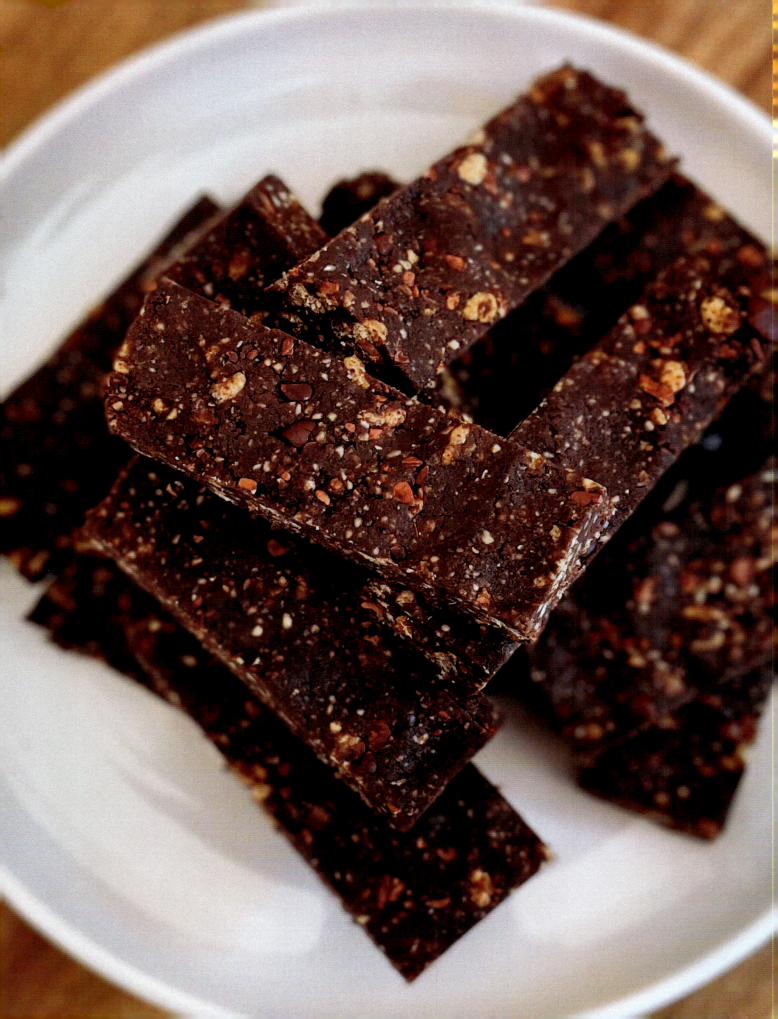

POST-WORKOUT SHAKES AND SNACKS

Carb Craver Choc Mint Protein Bars (V)

SERVINGS: 16 BARS

MACRO BREAKDOWN (per bar)

FAT: 5G

PROTEIN: 6G

CARBS: 12G

RECIPE HIGHLIGHTS

These bars have everything to replace store-bought protein bars and are void of artificial additives and sweeteners. Having a few of these bars after an intense workout will ensure you get a good dose of protein and quick absorbing carbs for proper recovery. Dates are perfect for quickly replenishing depleted glycogen and they also contain much needed minerals like magnesium and iron.

INGREDIENTS

- 1 cup medjool dates (deseeded)
- 1 cup raw cashews
- 1 cup whey or plant-based protein powder (plain or chocolate)
- ¼ cup cacao powder
- ½ teaspoon peppermint extract
- 1 teaspoon vanilla bean paste
- 2 tablespoon unsweetened almond milk
- ¼ teaspoon sea salt
- ¼ cup cacao nibs (plus extra to decorate the top of the bars)
- ½ cup puffed brown rice (place on a baking sheet and place in the oven for 15 minutes at 150 °C. This helps the puffed brown rice to be nice and crispy in the bars)

METHOD

1. Place medjool dates in a food processor and pulse until they are broken up into small pieces.
2. Add raw cashews and process until the dates and cashews are finely ground.
3. Add protein powder, cacao powder, peppermint extract, vanilla bean paste, unsweetened almond milk, and sea salt. Process until well-combined and a slightly sticky ball is formed.
4. Remove from food processor and place in a bowl. Add in puffed brown rice and cacao nibs.
5. Mix the puffed brown rice and cacao nibs through the date mixture using your hands or a palette knife.
6. Take a 20-cm square cake tin and line with plastic cling wrap. Place bar mixture into cake tin and flatten down with your hands so that the top is even.
7. Sprinkle with extra cacao nibs to decorate. Cover the top with plastic cling wrap.
8. Place into the freezer for an hour.
9. Remove from freezer and remove plastic wrap. Place on a large chopping board and cut into 16 bars. Each bar contains 6 g of protein. These can be kept in the fridge for up to seven days, or in the freezer for up to 3 months.

THE LEAN BODY SOLUTION

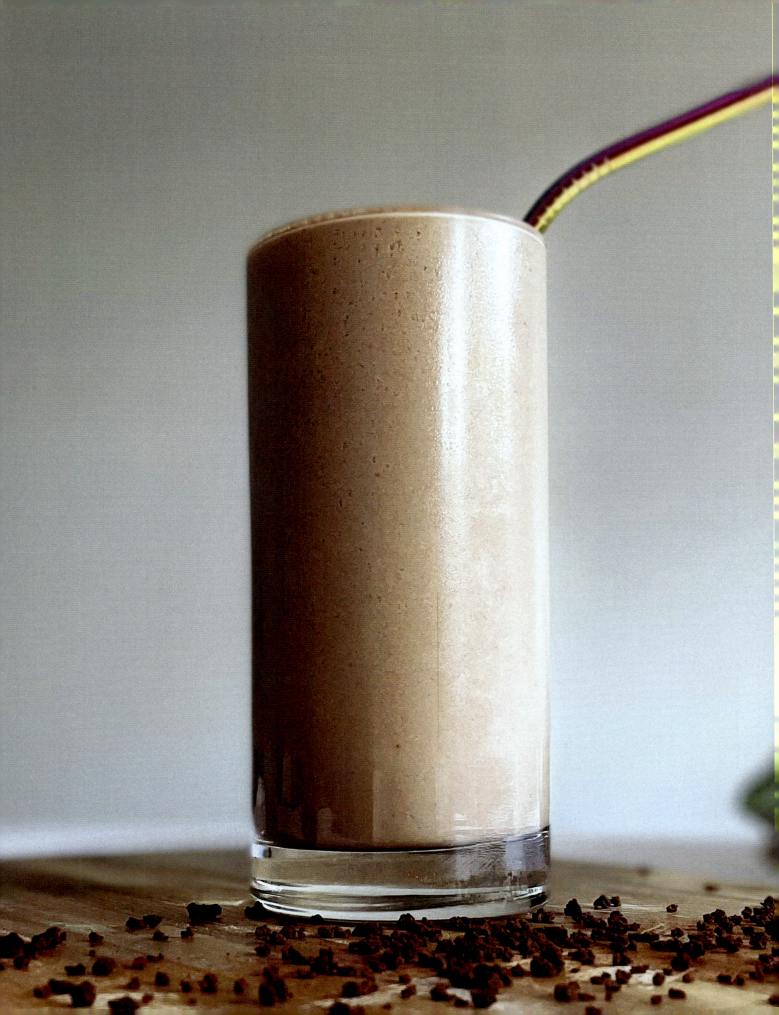

POST-WORKOUT SHAKES AND SNACKS

Espresso Protein Shakes & Smoothies (V)

SERVINGS: 1

RECIPE HIGHLIGHTS

The espresso smoothie is both a delicious and energising pre- or post-workout drink. If you get hooked on the taste and want to have it during other times of the day, simply ditch the banana and opt for the shake version.

MACRO BREAKDOWN (per serve)

For Espresso Shake (made on light milk)	For Espresso Smoothie
FAT: 4G	FAT: 5G
PROTEIN: 33G	PROTEIN: 40G
CARBS: 16G	CARBS: 25G

INGREDIENTS

For Espresso Shake
- 2 ice cubes
- 1 chilled shot (or double shot if you prefer) of espresso or 2–3 teaspoons of instant espresso/coffee
- 1 cup cold water or light milk
- 1 scoop chocolate or vanilla protein powder
- Stevia to taste

For Espresso Smoothie
- ½ banana
- 1 cup light milk or unsweetened almond milk (preferably vanilla flavour)
- ½ cup of 0%-fat Greek yoghurt
- 1 tbsp cacao powder
- 1 scoop chocolate protein powder
- 1 chilled shot (or double shot, if you prefer) of espresso or 1–2 teaspoons of instant espresso/coffee

METHOD

For Espresso Shake

1. In a shaker bottle, add ice cubes with a chilled shot (or double shot if you prefer) of espresso (or you can use 2–3 teaspoons of instant espresso if you like).
2. Add 1 cup of cold water or light milk.
3. Add one scoop of chocolate or vanilla protein powder.
4. Add Stevia to taste.
5. Put the lid on and hold down firmly. Shake vigorously until all the ice has dissolved. Enjoy!

For Espresso Smoothie

Place all ingredients in a blender then pulse and puree until smooth. For a thinner mixture, skip the ice. For a thicker mixture, add more ice.

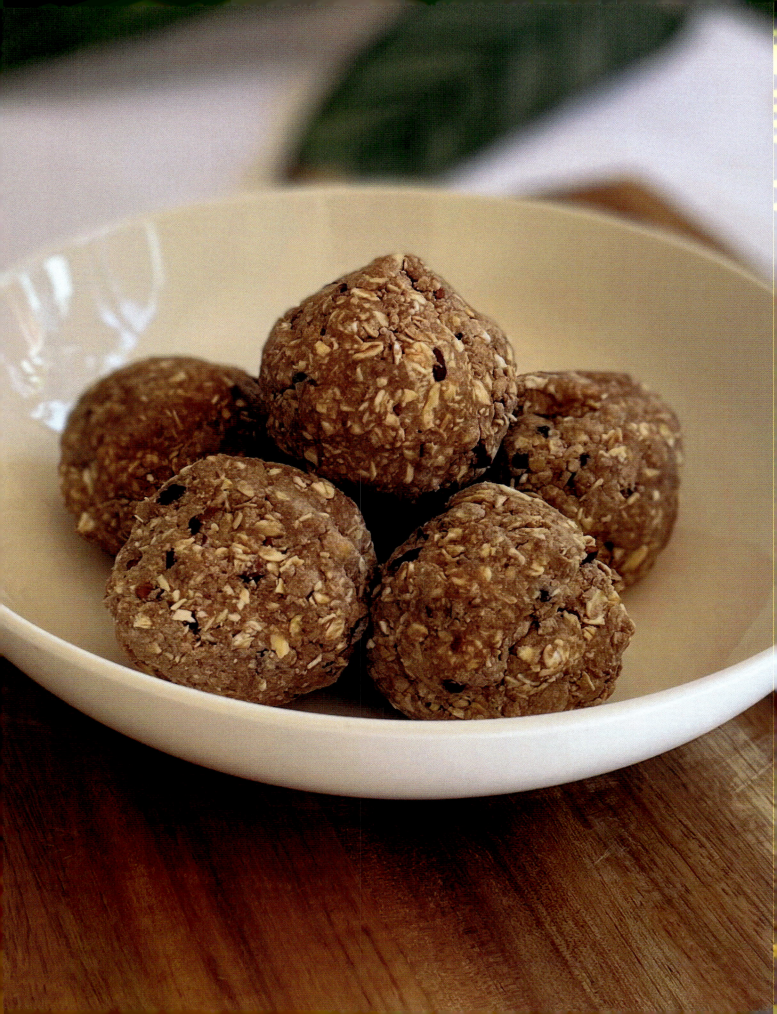

POST-WORKOUT SHAKES AND SNACKS

Choc Peanut Butter Protein Balls (V)

SERVINGS: 7 BALLS

MACRO BREAKDOWN (per ball)

FAT: 10G

PROTEIN: 12G

CARBS: 13G

RECIPE HIGHLIGHTS

These protein balls are perfect for when you need a portable post-workout snack. Some healthy fats are also included so you can have enough sustained energy until the next main meal. These protein balls are very tasty and of very high nutritional quality. You will never buy an overpriced store-bought version of these again.

INGREDIENTS

- 1 ½ cups oats + ½ cup extra oats
- 1 tbsp coconut oil
- 2 tbsp mini chocolate chips/cacao nibs
- 3 tbsp smooth peanut or almond butter
- 1 tsp pure vanilla extract
- 2 scoops chocolate protein powder
- ¼ tsp sea salt
- 1–2 tbsp almond milk

METHOD

1. Start by grinding 1½ cups of oats into a flour using a blender or coffee grinder, then set aside in a bowl.
2. In a small separate bowl, combine the peanut butter, oil, and vanilla. Mix together until well incorporated.
3. Combine the chocolate chips, protein powder, and sea salt with the oat flour.
4. Mix together the liquids from the second bowl with the solids of the first bowl and roll into about 7 small balls. If the balls are too sticky, roll in ½ cup remaining whole oats to coat the outside. If the mixture is too dry, add 1–2 tbsp unsweetened almond milk for more moisture, and then form into balls.
5. Place the rolled balls in the freezer and store until needed.

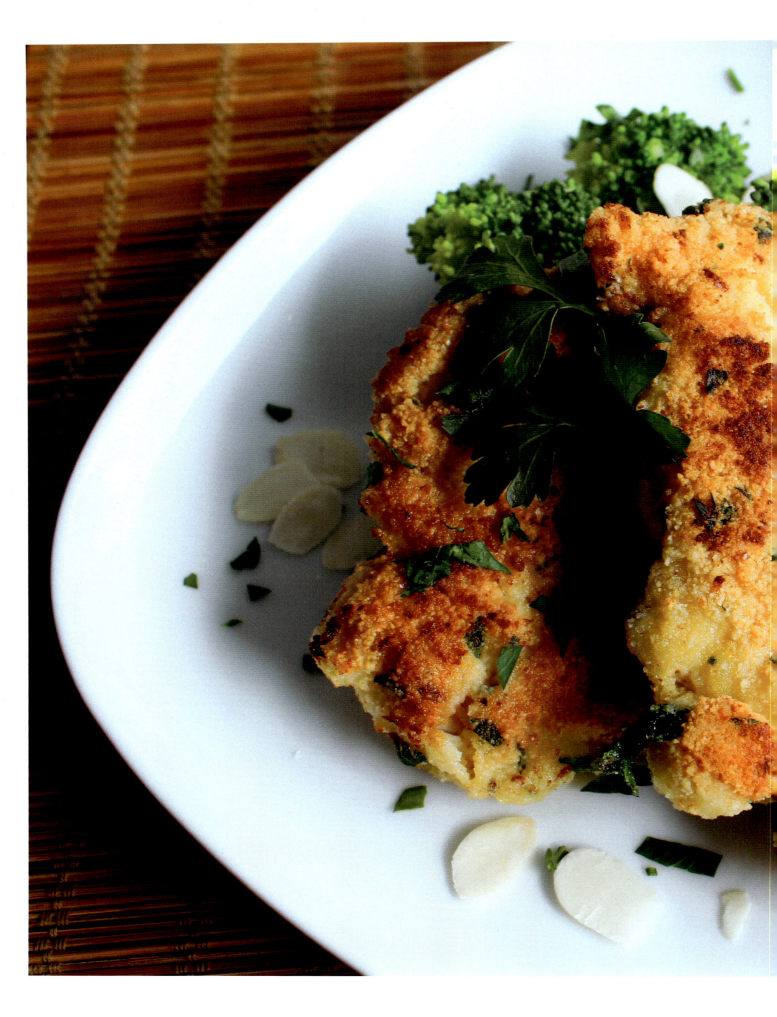

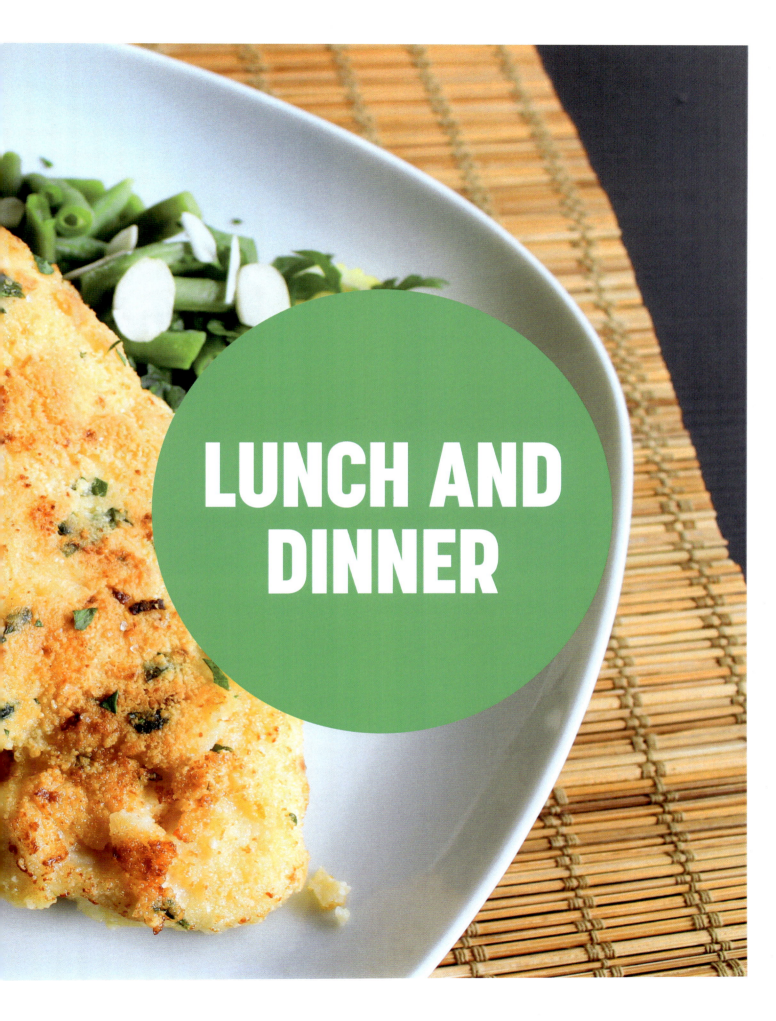

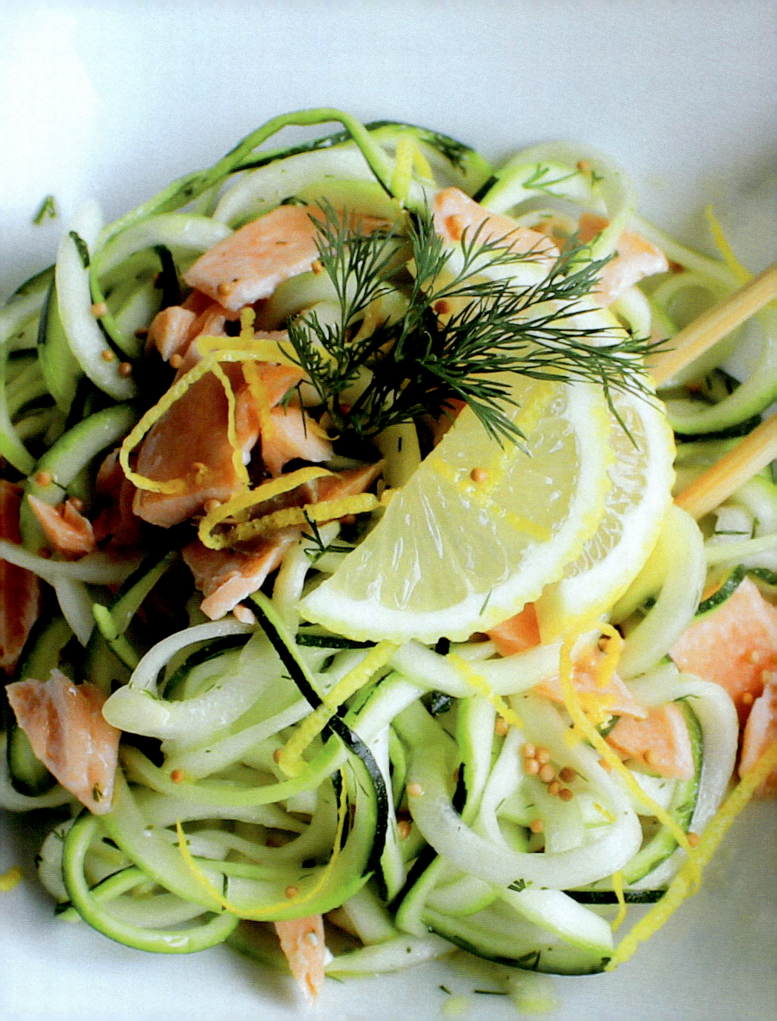

LUNCH AND DINNER

Hot Smoked Salmon with Zucchini Linguine

SERVINGS: 1

MACRO BREAKDOWN (per serve)

FAT: 41G

PROTEIN: 46G

CARBS: 14G

RECIPE HIGHLIGHTS

Salmon is not only a great source of protein, it's also an abundant source of omega-3 fatty acids, which are important for a healthy metabolism, good heart health, and brain function.

INGREDIENTS

- 1 large zucchini (use a mandolin or veggie spiral cutter or grater to create long 'linguine' threads of zucchini)
- ¼ cup chopped fresh dill
- 1 tbsp chopped fresh continental parsley
- 1 tbsp extra-virgin olive oil
- 1½ tbsp fresh lemon juice
- ½ tsp Dijon mustard
- 1 tsp finely grated lemon rind
- 185 g hot-smoked salmon fillet, skin removed, flaked
- Freshly ground black pepper

METHOD

1. Place the zucchini linguine into a bowl.
2. Mix together the dill, parsley, olive oil, lemon juice, Dijon mustard and lemon rind in a jug. Whisk well to combine.
3. Pour the herb mixture over the zucchini linguine and use your fingers to mix through the zucchini until it is well covered.
4. Season with freshly ground black pepper
5. Add the flaked salmon pieces and toss to combine. Serve in a bowl and enjoy!

If you would prefer this dish hot, simply toss the zucchini in a large pan with a smear of olive oil over medium heat. Wait until the dish is warmed through, then add the herb mixture and salmon.

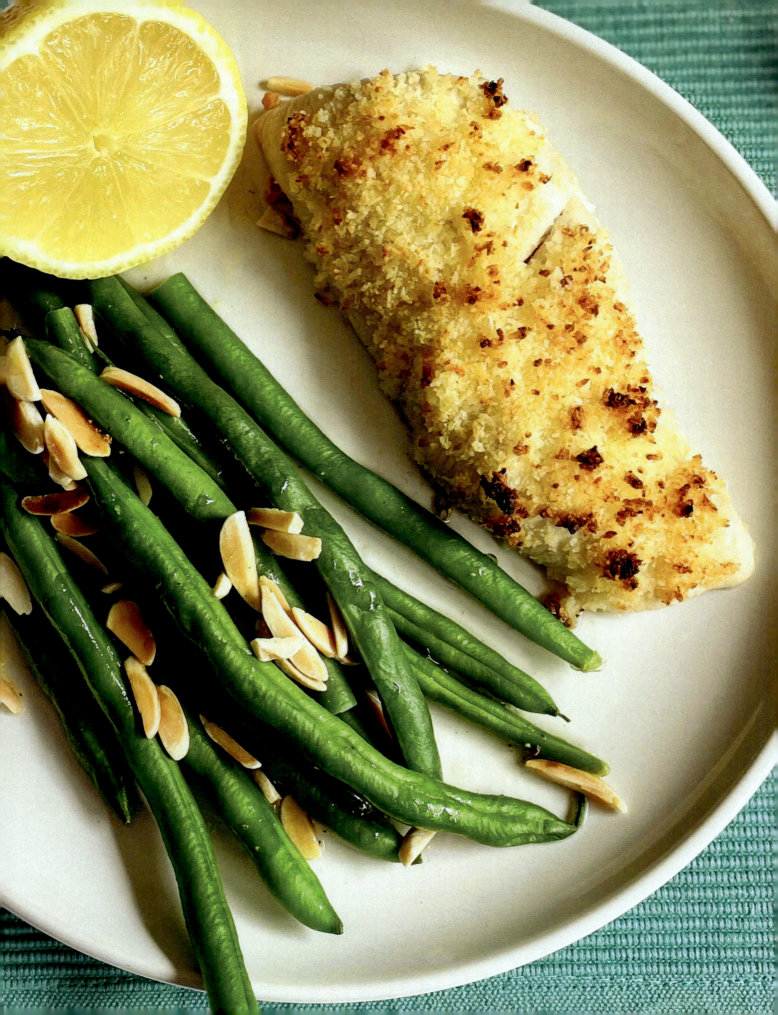

LUNCH AND DINNER

Coconut Chicken Schnitzel

SERVINGS: 4

RECIPE HIGHLIGHTS

This chicken recipe is both spicy and well-textured. If you're craving chicken schnitzel, but don't want all the usual crumbed carbs and unhealthy oil in the coating, then opt for this leaner high protein option instead. The taste is amazing and the greens provide plenty of vitamin K and folate as well.

MACRO BREAKDOWN (per serve)

FAT: 25G

PROTEIN: 31G

CARBS: 4G

INGREDIENTS

- 4 free range chicken breast halves
- 2 cloves garlic, minced
- 2/3 cup shredded coconut
- ½ tsp cayenne (optional)
- 2 tbsp of butter
- 250 g green beans
- 2 tsp olive oil
- 2 tbsp lemon juice
- 2 tbsp slivered almonds
- Pepper (to taste)

METHOD

1. Heat oven to 180° C. Lightly coat a 13x9-inch baking dish with olive oil spray and place the chicken breast halves on top.
2. Combine the garlic, coconut, cayenne (optional) and butter in a bowl and microwave until the butter softens. Stir the mixture thoroughly then spread evenly over the top side of the chicken.
3. Bake the chicken in the oven for 20–25 mins (or until desired tenderness).
4. Meanwhile, mix the lemon juice and oil together in a small jug. Season with pepper.
5. When chicken is close to cooked, add the green beans to a large saucepan of boiling water for 1–2 minutes or until bright green and tender crisp. Drain well.
6. Simultaneously heat a medium frying pan over medium heat. Add the slivered almonds and cook, stirring, for 1–2 minutes or until lightly toasted. Remove from heat.
7. Serve chicken with green beans sprinkled with almonds and drizzled with lemon oil dressing.

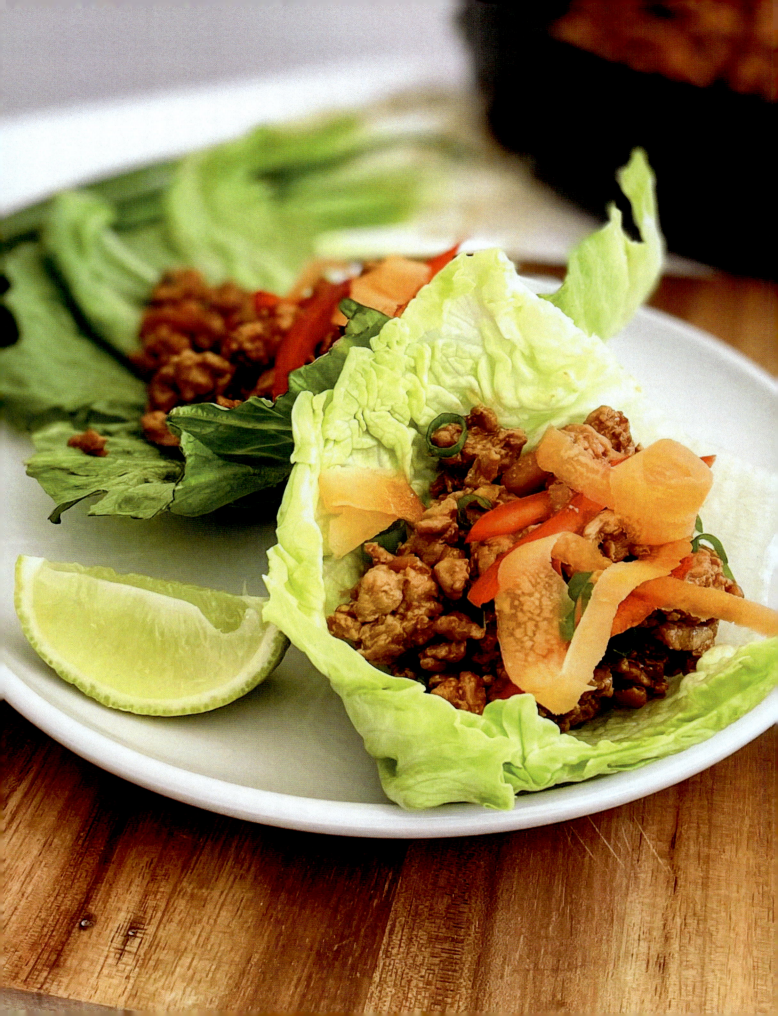

LUNCH AND DINNER

Sweet Chilli Chicken San Choy Bau

SERVINGS: 4

RECIPE HIGHLIGHTS

This is a perfect Asian dish without the over-use of oils. Macadamia oil is both flavoursome and a rich source of monounsaturated fats that can withstand high-heat cooking. This makes it a great oil to use in stir fry dishes like this one.

MACRO BREAKDOWN (per serve)

FAT: 13G

PROTEIN: 27G

CARBS: 13G

INGREDIENTS

- 1 tablespoon macadamia nut oil
- 500 g free-range organic chicken mince
- 1 long red chilli, seeds removed and finely chopped
- 2 centimetre piece of ginger, finely chopped
- ¼ cup tamari soy sauce (salt reduced)
- 3 tbsp sugar-free maple syrup (naturally sweetened)
- 227 g canned water chestnuts, drained, rinsed and roughly chopped.
- ½ tbsp cornflour, dissolved in 2 tablespoons water
- 3 kaffir lime leaves: cut out centre vein, roll into a cigar shape, and then slice very finely
- 1 iceberg lettuce, trimmed into cups
- Carrot, capsicum, and spring onion, sliced finely (to garnish)
- Light sweet chilli sauce and lime to serve

METHOD

1. Heat the oil in a wok or frying pan over medium-high heat. Add the chicken mince, chilli, and ginger and cook, stirring constantly for 2–3 minutes to break up any lumps.
2. Add the tamari and maple syrup, and cook for a further 1–2 minutes until combined.
3. Add the water chestnuts, stirring to combine. Check your seasoning at this point; add more tamari or maple syrup to balance the flavours of sweet and salty.
4. Add the cornflour mixture into the chicken mixture and stir well until slightly thickened and glossy.
5. Stir through the kaffir lime leaves. Take off the heat.
6. Fill the lettuce cups with the chicken mixture, then garnish with the carrot, capsicum, and spring onion.
7. Serve with sweet chilli sauce and lime wedges.

THE LEAN BODY SOLUTION

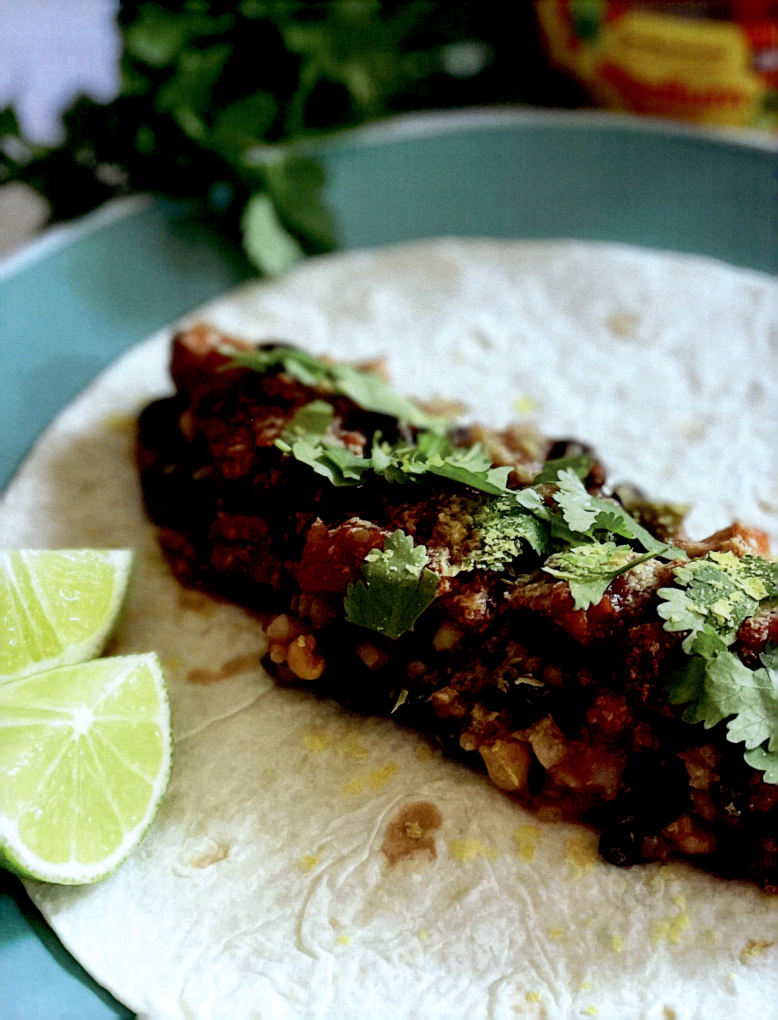

Zesty Chicken and Black Bean Burritos

SERVINGS: 8 BURRITOS

MACRO BREAKDOWN (per burrito)

FAT: 7G

PROTEIN: 25G

CARBS: 64G

RECIPE HIGHLIGHTS

It's not unusual to be very hungry in the hours after intense workouts. This recipe is sure to fill you up. Say goodbye to dirty burritos with this nutritious and tasty alternative. It's jam-packed with fibre-rich beans and veggies, as well as high-quality protein.

INGREDIENTS

- 2x 400 g cans of diced tomato
- 2x 400 g cans of black beans, rinsed
- 200 g chicken breast diced
- ½ cup dry brown rice
- 1 cup of frozen corn
- 2 cups of water or vegetable broth
- ¼ cup of salsa
- 1 capsicum, chopped (any colour)
- 1 medium onion, chopped
- 2 tbsp diced coriander leaves
- 1 tsp chilli pepper
- 3 tablespoons nutritional yeast
- 2 limes, sliced
- 8 whole wheat tortillas (40 g each)

METHOD

1. After rinsing the black beans, dump the beans, chicken, rice, chopped capsicum, onion, corn, chilli pepper, broth and seasoning into a slow cooker. Stir everything together until mixed well.
2. Set your slow cooker to medium and let the burrito mixture cook for 8 hours.
3. Fill whole wheat tortillas with mixture.
4. Top with lime, salsa, coriander, and nutritional yeast.

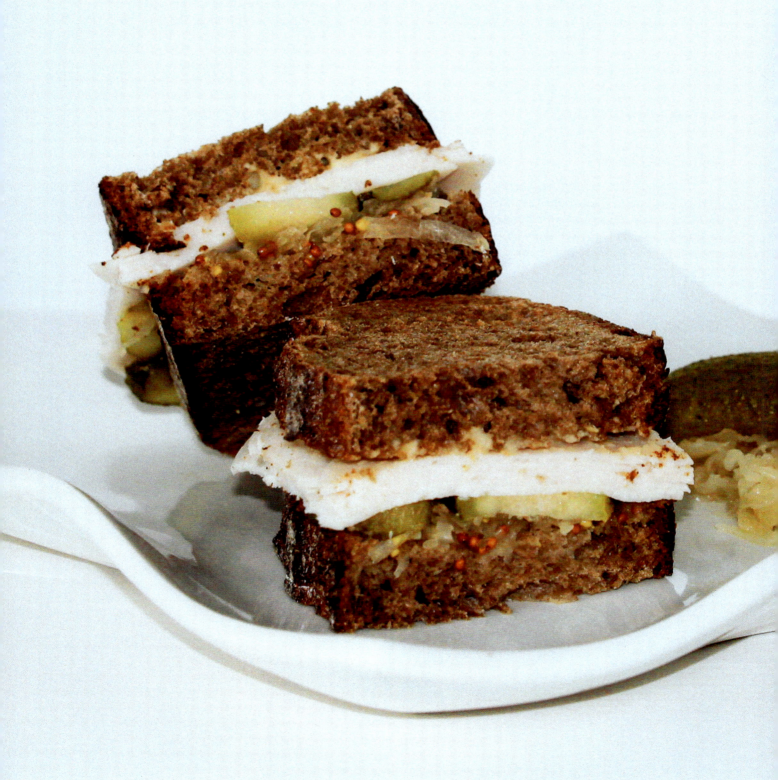

LUNCH AND DINNER

Reuben-Style Turkey Sandwich

SERVINGS: 1

MACRO BREAKDOWN (per serve)

FAT: 15G
PROTEIN: 38G
CARBS: 47G

RECIPE HIGHLIGHTS

This sandwich delivers a savoury and tangy flavour. It also contains a lot more fibre and B vitamins than traditional sandwiches. Rye bread is great for digestion, too, and you can eat this recipe either toasted or fresh.

INGREDIENTS

- 2 slices of rye bread
- 1 tbsp wholegrain mustard
- 2 tbsp hummus
- ⅓ cup sauerkraut
- 2 large, pickled cucumber slices, thinly sliced (lengthways)
- 100 g white meat turkey breast slices
- 1 slice light Swiss cheese

METHOD

1. Toast the rye bread and spread with mustard and hummus.
2. Top with sliced turkey, sauerkraut, and cucumber slices.
3. Drizzle with extra mustard if desired.
4. Toast in sandwich press or eat fresh.

THE LEAN BODY SOLUTION

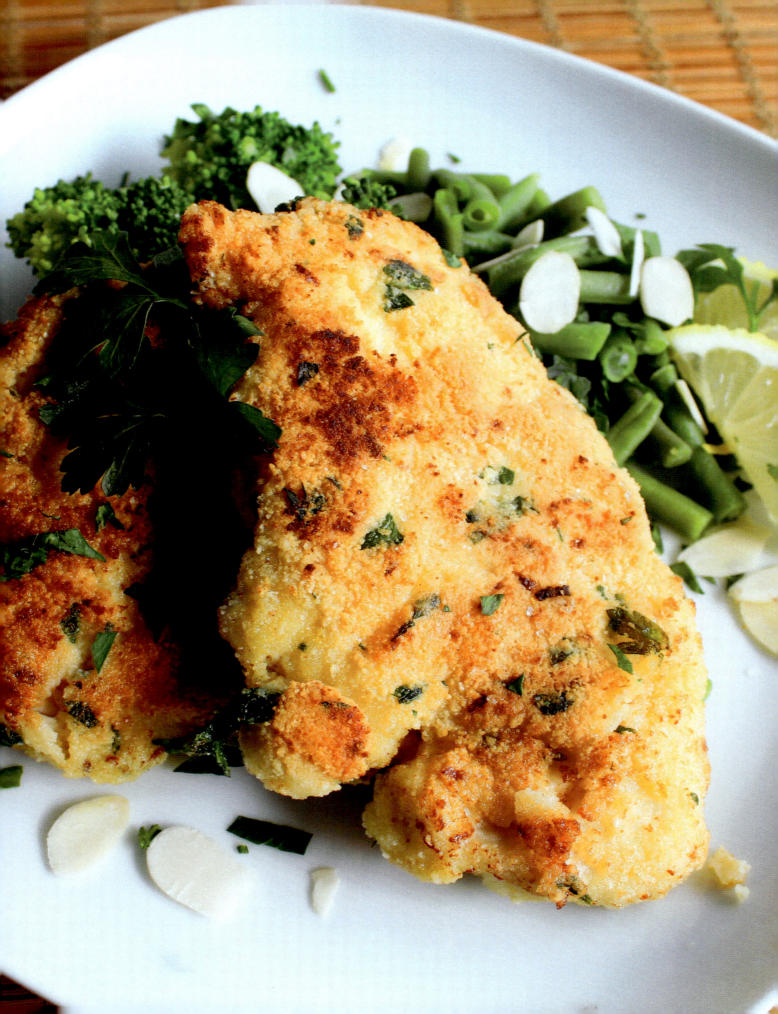

LUNCH AND DINNER

Almond Crusted Chicken

SERVINGS: 4

MACRO BREAKDOWN (per serve)

FAT: 21G

PROTEIN: 25G

CARBS: 4G

Prepared with 100 g steamed green beans and broccoli

RECIPE HIGHLIGHTS

For those dying for a taste similar to fried chicken without having to sacrifice the integrity of their diet, this recipe is perfect! It's low carb and packed with protein plus healthy fat. Pair this with greens as recommended and you have a very filling and lean meal.

INGREDIENTS

- 2 free-range chicken breast fillets, sliced in half widthways
- 1 tablespoon arrowroot
- 1 free range egg, beaten
- 1 cup almond meal
- ½ tbsp of lemon zest, finely grated
- 2 tbsp parsley chopped
- ¼ tsp salt and pepper
- 1 tbsp olive oil
- Steamed broccoli and green beans to serve

METHOD

1. In a bowl, combine almond meal, lemon zest, chopped parsley, salt, and pepper.
2. Lightly coat the chicken breast in the arrowroot, then dip into the egg mix followed by the almond mix.
3. Cook the 4 pieces of crumbed chicken over a low- to medium-heat in a pan, using 1 tablespoon olive oil, for three minutes each side (or until lightly golden and chicken is cooked through).
4. Serve alongside steamed green vegetables with a squeeze of lemon.

THE LEAN BODY SOLUTION

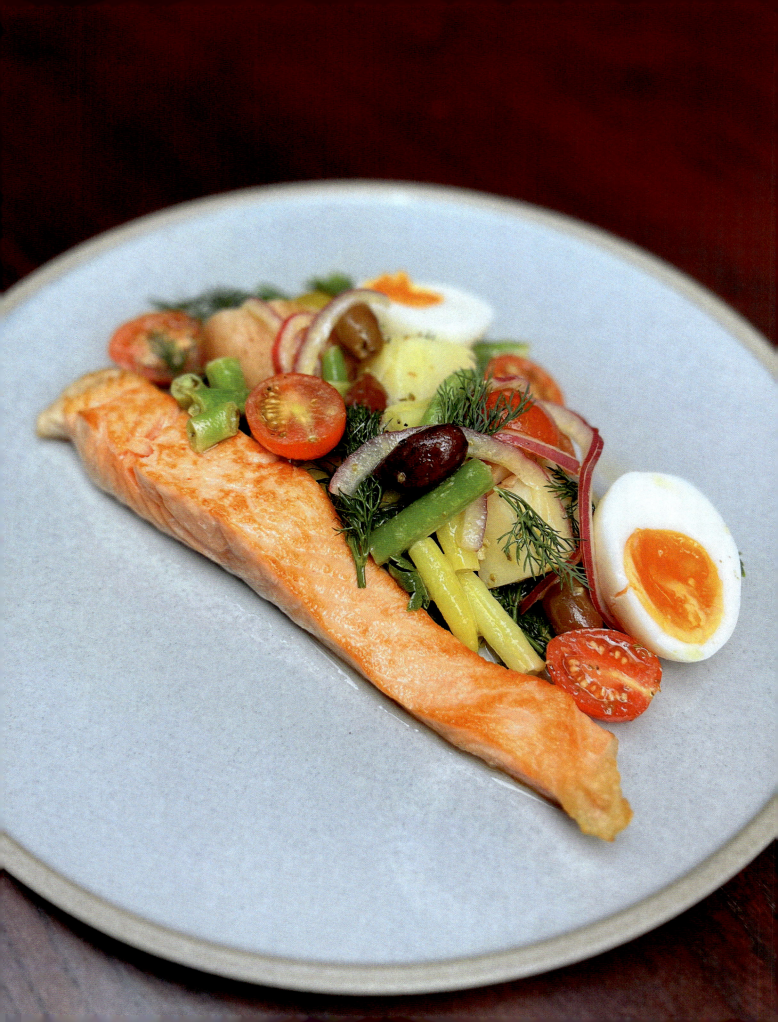

LUNCH AND DINNER

Niçoise Salad with Tasmanian Salmon

SERVINGS: 1

RECIPE HIGHLIGHTS

The ingredients in this recipe contain lots of vitamin C which supports the immune system and collagen formation. Whole eggs also boast a lot of vitamin B12 (in the yolk) which is essential for nerve function and DNA synthesis.

MACRO BREAKDOWN (per serve)

FAT: 45G

PROTEIN: 39G

CARBS: 24G

INGREDIENTS

Salmon
- 1 fillet (~120 g) fresh Tasmanian salmon, skinned and pin-boned, served whole or cut into 2-cm cubes
- Extra-virgin olive oil

Salad
- 1 soft boiled organic egg, cut in half
- 2 vine-ripened tomatoes, blanched and cut into quarters (or 15-20 halved cherry tomatoes)
- ¼ small red onion, sliced into thin rounds
- ¼ cup black kalamata olives
- ½ small red potato, steamed, peeled, and cut into bite sized pieces
- Handful Italian parsley
- 1 cup green beans, blanched and sliced lengthwise
- Freshly ground black pepper and sea salt

Lemon Dressing
- 1 tbsp lemon juice
- 1 tsp good-quality seeded mustard
- 2 tsp fresh thyme leaves
- ½ tbsp extra-virgin olive oil

METHOD

1. Season salmon pieces with salt and black pepper.
2. Wipe a smear of olive oil over a heavy-based pan. Heat over high heat. Add the salmon pieces and gently toss them so they are brown on the outside and cooked until medium rare.
3. To make lemon dressing: combine lemon juice, mustard, and thyme. Whisk in oil and then season to taste.
4. To make salad: combine egg, tomatoes, onion, olives, potato, parsley, and beans in a bowl. Dress with lemon dressing
5. Serve the salmon fillet with the salad or toss the salmon pieces through the salad then serve.

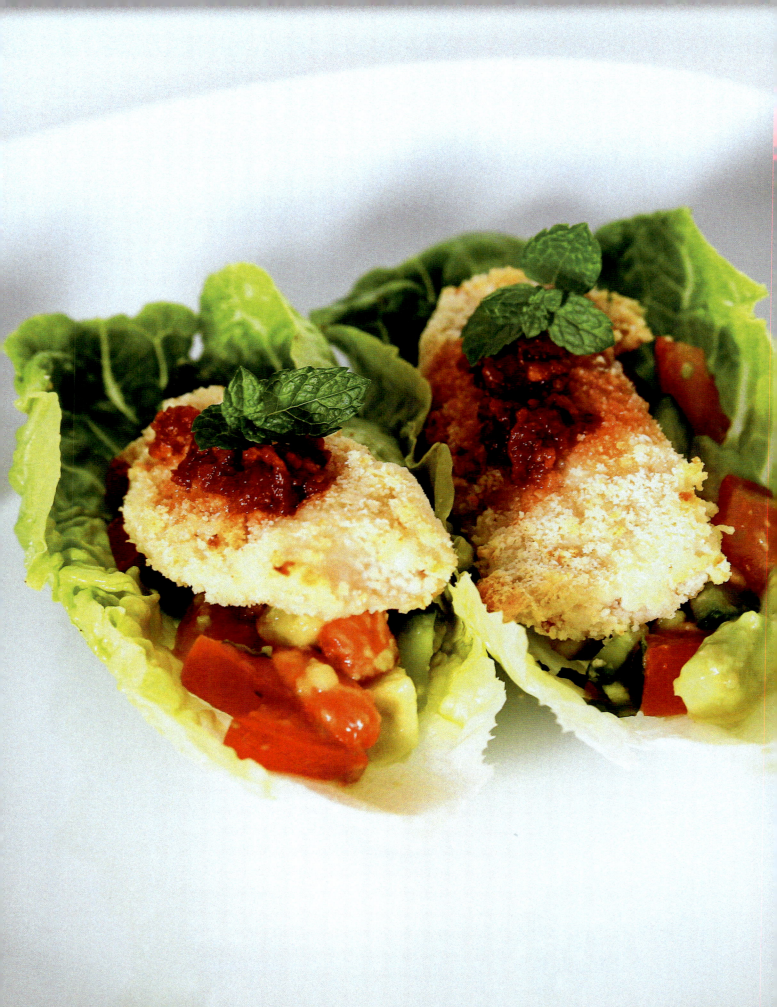

LUNCH AND DINNER

Lower-Carb Fish Tacos

SERVINGS: 2

RECIPE HIGHLIGHTS

The lower-carb alternative shell makes this recipe a lot leaner than a typical taco. The good dose of avocado supplies healthy fats and fibre for satiety, while the arrowroot used in place of fish crumbing also enhances the fish's texture.

MACRO BREAKDOWN (per serve)

FAT: 30G

PROTEIN: 37G

CARBS: 15G

INGREDIENTS

- 2 flathead fillets, pin-boned (this amount will depend on the size of the fillets)
- 1 egg, whisked
- 2 tbsp arrowroot (tapioca flour)
- ½ cup almond meal
- 1 tbsp olive oil
- 1 butter crunch lettuce: leaves pulled off, trimmed, and placed into cold, icy water (this makes it nice and crunchy!)
- ½ avocado
- 1 tomato, diced into small pieces
- ½ Lebanese cucumber, diced into small pieces
- Large handful coriander leaves, chopped finely
- Small handful mint leaves, chopped finely
- ½ lime, juiced
- Sea salt and cracked pepper
- To serve: extra lime wedges, sweet chilli sauce and/or sambal oelek

METHOD

1. Place avocado, tomato, cucumber, coriander leaves, mint leaves, lime juice and salt and pepper in a small bowl. Mix until all ingredients are well combined. Taste and adjust seasoning as necessary.
2. Drain lettuce leaves.
3. Cut flathead fillets into small strips.
4. Place arrowroot on one plate, whisked egg in a bowl, and almond meal on another plate.
5. Dust the flathead strips in arrowroot to coat. Place the flathead strips into the whisked egg and coat. Roll the flathead fillets in the almond meal to cover completely.
6. Heat the olive oil in a large frying pan over medium-high heat. Cook the flathead fillets until golden and crispy on all sides. Be very gentle when turning as flathead is a very delicate fish and they can easily break.
7. To serve, place the lettuce leaves on a plate, scoop a spoon of the avocado and vegetable mixture onto the lettuce, top with a few pieces of flathead.
8. Squeeze fresh lime juice over the flathead, and then top with sweet chilli sauce or sambal oelek.

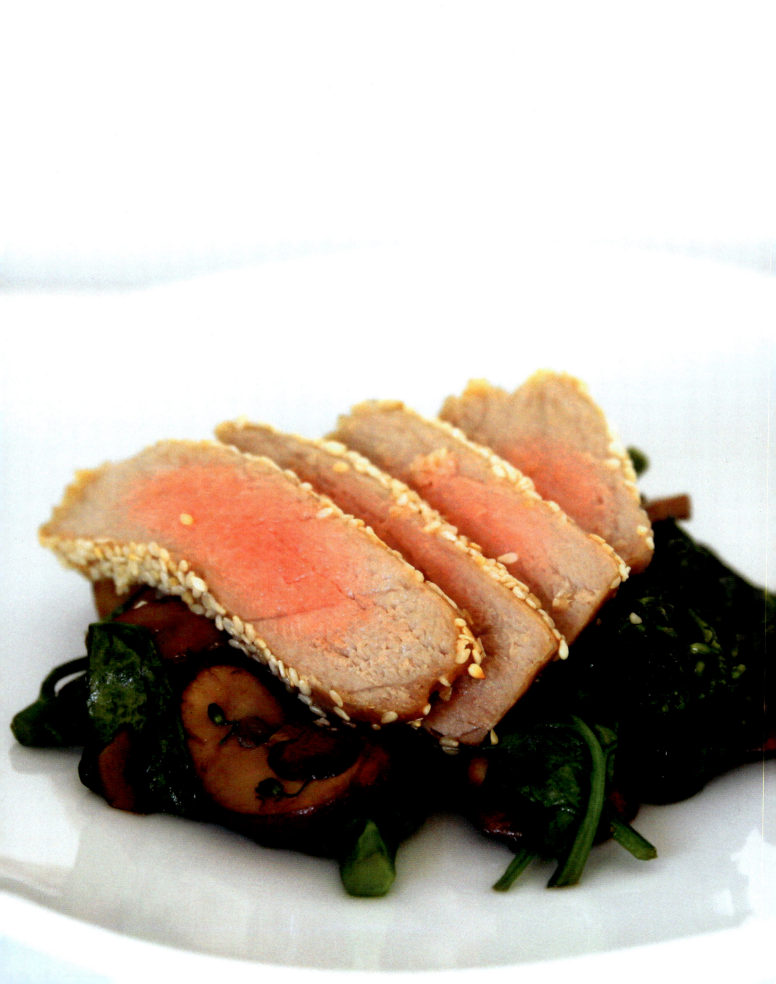

LUNCH AND DINNER

Seared Yellowfin Tuna with Fried Greens & Mushrooms

SERVINGS: 1

RECIPE HIGHLIGHTS

Sashimi grade yellowfin tuna is a rich source of high-quality protein, which is essential for tissue repair and muscle growth. The accompanying mixed medley of vegetables are packed with fibre, vitamins, and minerals.

MACRO BREAKDOWN (per serve)

FAT: 19G

PROTEIN: 60G

CARBS: 12G

INGREDIENTS

Tuna
- 180 g sashimi-grade yellowfin tuna
- 1 tbsp sesame seeds
- 2 cups mixed mushrooms, sliced (enoki, oyster, shiitake, and button mushrooms are a nice blend)
- 2 cups green, washed and roughly chopped (spinach, kale, or water spinach are all great options)
- ½ bunch broccolini, trimmed and cut
- 1 tsp perilla oil

Dressing
- 1 tbsp tamari soy sauce
- 1 tbsp mirin (Japanese rice wine)
- 1 tsp white miso paste

METHOD

1. To make the dressing; place the tamari, mirin, and white miso paste in a jar. Shake well until the miso paste has dissolved. Taste to check flavour. Adjust to suit your tastes.

2. Pour the sesame seeds onto a plate. Press both sides of the tuna into the sesame seeds until coated. Set aside.

3. Put a teaspoon of perilla oil in a frying pan and heat over medium-high heat. Add the mushrooms and cook until soft. Add the broccolini and stir. Cook until just tender. Add the greens and stir until wilted. Pour the dressing over the vegetables and take off the heat.

4. Heat a frying pan over high heat. Add one teaspoon of perilla oil and heat. Place the tuna into the frying pan and cook for one minute. Turn and cook for another minute (this will result in your tuna being seared on the outside, but still raw on the inside; leave for longer if you prefer your tuna a little more cooked).

5. Take tuna out of the frying pan. Using a sharp knife, cut thick strips on the diagonal.

6. Place the vegetables in the bottom of a bowl. Pour over any juices from the dressing. Place on the tuna strips and serve.

THE LEAN BODY SOLUTION

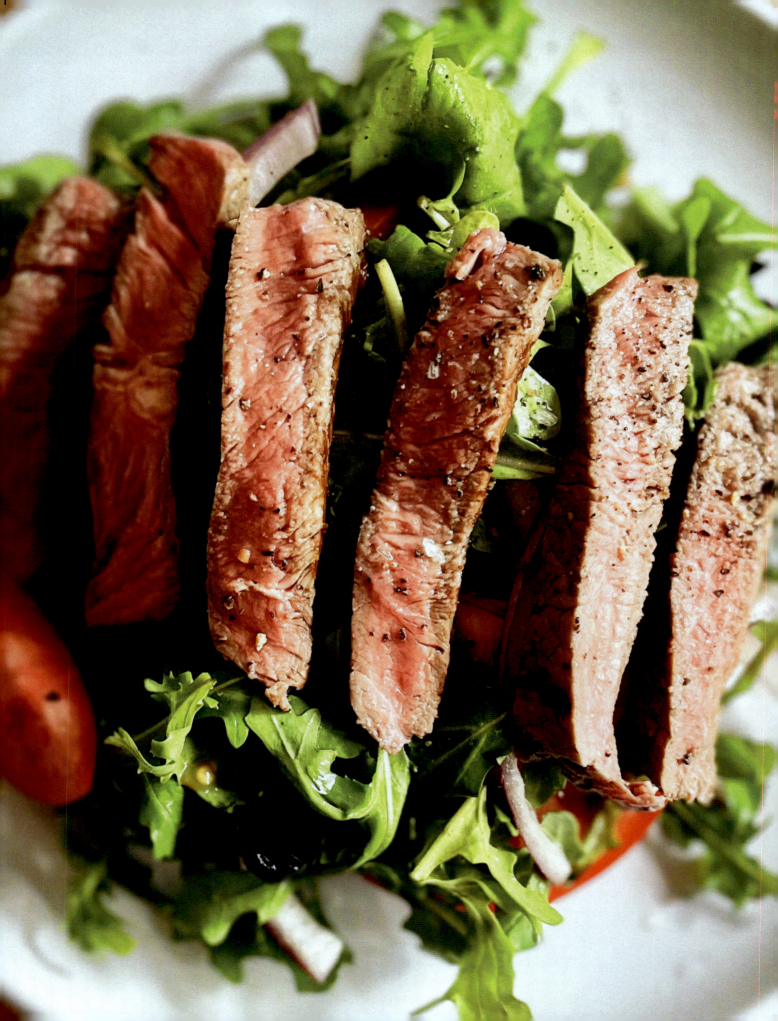

LUNCH AND DINNER

Easy Rocket & Steak Salad

SERVINGS: 4

MACRO BREAKDOWN (per serve)

FAT: 11G

PROTEIN: 65G

CARBS: 9G

RECIPE HIGHLIGHTS

This easy rocket and steak salad provides a balanced combination of protein, fibre, vitamins, minerals, and antioxidants. Steak is a great source of high-quality protein and iron, while the rocket (or arugula leaves) contributes with a peppery and distinctive flavour. These leaves are rich in vitamins A, C, and K, as well as folate, calcium, and potassium.

INGREDIENTS

- 1 kg lean sirloin or top round steak (broiled or grilled and cut thin)
- 8 cups rocket (arugula leaves)
- ½ cup black olives, sliced
- 1 red onion, sliced
- 6 fresh tomatoes, thinly sliced
- ¼ cup red wine vinegar
- Sea salt and black pepper to taste
- Additional cherry tomatoes (optional)

METHOD

1. Prepare the steak by either roasting in the oven or grilling until cooked to preferences. Then set aside.
2. While the steak is cooling, in a large salad bowl add rocket (arugula), olives, onion and tomatoes.
3. Next, cut the steak into thin strips and lay over the salad. Top with red wine vinegar, sea salt and black pepper, as well as sweet cherry tomatoes (optional).
4. Serve immediately or keep refrigerated and covered for 3–4 days.

THE LEAN BODY SOLUTION

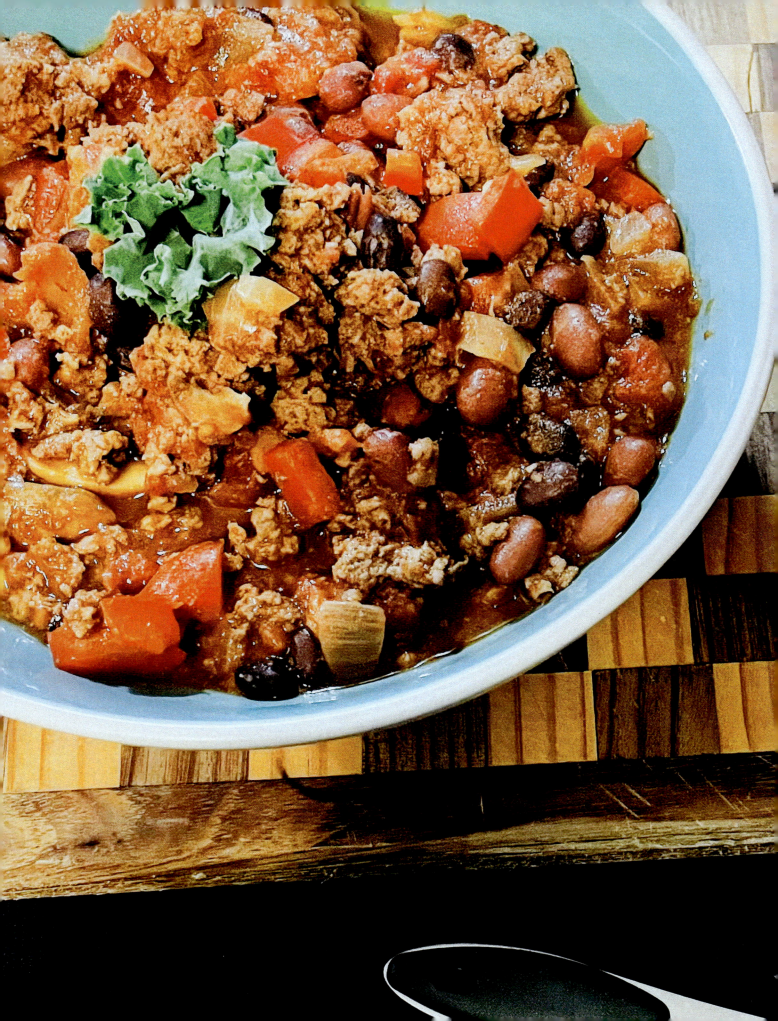

LUNCH AND DINNER

Beefy Mushroom Chilli

SERVINGS: 4

RECIPE HIGHLIGHTS

This dish has a lot of spice and flavour but it's also packed with nutritious ingredients. The diced onion and tomato add flavour whilst providing plenty of vitamin C. The assortment of vegetables and beans also provide filling fibre, while the ground beef is a great source of protein, iron, and zinc.

MACRO BREAKDOWN (per serve)

FAT: 19G

PROTEIN: 40G

CARBS: 30G

INGREDIENTS

- 1 tbsp extra-virgin olive oil
- 1 large, onion (red or white), diced
- 2 garlic cloves, minced
- 2 medium red or yellow capsicum, diced
- 100 g mushroom (any variety)
- 500 g extra lean ground beef (90/10 variety)
- 1 tsp chilli powder
- ½ tsp cumin
- ½ tsp oregano
- 1x 800 g can diced tomatoes with juice
- 1x 400 g can kidney beans
- 1x 400 g can black beans
- hot sauce of your preference (optional)
- Salt and black pepper to taste

METHOD

1. In a large pot, mix together olive oil, onions, capsicum, and garlic, and cook over medium heat for 5–7 minutes.
2. Slice mushrooms very thin and add those to the pot along with ground beef. Cook for 5–10 additional minutes until the beef is well done (add small amounts of water to the pot if needed to prevent sticking).
3. Add remaining ingredients and turn heat to high.
4. Bring mixture to a boil and cook for 20 minutes or until all vegetables are very soft.
5. Let soup cool; taste. Add hot sauce, if preferred, along with salt and black pepper to taste.

THE LEAN BODY SOLUTION

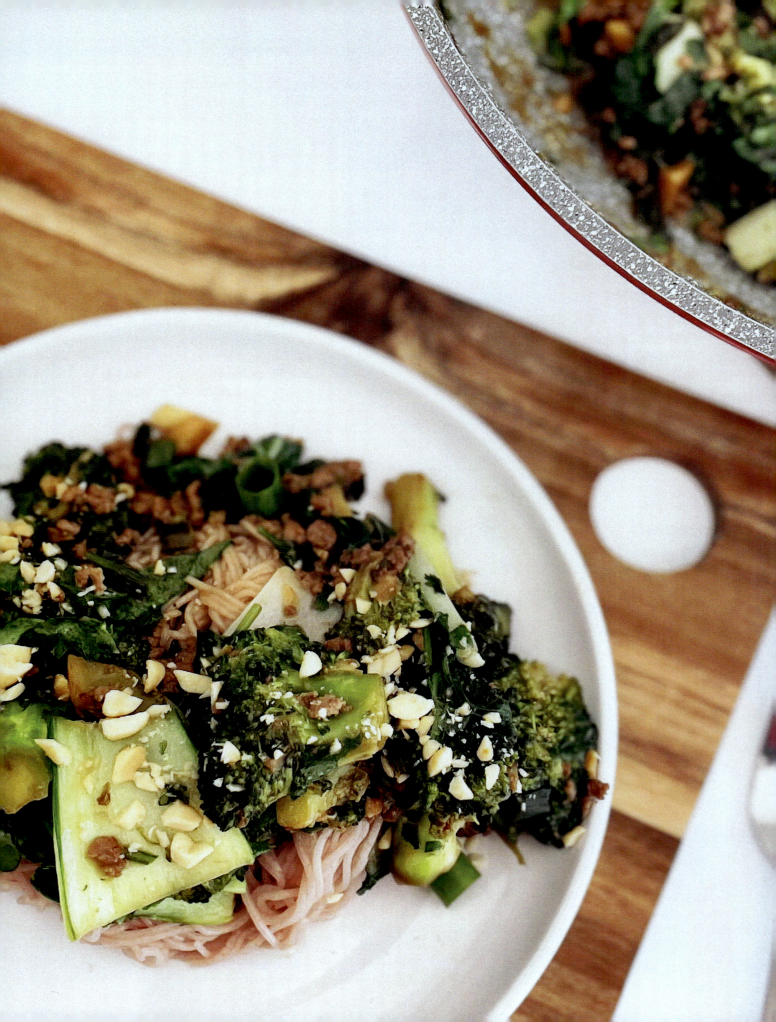

LUNCH AND DINNER

Wok'd Mushroom Beef Noodles

SERVINGS: 4

MACRO BREAKDOWN (per serve)

RECIPE HIGHLIGHTS

This hot wok Asian-style dish is perfect if you need a filling feed after intense training. It offers more complex carbs in the form of brown rice noodles and a good amount of protein in the beef. This dish is full of vitamin C and the inclusion of ginger and garlic adds both aromatic and immune-boosting properties. The taste is not forgotten either with raw peanuts rounding out the recipe with a crunchy texture.

FAT: 26G

PROTEIN: 26G

CARBS: 45G

INGREDIENTS

- *2 tbsp olive oil*
- *1 bunch of spring onion*
- *2 cuttings of ginger*
- *4 cloves garlic*
- *2 heads broccoli*
- *2 bunches Asian greens*
- *1 bunch coriander*
- *250 g beef mince*
- *1 cup cream of mushroom soup*
- *2 tbsp light soy sauce*
- *200 g brown rice noodles (mai fun or angel hair)*
- *½ cup raw peanuts*

METHOD

1. Heating a pot of water to boiling. Drop in brown rice noodles to begin cooking. They should take about 10 minutes of boiling before soft.
2. On a separate burner, pour 1 tbsp of olive oil in a large wok over medium heat.
3. While the wok is getting hot, pull out the vegetables. Crush the garlic cloves and dice the ginger ahead of time. Chop broccoli and onion; add these to the wok pan first. The wok should be near a sizzling temperature by this point.
4. Don't forget to check the brown rice noodles. Once they're completely softened, drain water.
5. Add the garlic and ginger to the pan. Stir frequently to prevent the veggies from sticking (you may add 1 tbsp of the soy sauce if needed).
6. Once the vegetables have begun to soften, add beef mince and the other tbsp of olive oil. Stir continuously to cook beef until completely browned.
7. Once meat is completely cooked, add the remaining soy sauce and mushroom sauce, and adjust the heat until the mixture is bubbling.
8. Finally, cut Asian greens and coriander; stir into wok for 1–2 minutes (just until greens have been softened).
9. Remove the wok from heat. Plate bowls in this order: fill a bowl with cooked brown rice noodles, top with cooked beef and vegetable mixture, and garnish with chopped peanuts.

THE LEAN BODY SOLUTION

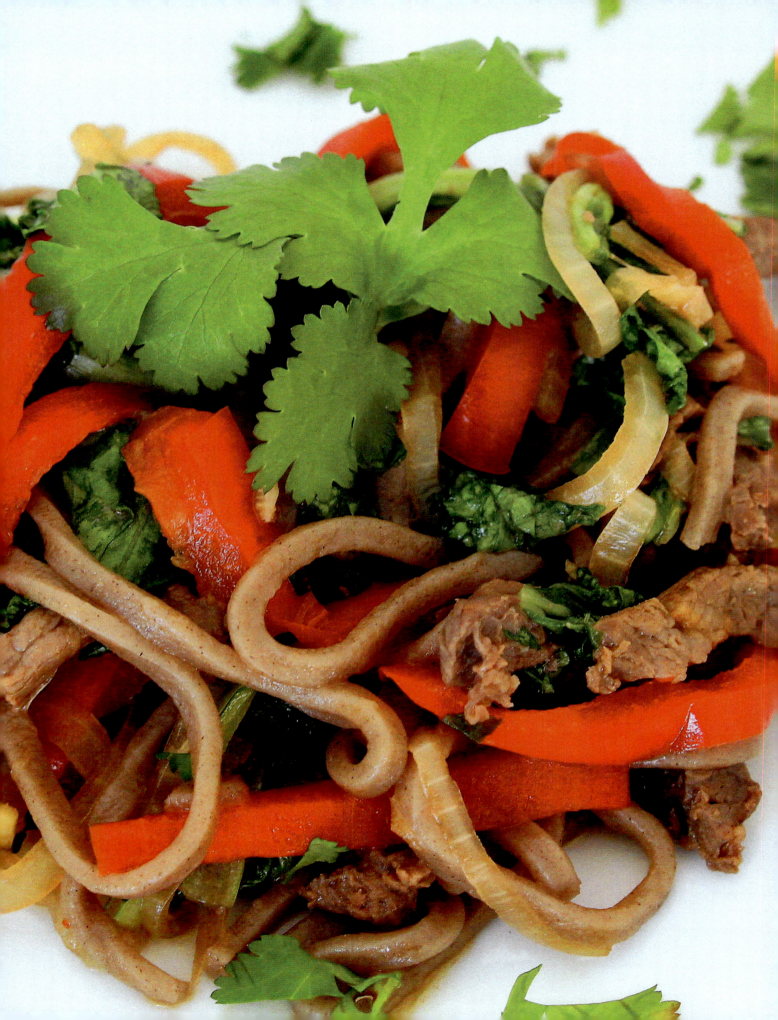

LUNCH AND DINNER

BBQ Beef Stir-Fry

SERVINGS: 4

MACRO BREAKDOWN (per serve)

FAT: 11G

PROTEIN: 13G

CARBS: 31G

RECIPE HIGHLIGHTS

If you need more carbs to support more intense training, then this recipe is for you! The combination of vegetables also adds colour and crunch to this stir-fry, while the inclusion of garlic and ginger adds both aromatic flavour and immune-boosting properties.

INGREDIENTS

- *2 knobs ginger*
- *1 medium onions*
- *2 red capsicum*
- *2 bunches Asian greens*
- *1 bunch coriander*
- *150 g brown rice noodles*
- *2 tbsp BBQ sauce*
- *4 tbsp soy sauce (salt reduced)*
- *2 tbsp brown sugar*
- *2 tbsp water*
- *250 g lean beef strips*

METHOD

1. First, start heating up a large pot of water over high heat. Keep it covered until it's at a boil; then drop in brown rice noodles. They'll be soft after about 10 minutes.
2. On the side, in a small bowl, mix together BBQ sauce, soy sauce, brown sugar. And water. Put in the meat to allow it to marinate.
3. Take out all of your vegetables; crush garlic cloves. Chop capsicum, onion, and ginger. Finally, cut Asian greens and coriander.
4. Now is a good time to check the brown rice noodles. Once soft, drain water and remove from heat. Set on the side.
5. Heat 1 tbsp of the olive oil in a large wok; while heating, add garlic, ginger, onion, and capsicum. Then add Asian green and coriander.
6. When the vegetables have begun to soften, add beef strips, along with remaining olive oil and BBQ soy sauce mixture. Keep stirring the beef continuously until completely cooked.
7. Finally, remove the wok from heat. Serve the noodles, top with meat, then sauce, and enjoy!

THE LEAN BODY SOLUTION

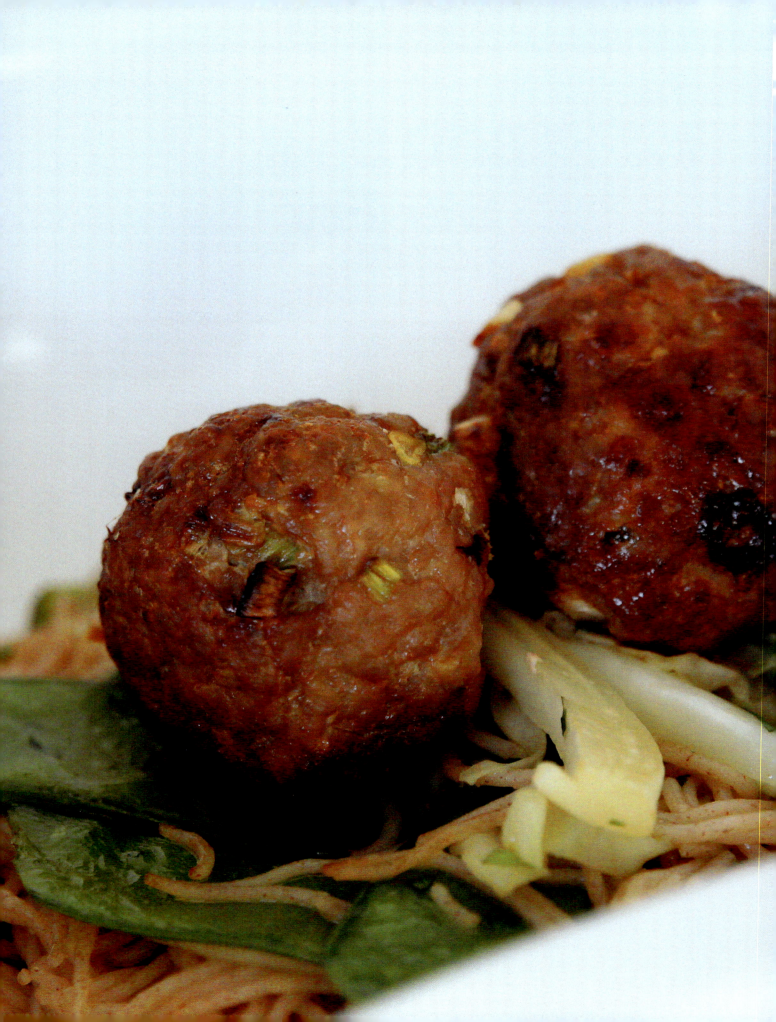

LUNCH AND DINNER

Sweet 'n' Sticky Pork Meatballs

SERVINGS: 4

MACRO BREAKDOWN (per serve)

FAT: 12G

PROTEIN: 29G

CARBS: 44G

RECIPE HIGHLIGHTS

Best consumed within the workout window, this nutritious pasta is sure to keep you full and handle your hunger. It includes lots of vegetables like cabbage, spring onions, and coriander, along with peas and brown rice noodles to keep you satisfied.

INGREDIENTS

- 400 g extra-lean pork mince
- 2 bunches spring onions
- 2 tbsp sweet soy sauce
- 2 cups green cabbage, chopped
- 4 cloves garlic, diced
- 2 packs brown rice noodles (160 g total)
- 2 bags snow peas (about 2 cups)
- 2 tbsp olive oil
- 2 red chilies, diced
- 1 tbsp fish sauce
- 1 bunch coriander

METHOD

1. Start by bringing a large pot of water to a boil. Once boiling, add brown rice noodles. Cook for about 10 minutes while you prepare other parts of the recipe.
2. Add pork mince to a large bowl with soy sauce, spring onions, diced garlic, and red chilies. Mix all the ingredients together thoroughly. Form into meatball-sized round balls with your hands.
3. Heat olive oil and fish sauce in a large flat pan over medium heat.
4. Once hot and on the point of sizzling, add meatballs. Allow to brown in the sauce, rolling periodically to cook them all the way through.
5. After meatballs are cooked through (cut one open to check middle for any red area left), add snow peas and coriander to the hot oil; cook just for 1–2 minutes until soft.
6. Once brown rice noodles are cooked, drain. Toss noodles with meatballs, snow peas, coriander, and remaining sauce in the pain. Enjoy delicious pasta-style meatballs!

THE LEAN BODY SOLUTION

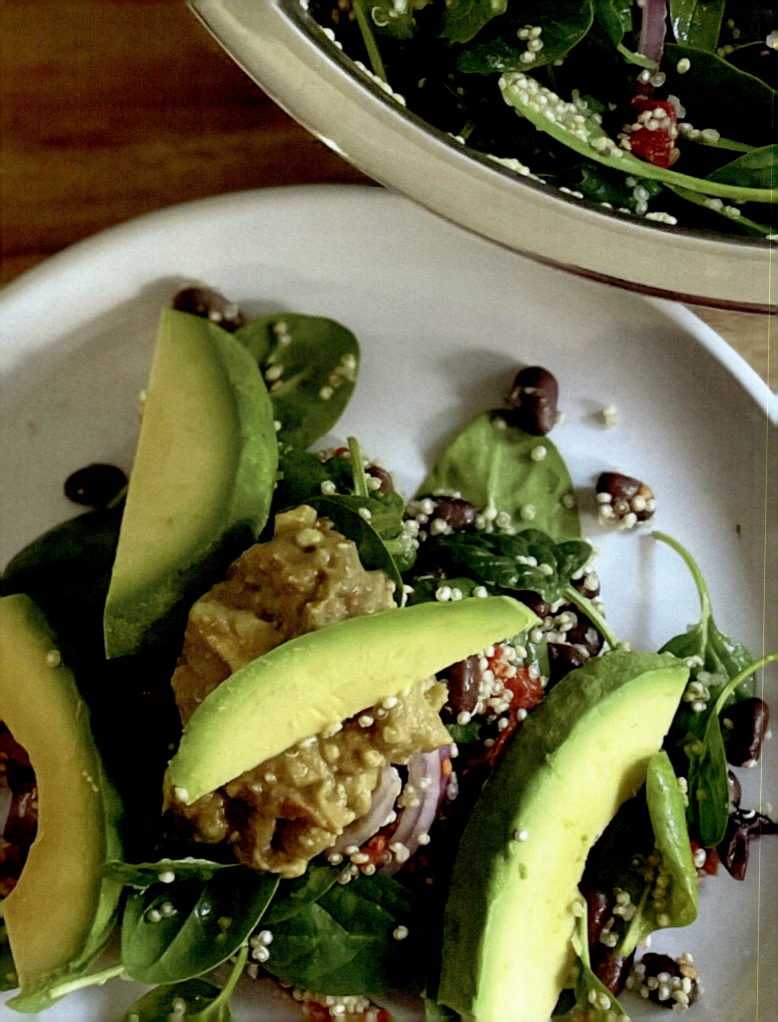

LUNCH AND DINNER

Spinach, Black Bean, and Quinoa Salad (V)

SERVINGS: 4

MACRO BREAKDOWN (per serve)

FAT: 7G

PROTEIN: 6G

CARBS: 26G

RECIPE HIGHLIGHTS

Many people believe that all salads are light and not very filling—this recipe will change one's mind quickly! The black bean and quinoa create a highly nutritious and satisfying filling, while the red onion and lemon juice give it a tangy full flavour. This recipe accommodates those who are vegetarian or plant-based eaters.

INGREDIENTS

- ½ cup dry quinoa (white or red work well)
- 1 can of black beans, rinsed and drained
- 2 cups spinach
- ¼ red onion, sliced
- ½ cup sun-dried tomatoes (optional)
- 1 ripe avocado
- 2 tbsp lemon juice
- 4 tbsp mild salsa
- Sea salt and black pepper to taste

METHOD

1. Cook the quinoa ahead of time (use a 1:2 quinoa to water ratio) by boiling water and simmering the quinoa for 10–15 minutes.
2. Create a dressing by mashing half of the avocado in a bowl, and then combining with the lemon juice and salsa.
3. In a large salad bowl, combine the quinoa, spinach, black beans, sliced red onion and sun-dried tomatoes (optional).
4. Top with the avocado-lemon dressing and slices of the remaining avocado.
5. Serve immediately or store in the refrigerator for 3–4 days (keeping the dressing separate will help extend the storage life).

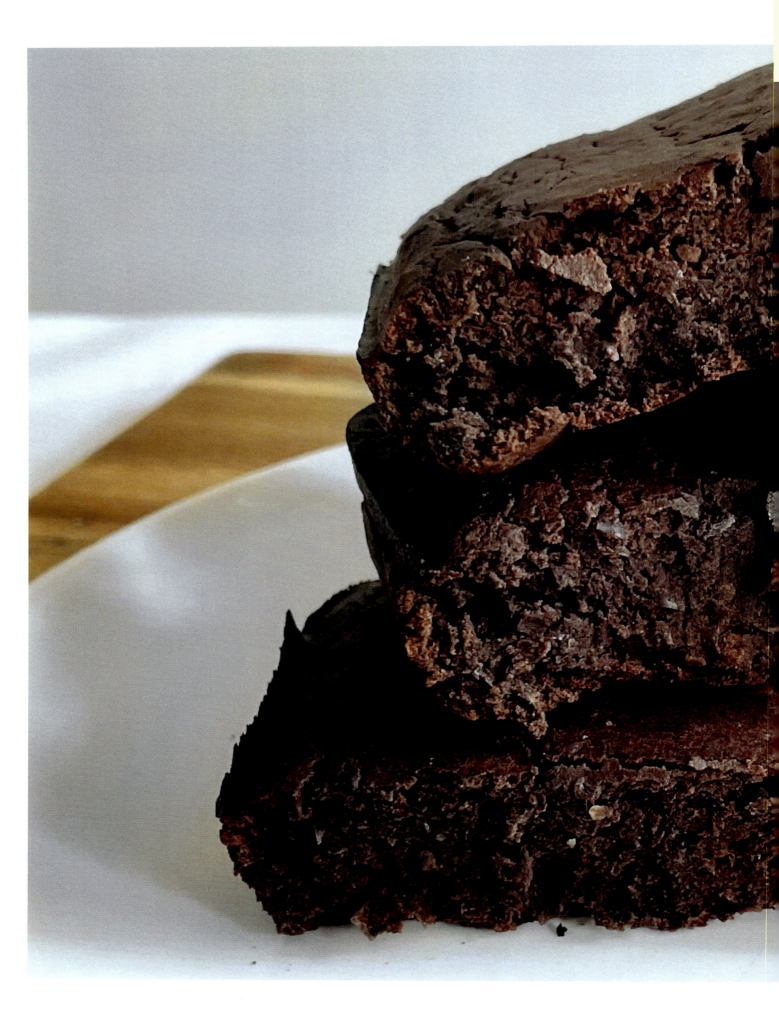

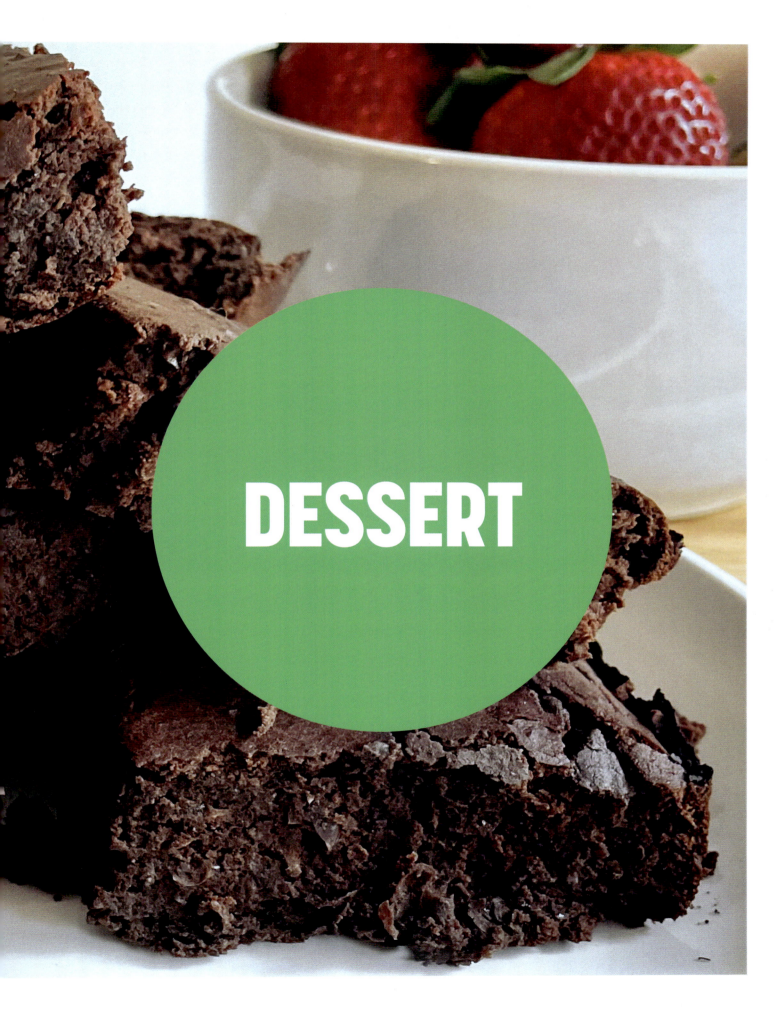

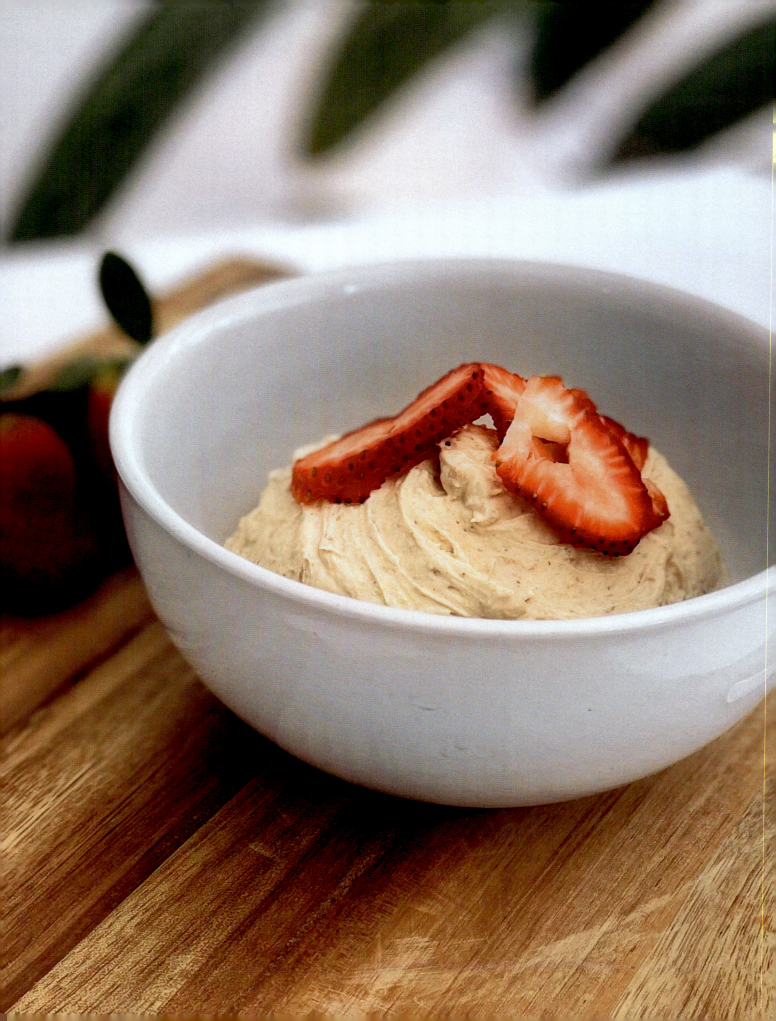

DESSERT

French Vanilla Almond Mousse (V)

SERVINGS: 1

RECIPE HIGHLIGHTS

This delicious creamy 'dessert' is full of protein and low in sugar. It's a perfect way to fix a craving for something sweet, but still keep on track with one's nutrition goals.

MACRO BREAKDOWN (per serve)

FAT: 6G

PROTEIN: 50G

CARBS: 15G

INGREDIENTS

- 1 cup Greek yoghurt (plain, 0–3% fat varieties)
- 1 tablespoon natural almond butter
- 1 scoop vanilla protein powder
- 1 teaspoon stevia
- ¼ teaspoon of almond extract or vanilla extract (optional; adjust to taste)

METHOD

1. Mix or whisk all ingredients together to remove all lumps.
2. Refrigerate for at least an hour before serving.

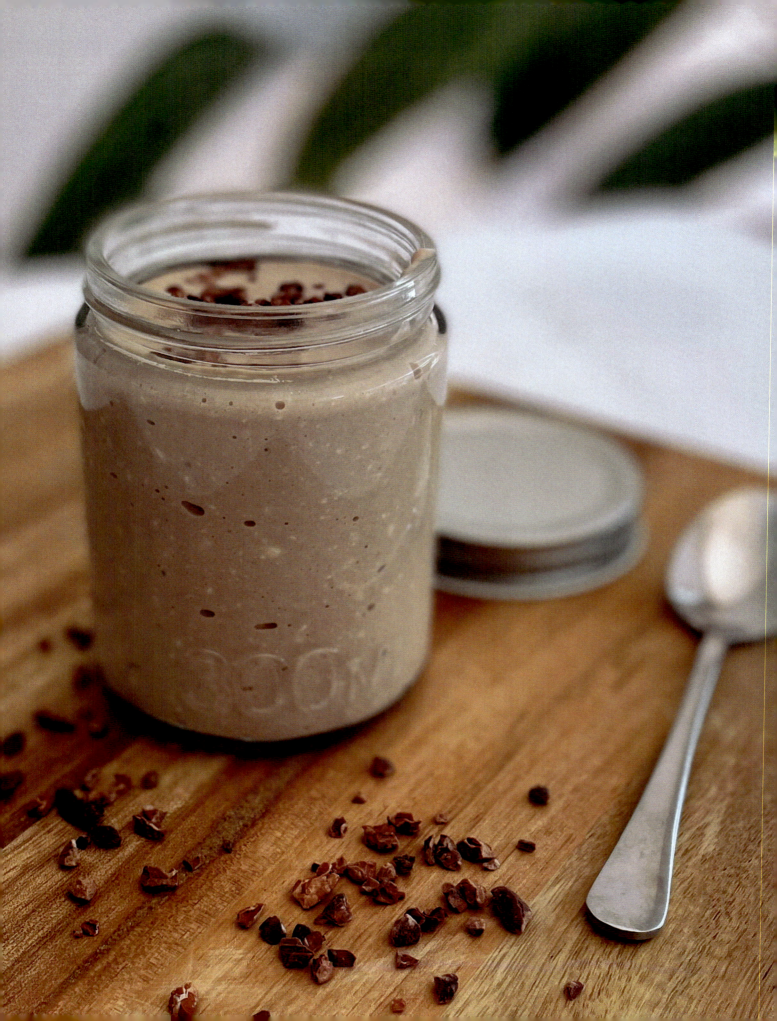

DESSERT

Chocolate Protein Mousse (V)

SERVINGS: 1

RECIPE HIGHLIGHTS

This recipe is super fast to prepare, delicious, and packed with protein. Cottage cheese is an excellent slow-release protein and its taste is perfect in this rich mousse.

MACRO BREAKDOWN (per serve)

FAT: 6G

PROTEIN: 51G

CARBS: 19G

INGREDIENTS

- 125 g low-fat cottage cheese
- 150 g nonfat Greek yoghurt (plain, 0–3% fat varieties)
- 1 scoop chocolate protein powder
- Sprinkle of cacao nibs to taste

METHOD

1. Using a countertop blender (or stick blender), whiz all ingredients together until smooth.
2. Place mixture into small serving bowls and chill.

For a more intense chocolate flavour, add 1–2 teaspoons of sugar-free drinking chocolate (naturally sweetened).

THE LEAN BODY SOLUTION

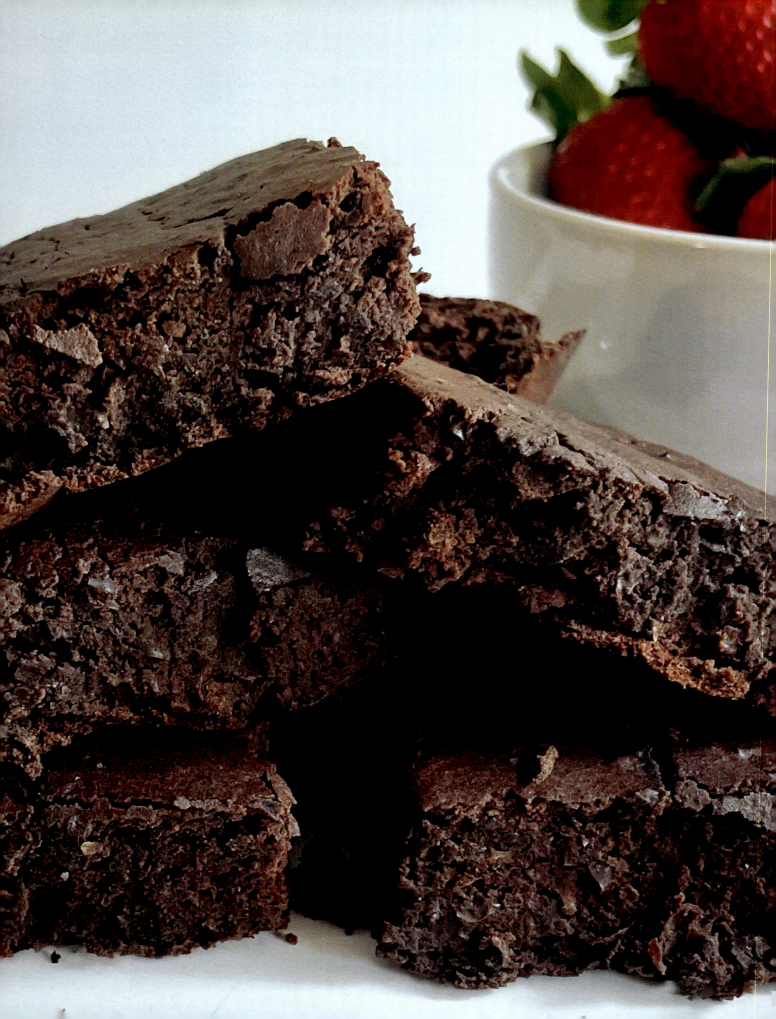

DESSERT

Cocoa Black Bean Brownies (V)

SERVINGS: 6 BROWNIES

MACRO BREAKDOWN (per brownie)

FAT: 6G

PROTEIN: 7G

CARBS: 14G

RECIPE HIGHLIGHTS

Say goodbye to sugary brownies that spike your blood-sugar levels and leave you feeling empty. This filling alternative is just as tasty and will not inflate a spare tyre around your waistline.

INGREDIENTS

- 1 x 420 g can of black beans (rinsed and drained)
- 1 whole egg
- 2 egg whites
- 1 tbsp ground flaxseed + 1 tbsp hot water
- 1½ tbsp coconut oil
- ¼ cup sugar-free maple syrup (naturally sweetened)
- 3 tbsp dark cocoa powder
- 2 tbsp stevia powder
- ½ tsp sea salt
- 1 tsp pure vanilla extract

METHOD

1. Preheat oven to 175 °C. Put black beans into a food processor to mash well into a paste.
2. Before adding the other ingredients, add 1 tbsp hot water to 1 tbsp ground flaxseed in a small bowl and set aside. After about 3 minutes, the flaxseed mixture should be slightly thickened.
3. Add this and remaining ingredients to the food processor and process.
4. Once the mixture is well incorporated in the processor without any chunks (should be smooth), scrape mixture into a greased 8 x 8 pan; bake for about 30 minutes. Before removing, ensure the brownie mixture is fully cooked by placing a toothpick into it to make sure it comes out clean.
5. Cut evenly into 6 brownies and store in the freezer if not immediately consumed.

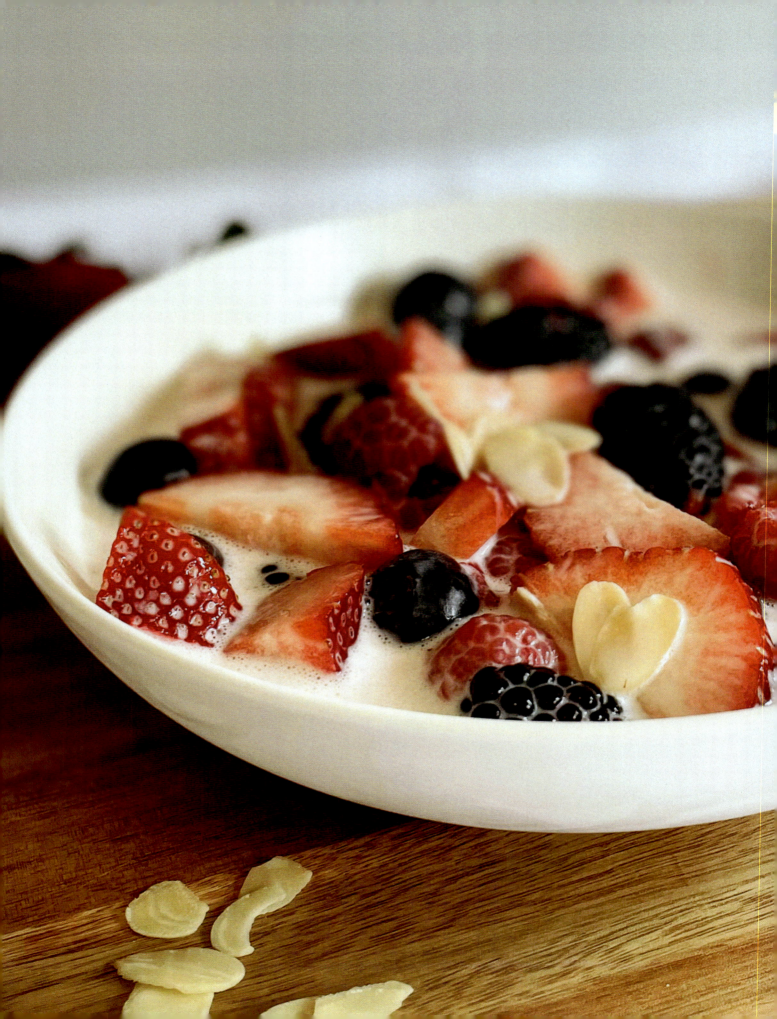

DESSERT

Protein Coconut Fruit Salad (V)

SERVINGS: 1

MACRO BREAKDOWN (per serve)

FAT: 11G

PROTEIN: 37G

CARBS: 30G

RECIPE HIGHLIGHTS

Traditional fruit salads are made up entirely of fruit and added sugar. This one is more filling and includes healthy fats (almonds) along with lots of protein. The assortment of berries adds natural sweetness, along with a wide range of vitamins, minerals, and antioxidants.

INGREDIENTS

- ½ scoop (~15 g) vanilla protein powder
- 1 cup low-fat Greek yoghurt
- ¼ cup unsweetened coconut milk
- 1 cup strawberries (sliced)
- ⅓ cup blackberries
- ⅓ cup raspberries
- ⅓ cup blueberries
- 2 tbsp flaked almonds

METHOD

1. Place the protein powder, Greek yoghurt, and coconut milk in a blender. Blend on high until smooth (if too thick, keep adding tablespoons of water and blend again).
2. Place all berries in a large bowl, then pour the blended mixture over the berries. Stir in flaked almonds.
3. Place in the refrigerator for 15–20 minutes until chilled, then enjoy!

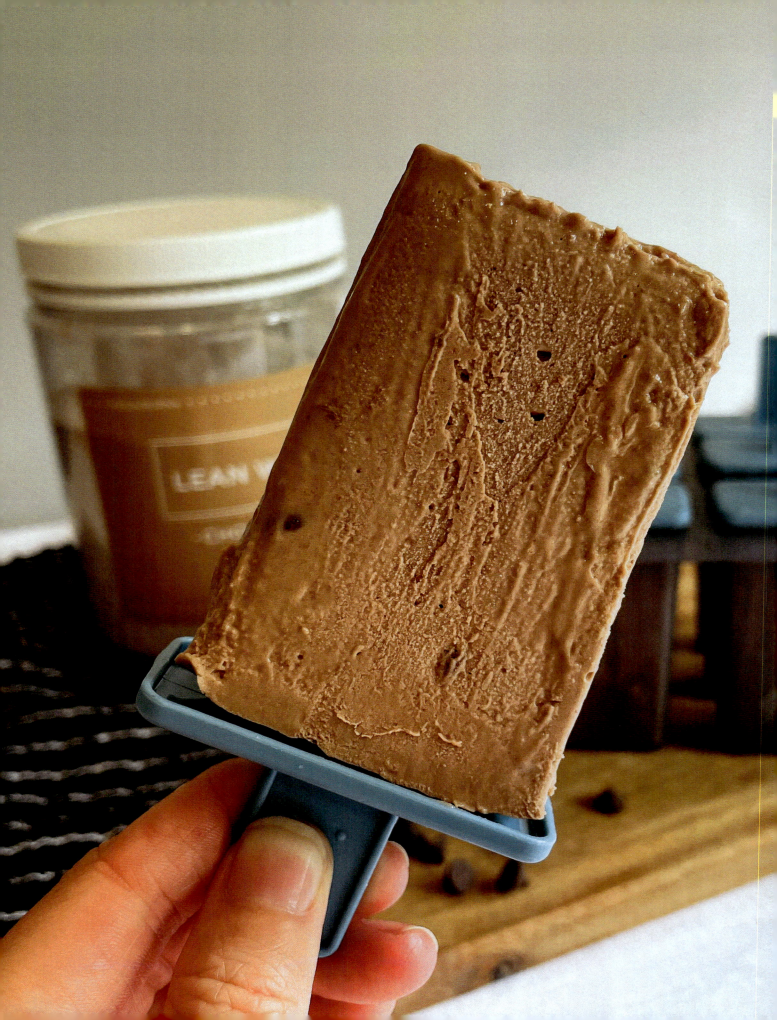

DESSERT

Choc Mint Protein Paddle Pops (V)

SERVINGS: 6

MACRO BREAKDOWN (per paddle pop)

FAT: 13G

PROTEIN: 16G

CARBS: 5G

RECIPE HIGHLIGHTS

These higher-protein paddle pops are very handy if you're craving something sweet after dinner but can do without all the sugar of conventional paddle pop ice creams.

INGREDIENTS

- ¾ cup light cream
- ⅔ cup low-fat, high-protein yoghurt
- 2 tbsp stevia
- 1 tsp peppermint essence
- 2 scoops (~50 g) chocolate protein powder
- 100 g protein chocolate (e.g. Vitawerx), melted
- ¼ cup (~50 g) sugar-free choc chips (naturally sweetened)

METHOD

1. Combine all ingredients, except choc chips, in a food processor until smooth and well combined. Add choc chips at the last minute so they are evenly distributed through ice-cream mixture.

2. Pour mixture evenly into 6 ice-cream stick moulds, leaving a little bit of room at the top so you can then insert the stick. Tap the dish lightly on the countertop to even out the ice-cream mixture.

3. Place in the freezer for 4 hours, or until fully frozen. Remove the ice creams carefully from the mould to serve (it may need to be run carefully under hot water to help release it), or store in the freezer for up to 2 weeks.

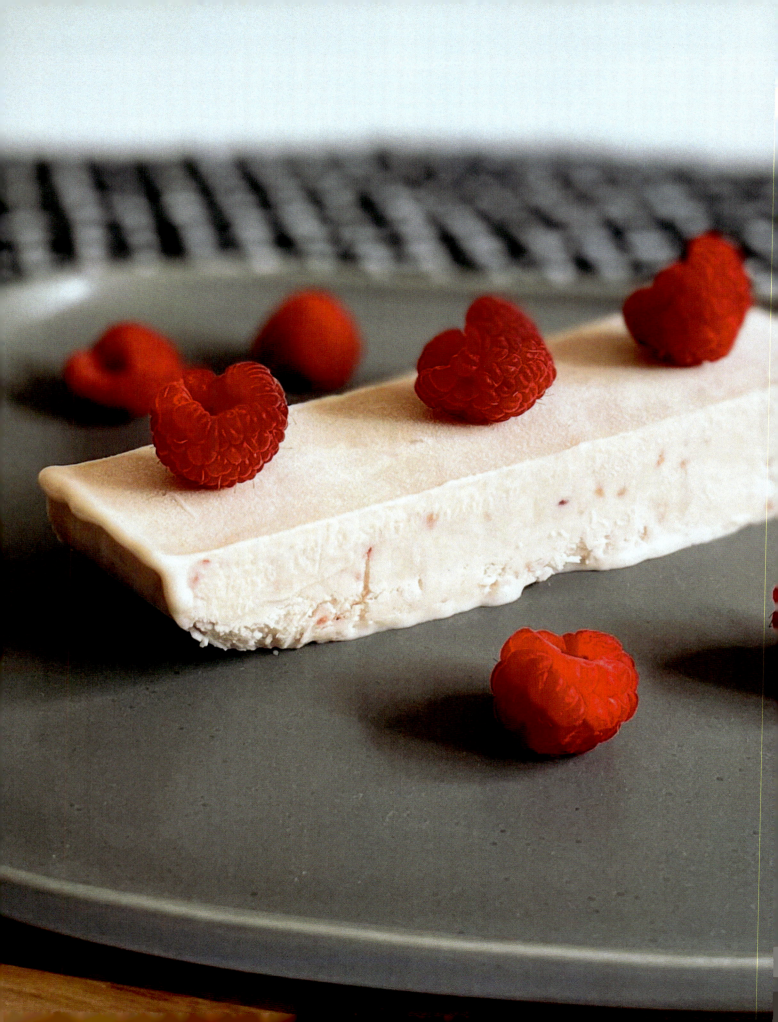

DESSERT

White Choc Raspberry Protein Ice Cream Bars (V)

SERVINGS: 4 BARS

MACRO BREAKDOWN (per serve)

RECIPE HIGHLIGHTS

Not many ice-cream bars can taste this good while packing this much protein! Each bar includes more 20 g of protein and can be enjoyed as a dessert or even as a snack on a hot summer's day.

FAT: 17G

PROTEIN: 21G

CARBS: 9G

INGREDIENTS

- ¾ cup light cream
- ⅔ cup low-fat, high-protein yoghurt
- ⅓ cup frozen raspberries
- 2 tbsp stevia
- ½ tbsp vanilla paste
- 50 g whey protein powder (vanilla or vanilla/raspberry flavour)
- 100 g white protein chocolate (e.g. Vitawerx), melted

METHOD

1. Combine all ingredients in a food processor until smooth and well combined.

2. Pour mixture into either a silicone ice cream dish, or a plastic wrap lined loaf tin; approximately 20x15 cm is an appropriate size. Tap the dish lightly on the countertop to even out the ice cream mixture. Cover and freezer for 4 hours, or until fully frozen.

3. Remove ice cream from dish and cut into 4 equal sized bars. Serve immediately or return to the freezer for up to 2 weeks.

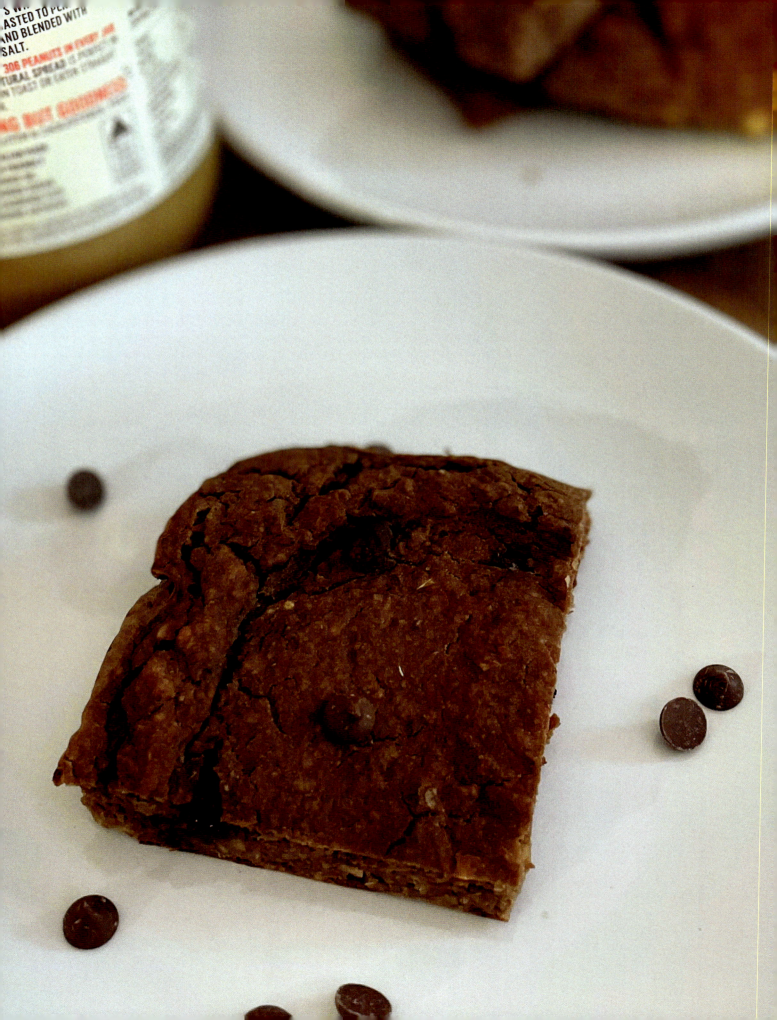

DESSERT

Peanut Butter and Choc Chip Brownies (V)

SERVINGS: 6 BROWNIES

MACRO BREAKDOWN (per serve)

FAT: 7G

PROTEIN: 14G

CARBS: 13G

RECIPE HIGHLIGHTS

These brownies combine protein powder with chickpeas for a high-protein base. The addition of unsweetened almond milk adds creaminess without excess sugar, while the powdered peanut butter provides vitamin E and niacin.

INGREDIENTS

- *1 cup drained chickpeas*
- *¼ cup unsweetened almond milk*
- *2 tbsp natural peanut butter*
- *2 tbsp powdered peanut butter*
- *¼ cup sugar-free maple syrup (naturally sweetened)*
- *1 banana*
- *1 tsp baking powder*
- *½ tbsp vanilla paste*
- *2 scoops chocolate flavoured protein powder of choice*
- *¼ cup sugar-free dark chocolate chips (naturally sweetened)*

METHOD

1. Preheat oven to 180 °C.
2. Combine all ingredients, except for protein powder and chocolate chips, in a food processor until well combined.
3. Fold through protein powder, then stir through the chocolate chips.
4. Pour mixture into a lined baking tin.
5. Bake for 20–25 minutes or until just golden, and a skewer comes out clean.
6. Let cool in pan, then cut into 6 squares.

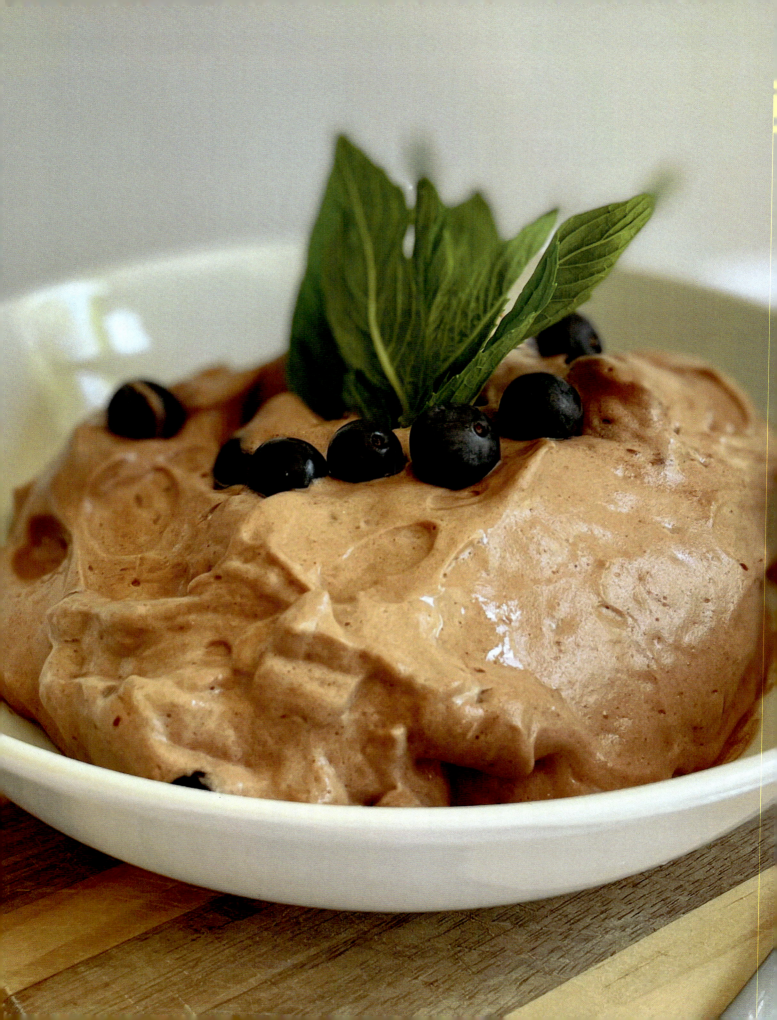

DESSERT

Choc Mint Protein Mousse (V)

SERVINGS: 1

MACRO BREAKDOWN (per serve)

FAT: 2G

PROTEIN: 27G

CARBS: 8G

RECIPE HIGHLIGHTS

This tasty and easy dessert is scarce of sugar and has plenty of lean protein. The addition of peppermint extract provides a cool and invigorating flavour while also offering potential digestive benefits. The antioxidative properties of the blue berries and cocoa shouldn't go unnoticed either.

INGREDIENTS

- *1 scoop chocolate protein powder*
- *1 tsp peppermint extract*
- *1 tbsp cocoa powder*
- *¼ cup unsweetened almond milk*
- *1 tsp guar/xanthan gum*
- *1 tbsp sweetener (stevia)*
- *1 cup of ice*
- *Blueberries (~20 g), to serve*

METHOD

1. Combine all ingredients, except blueberries, in a blender or food processor until smooth and well combined.
2. Pour mixture into a bowl and top with blueberries. Serve immediately.

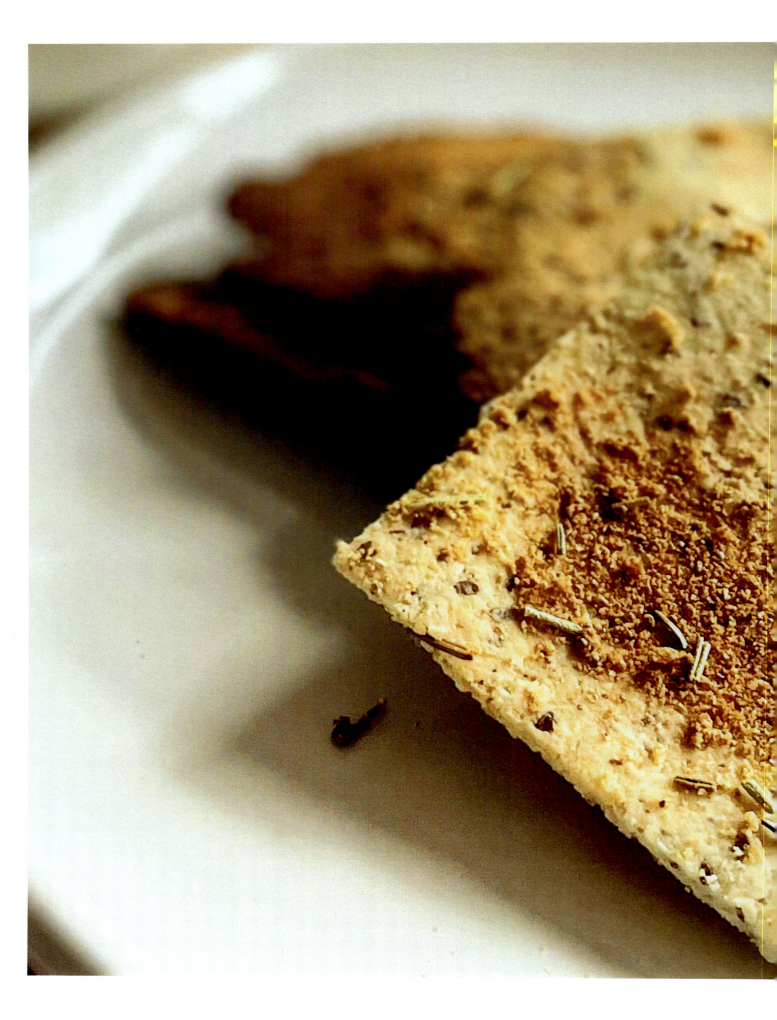

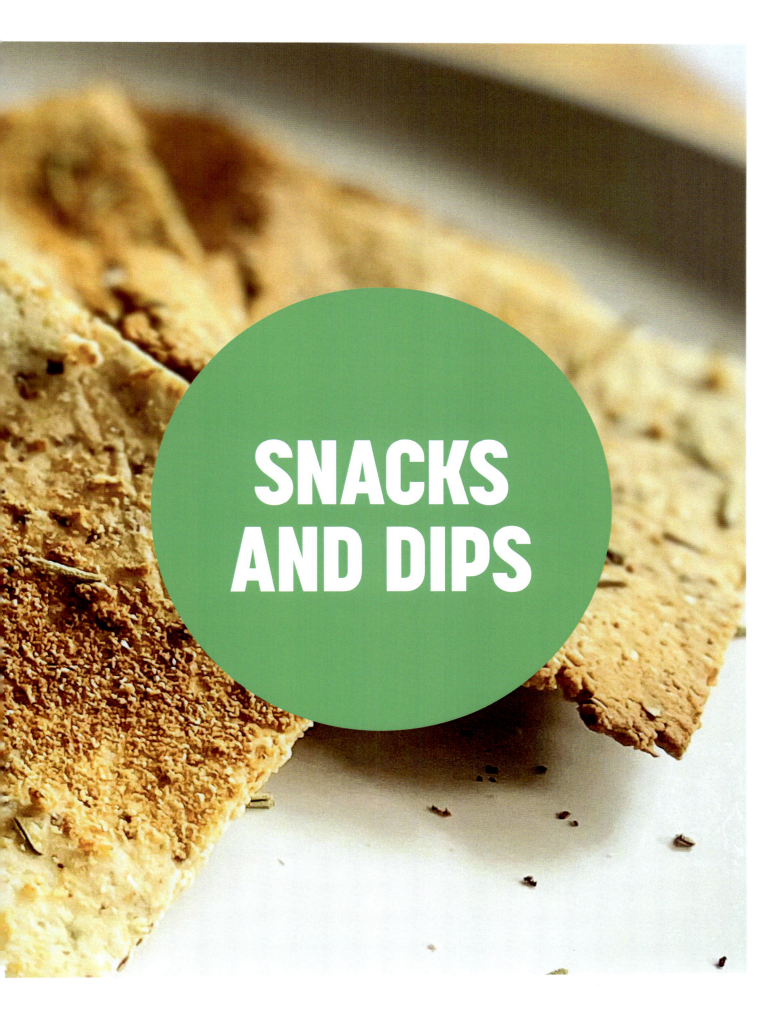

SNACKS AND DIPS

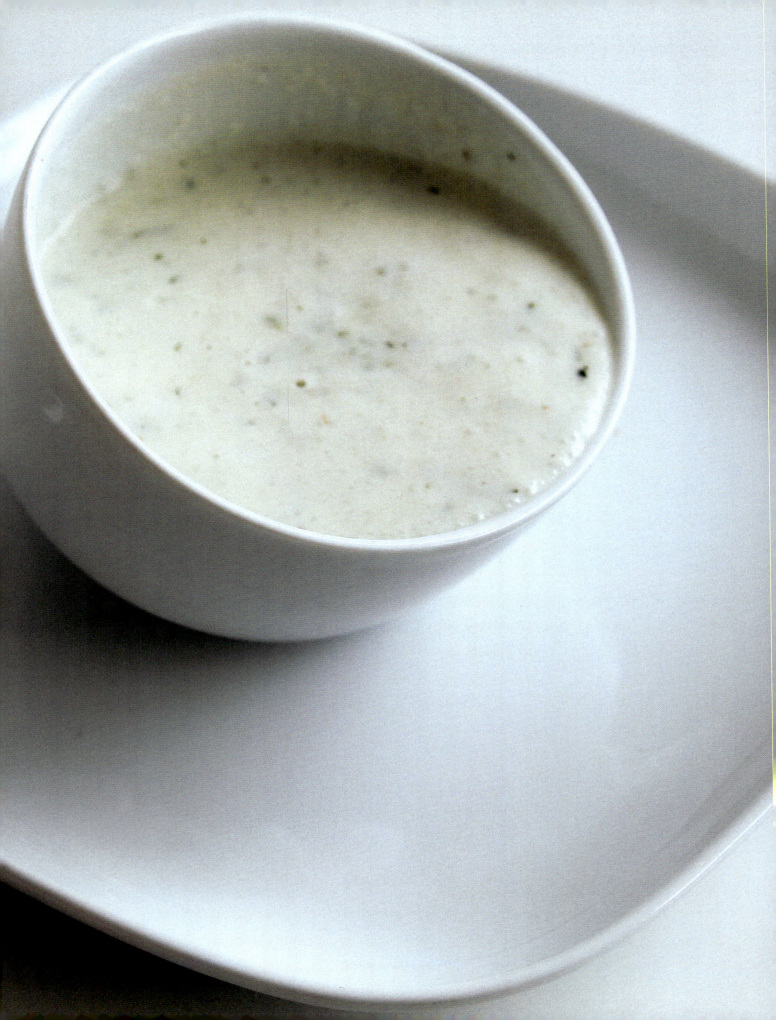

SNACKS AND DIPS

Greek Dill Tzatziki Sauce/Dip (V)

SERVINGS: 6 (½ CUP)

MACRO BREAKDOWN
(per serve: ½ cup)

FAT: 0.8G

PROTEIN: 4G

CARBS: 8.6G

RECIPE HIGHLIGHTS

Due to its yoghurt base, this traditional Greek sauce will deliver protein as well as beneficial bacteria for a healthy digestive tract. The array of mixed herbs also offer digestive and anti-inflammatory properties, along with enhanced flavour.

INGREDIENTS

- *2 cucumbers, halved, seeded, shredded*
- *¼ tsp salt*
- *2 cups low-fat plain yoghurt (dairy or coconut are acceptable)*
- *1 tbsp extra-virgin cold-pressed olive oil*
- *1 tbsp dried basil*
- *2 tsp dried oregano*
- *2 tbsp chopped dill (preferably fresh)*
- *2 tsp honey*
- *1 tsp fresh minced garlic*

METHOD

1. Halve and seed the cucumber and then shred into a medium-sized bowl using a cheese grater.
2. Sprinkle shredded cucumber with salt; toss in bowl. Afterward, place in a sieve, allowing juices to drain from the cucumber for 30 minutes.
3. Place cucumber and the rest of the ingredients into a food processor (sauce) or bowl and whip (dip) to desired consistency.
4. Place in mixture in a sealed bowl and refrigerate for 3 hours to allow flavours to blend and mixture to cool. Use as a sauce for meats, wraps, and sandwiches, or as a dip for savoury snacks.

THE LEAN BODY SOLUTION

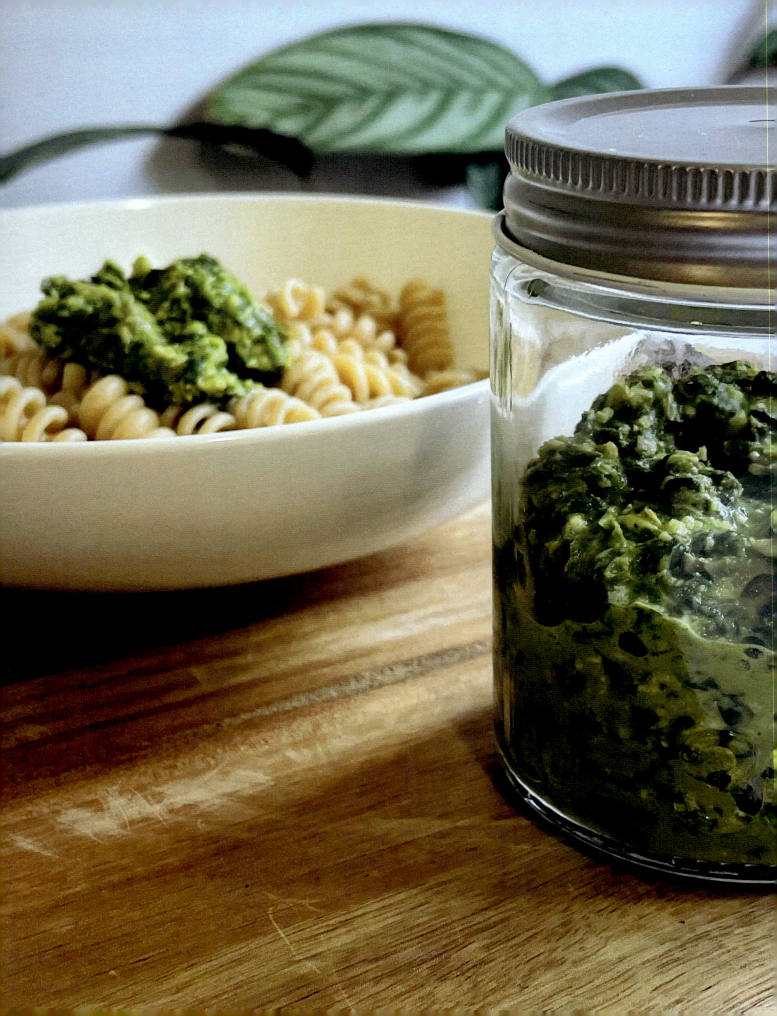

SNACKS AND DIPS

Zesty Pesto (V)

SERVINGS: 4 (²/₃ CUP)

MACRO BREAKDOWN
(per serve: ²/₃ cup)

FAT: 6G

PROTEIN: 3G

CARBS: 2.5G

RECIPE HIGHLIGHTS

Walnuts are a nutritious nut rich in heart- and brain-healthy omega-3 fatty acids. They also deliver a good amount of minerals like copper and manganese, while contributing a satisfying crunch to the pesto. The cannellini beans offer a creamy texture and contain a good amount of fibre to help with satiety.

INGREDIENTS

- *2 cups fresh basil leaves*
- *¼ cup walnuts*
- *2 tbsp fresh lemon juice*
- *1 clove fresh garlic*
- *¼ tsp lemon zest*
- *¼ tsp turmeric powder*
- *¼ cup white cannellini beans*
- *¼ tsp salt*
- *2 tbsp to ¼ cup water*

METHOD

1. Combine all ingredients, except water, in a food processor or high-speed blender.
2. Blend on high and add water while blending to reach desired consistency. The final texture should be smooth and thick.
3. Place in the refrigerator to cool and then serve over pasta or salad.

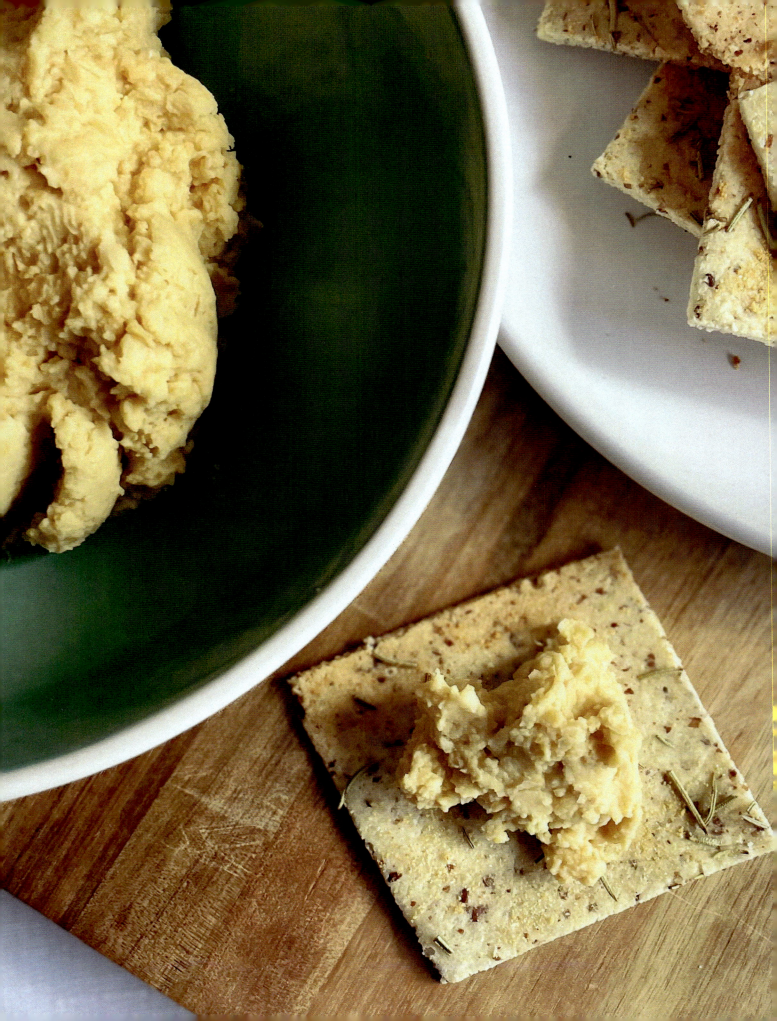

SNACKS AND DIPS

Simple & Classic Hummus (V)

SERVINGS: 14 (2 TBSP)

MACRO BREAKDOWN (per serve: 2 tbsp)

FAT: 4.6G

PROTEIN: 3.4G

CARBS: 12.8G

RECIPE HIGHLIGHTS

Many store-bought hummus varieties are full of preservatives or additives to prolong the shelf life and enhance flavour. This homemade hummus, on the other hand, allows you to avoid these preservatives and have a full-flavoured natural and wholesome dip.

INGREDIENTS

- 1x 420 g can chickpeas
- ½ tsp sea salt
- Juice of 1 lemon
- 1 clove garlic, minced
- ¼ tbsp tahini
- 1 tbsp olive oil
- 1 tsp cayenne powder for spiciness (optional)

METHOD

1. Open the can of chickpeas; rinse 1–2 times with water, then drain.
2. In a food processor, add chickpeas, sea salt, lemon juice, garlic clove, and tahini.
3. Add the olive oil while blending on low speed. Stop and scrape the sides of the food processor if needed.
4. Continue blending until a creamy texture is reached. If needed, add small amounts of olive oil.
5. Use as a dip or as a spread for sandwiches.

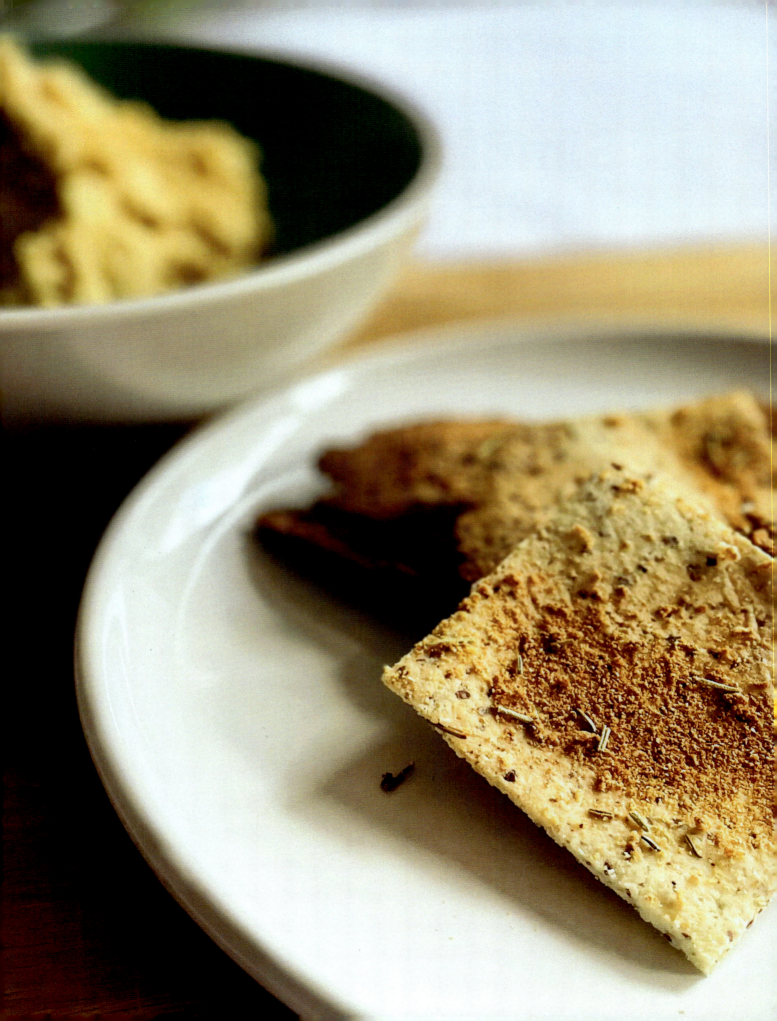

SNACKS AND DIPS

Homemade Almond Crackers with Hummus (V)

SERVINGS: 4 (8–10 CRACKERS)

MACRO BREAKDOWN
(per serve: 8–10 square crackers)

FAT: 28G

PROTEIN: 13G

CARBS: 5G

RECIPE HIGHLIGHTS

Most crackers are full of processed carbohydrates and leave you craving more food. These almond crackers, however, deliver plenty of healthy fats and minimal carbs so you will feel fuller longer. They also taste amazing and make the perfect crunchy pairing for healthy dips or protein sources like tuna fish and cottage cheese.

INGREDIENTS

- 1 cup almond meal (almond flour works, too)
- 1 tbsp flaxseed, ground
- 2 tbsp warm water
- ½ tsp salt
- 1 tbsp fresh rosemary, finely chopped
- ½ tsp garlic powder
- 1 container of Simple & Classic Hummus or top with canned tuna for extra protein

METHOD

1. Preheat the oven to 160 °C.
2. In a medium bowl, add almond flour, water, ground flaxseed, and salt; stir together until the mixture turns into dough. Then form the dough into 2 equal-sized balls. Complete the flattening steps below for both balls of dough.
3. Using a piece of parchment paper, cover the ball and use a rolling pin or a wine bottle to roll it out to about ⅛" (0.3 cm) thick and roughly square, smoothing the wrinkles out as it becomes thinner.
4. Once flat, flip the dough over and repeat the same process with another piece of parchment paper to flatten the dough even more.
5. Once flattened on both sides and even, sprinkle with the rosemary and garlic powder. Press seasoning just slightly so it sticks to the dough.
6. Cut the dough into 1–2" (4–5 cm) squares.
7. Bake until only slightly brown for about 15 minutes, then let cool for 5 minutes.
8. Serve immediately with hummus or tuna fish, or keep crackers in an airtight container for 2–3 days.

THE LEAN BODY SOLUTION

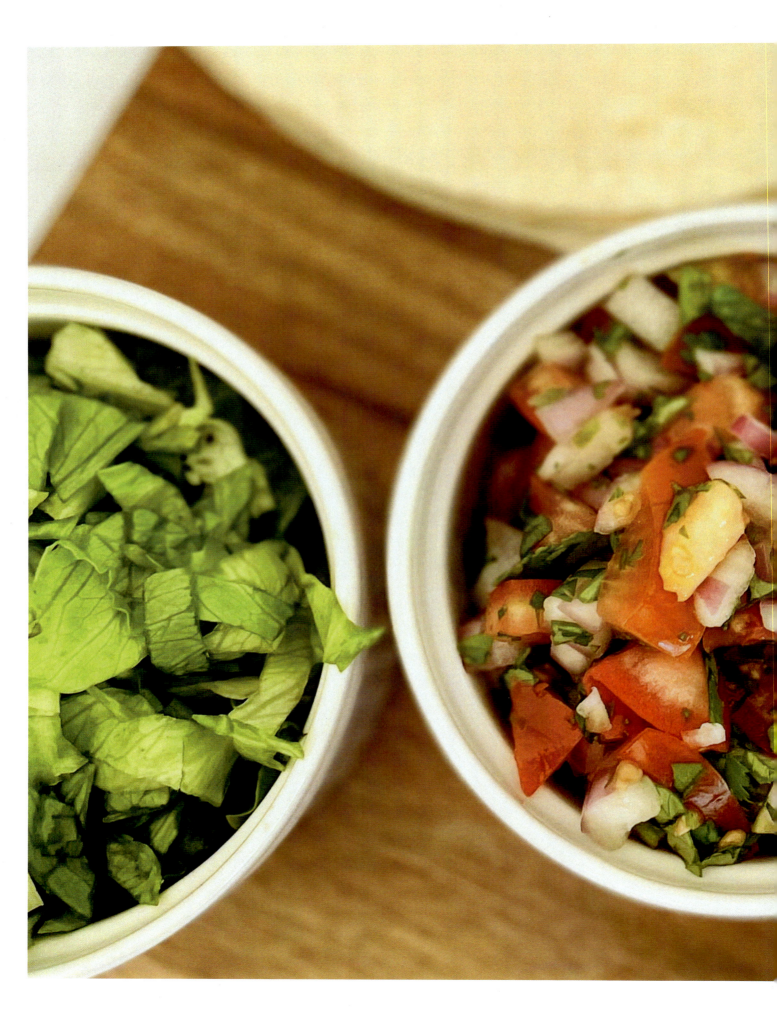

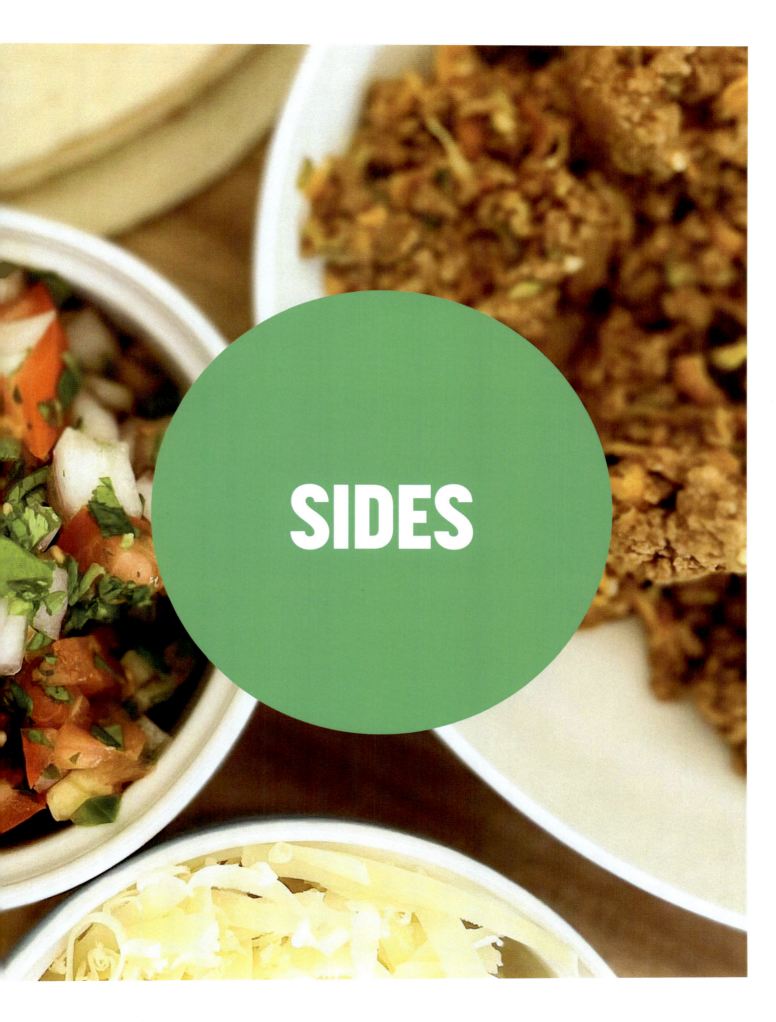
SIDES

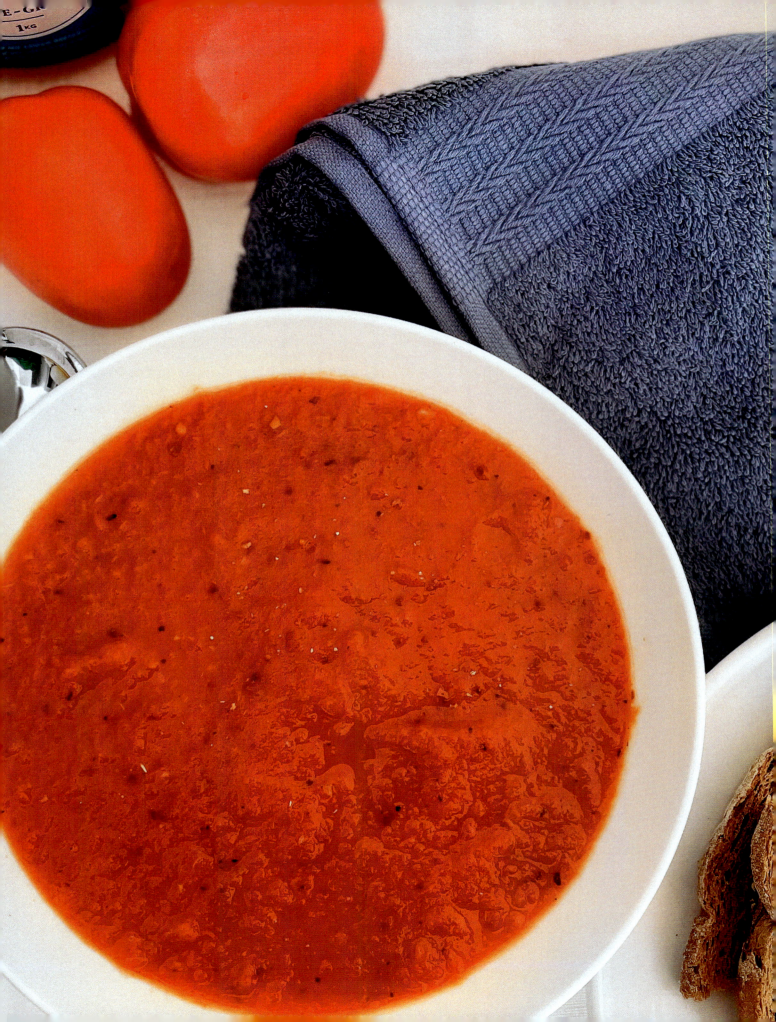

Spicy Red Pepper & Tomato Soup (V)

SERVINGS: 8

MACRO BREAKDOWN (per serve)

		with black beans
FAT: 2.5G		FAT: 3G
PROTEIN: 3G		PROTEIN: 7G
CARBS: 20G		CARBS: 30G

RECIPE HIGHLIGHTS

One serve of this spicy soup will provide you with two-thirds of your daily requirement for vitamin C! If you need to create a more filling serve, fibrous black beans can be added to this meal as well. This soup is also suitable if you're vegetarian or a plant-based eater.

INGREDIENTS

- 2x 300 g jars roasted red peppers, drained
- 4x 400 g cans tomatoes—whole or diced (reduced salt if possible)
- 1½ cups chicken broth
- 1 brown onion, chopped
- 2 cloves garlic, chopped
- 1 tablespoon extra-virgin olive oil
- ¼ teaspoon red chilli flakes (to taste)
- Salt and pepper (to taste)
- 2 teaspoons granulated sugar (optional)
- 1x 400 g can black beans, drained and rinsed (optional)

METHOD

1. In a Dutch oven or large soup pot, add olive oil and sauté onion on medium heat until the onions are soft and translucent.
2. Add garlic and sauté another 2 minutes.
3. Add canned tomatoes, drained peppers, and sugar. Add black beans (optional). Simmer for 8–10 minutes and season with salt and pepper to taste (note: taste test as canned tomatoes can be salty).
4. Add 1 cup chicken broth and red chilli flakes (optional). Heat to a simmer then reduce heat to low.
5. Puree the soup with a stick blender (or in batches in a food processor/regular blender) until the soup is smooth.
6. Reheat the soup and add more broth if desired. Also taste test for seasoning and adjust accordingly.
7. Serve as side with a main meal. Refrigerate leftovers in airtight containers (or freeze in Ziploc freezer bags).

SIDES

Homemade Sauerkraut (V)

SERVINGS: 6-7 (1 CUP)

MACRO BREAKDOWN
(per serve: 1 cup)

FAT: 6G

PROTEIN: 3G

CARBS: 2.5G

RECIPE HIGHLIGHTS

Sauerkraut is a fermented food that results in the growth of beneficial bacteria. These probiotics help promote a healthy gut by enhancing digestibility and increasing the availability of nutrients. The probiotics found in sauerkraut also have the potential to alleviate symptoms of bloating and gas.

INGREDIENTS

- 1 large head green cabbage
- 4 teaspoons sea salt
- 1 white onion
- 1 tbsp fresh thyme or other seasoning (optional)

METHOD

1. Cut the cabbage in half, separating the core. On each half, cut out the bottom bulb by slicing in a V style to remove the extra-hard parts of the cabbage. Cut the halves in half again to make 4 equal-sized parts.

2. Put the 4 pieces into a food processor to shred or cut them into thin strips manually. If cutting manually, you'll want to keep one flat side of the quartered piece down and carefully cut from the top down to make thin, long strips. Place the shredded cabbage into 1 or 2 large bowls as you go.

3. Slice the onion into similar strips of shorter length. Add these to the cabbage, along with thyme or other preferred seasonings. Next, add salt on top of the cabbage/onion mixture in each bowl.

4. With clean hands, start massaging the salt into the cabbage and onion. Squeeze tightly to help release the vegetable juices as you go and continue for 3–5 minutes to keep releasing liquids.

5. Next, put the contents into a large fermentation vessel (large 1 gallon jar or ceramic crock pots work well). Compress the vegetables into the bottom of the vessel using your hands or kitchen tool. The goal is to have the released juices submerge the cabbage and onion.

SIDES

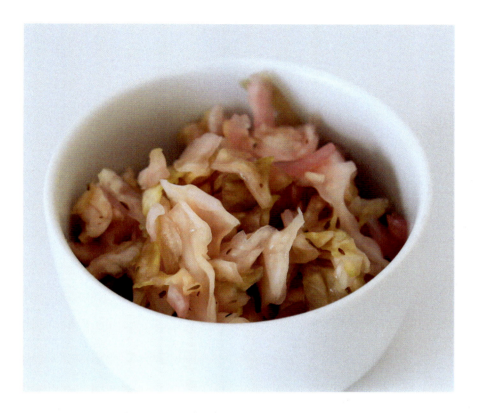

6. The next step is to add weight that will continually provide pressure to the mixture. This can be done by putting glass jars full of water on top of the vegetables. You can use anything that's heavy and clean, which you don't mind keeping pressed against the mixture for 7–10 days.

7. After adding weight, cover the mixture with a clean cloth to keep out dust. Place where it can be checked on day to day.

8. Let sit. Once a day, adjust the weight and vegetables so that ideally they are submerged by the juices.

9. After about 7 days, the mixture should start to taste slightly soured; it's ready to eat. Waiting longer will intensify the flavour. Once it's right, place in the refrigerator in an airtight container. The flavour will continue to change, but much slower in the refrigerator. Sauerkraut makes a great addition to meats, especially sausages and on sandwiches.

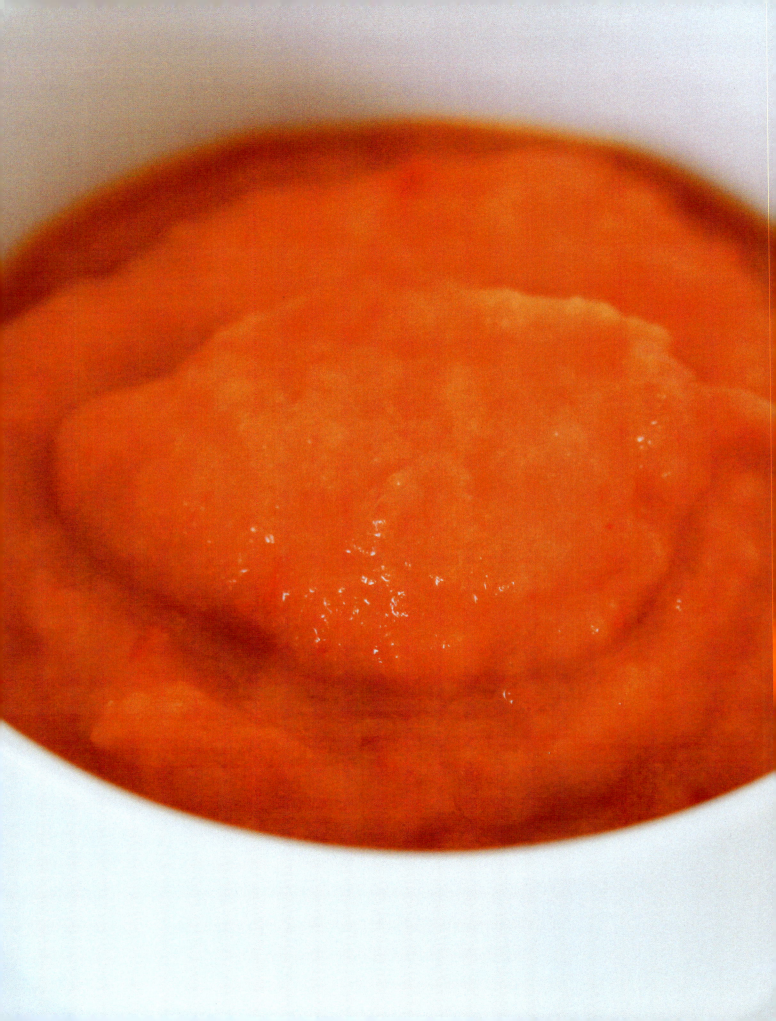

SIDES

Sofrito (V)

SERVINGS: 4 (¾ CUP)

MACRO BREAKDOWN
(per serve: ¾ cup)

FAT: 7.3G

PROTEIN: 2G

CARBS: 18G

RECIPE HIGHLIGHTS

The assortment of vegetables in sofrito contain many antioxidants to help reduce inflammation and support overall cellular health. They also contain a good amount of dietary fibre to help regulate blood sugar levels and promote satiety. The combination of ingredients in sofrito adds a burst of flavour to dishes without the need for excessive sugars or added flavours.

INGREDIENTS

- 2 red onions (diced)
- 4 large carrots (diced)
- 2 diced capsicum (red or green)
- 4 garlic cloves (minced)
- 2–3 chilli peppers (optional)
- 2 tbsp olive oil
- ½ tsp sea salt

METHOD

1. Heat the olive oil in a frying pan over medium heat. Add the diced vegetables and salt. Cook until vegetables are soft.
2. Continue cooking for 5–7 more minutes while stirring constantly at this point so the vegetables don't stick to the pan. The vegetables should begin to fry a little bit and take on a caramelised look. Remove from heat and allow to cool.
3. Once the mixture is cooled, transfer to a blender or food processor and blend just until you get a smooth texture. The final product should be like a thick soup, but not too runny.
4. Add sofrito any Latin-style dishes for more flavour. Keeps well in an airtight container for up to 1 week.

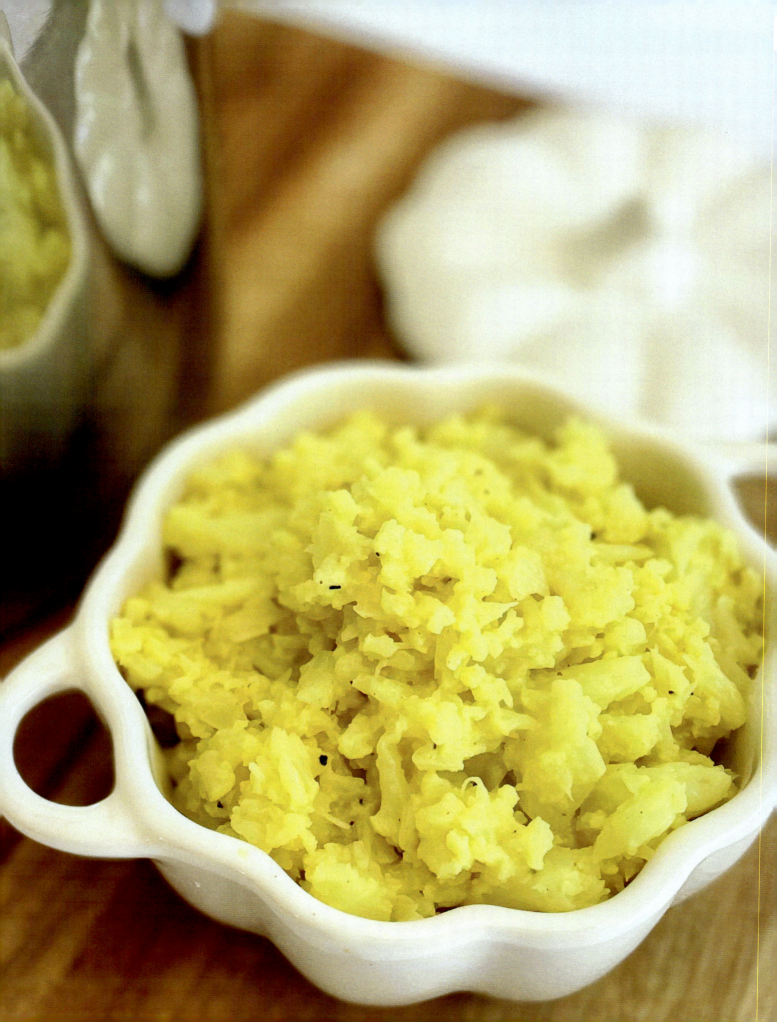

Tasty Cauliflower Mash (V)

SERVINGS: 3 (¾ CUP)

MACRO BREAKDOWN
(per serve: ¾ cup)

FAT: 6.1G

PROTEIN: 1.3G

CARBS: 6.5G

RECIPE HIGHLIGHTS

Mashed potatoes contain starchy carbohydrates and usually excess amounts of fat. This recipe's texture and taste is so similar to mashed potatoes, yet you'll hardly know the difference—except around your waistline! Make the switch and you'll be fuller (and leaner) for longer.

INGREDIENTS

- 1 head cauliflower
- ½ can light, unsweetened coconut milk
- ½ tsp turmeric
- Sea salt and pepper to taste

METHOD

1. Break the cauliflower apart into small florets, using a knife if needed.
2. Place florets into a large pot with enough water to cover all florets.
3. Put pot over high heat and bring to a boil. Continue cooking until the cauliflower is soft enough to be easily pierced with a fork. Drain the water.
4. Add the coconut milk and turmeric. Using a masher or wooden spatula, smash the softened cauliflower into smaller pieces. Reduce heat to medium and cook for 15–20 minutes, stirring occasionally to prevent burning. The mixture should be a creamy mashed potato-like texture.
5. Add in sea salt and pepper to taste and serve immediately or store in the fridge for 4–5 days.

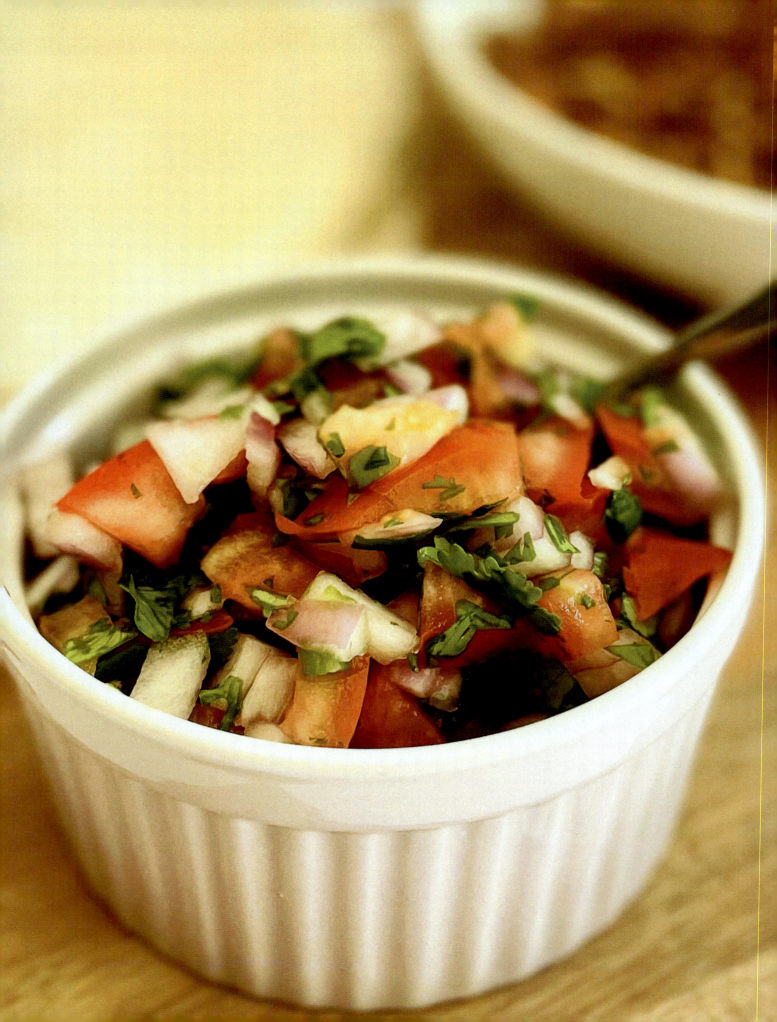

SIDES

Simple & Spicy Pico de Gallo (V)

SERVINGS: 4 (½ CUP)

MACRO BREAKDOWN
(per serve: ½ cup)

FAT: 0.3G

PROTEIN: 1.3G

CARBS: 8.1G

RECIPE HIGHLIGHTS

This side is rich in vitamin C and antioxidant properties. The hot peppers not only give pico de gallo a spicy kick, they also contain capsaicin, a compound that promotes satiety and can have potential pain-relief properties.

INGREDIENTS

- *2 large, fresh tomatoes*
- *1 bunch coriander*
- *1 red or white onion*
- *1 lime*
- *1 jalapeño pepper or other hot pepper*
- *1 pinch sea salt*

METHOD

1. First, destem the coriander and rinse under cold water. Finely chop coriander, tomatoes, and onion.
2. Next, remove the seeds from the jalapeno pepper. Dice and add to the bowl.
3. Cut and squeeze the lime juice over the bowl and cover with 1 pinch of sea salt; mix thoroughly until well combined.
4. Use pico de gallo in any place where salsa is normally used. Store in an airtight container in refrigerator.

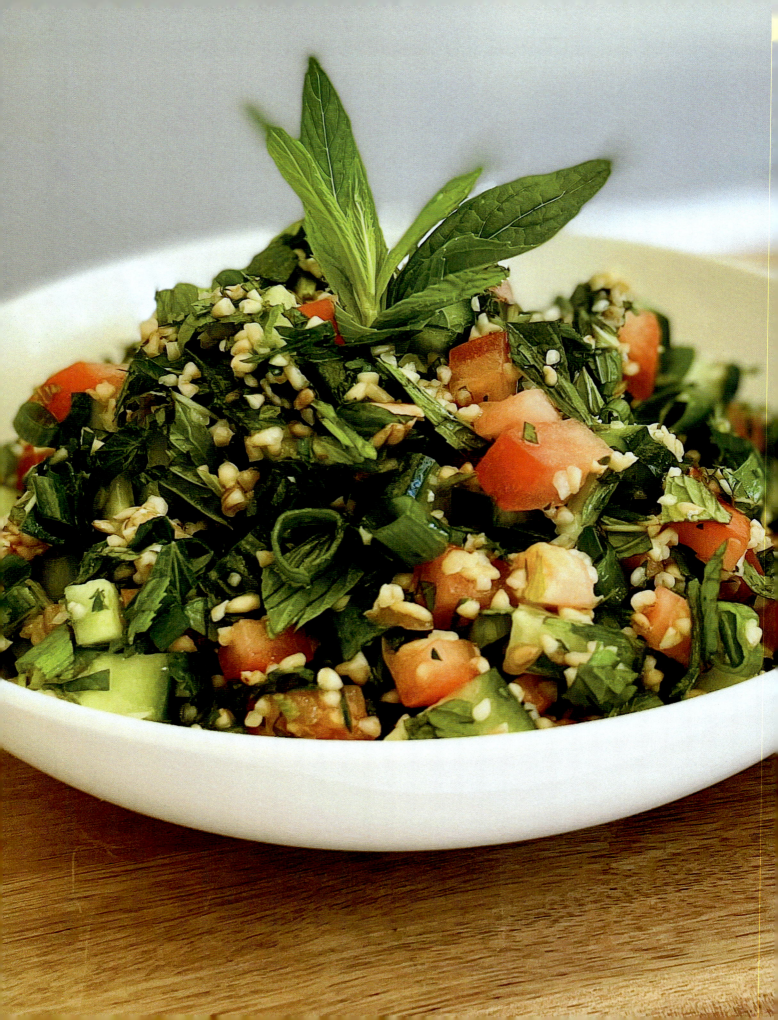

SIDES

Tasty Tabouli Salad (V)

SERVINGS: 3 (1 CUP)

MACRO BREAKDOWN
(per serve: 1 cup)

FAT: 9G

PROTEIN: 4G

CARBS: 10G

RECIPE HIGHLIGHTS

The inclusion of bulgur wheat in this salad provides a good amount of dietary fibre and essential minerals like manganese, magnesium, and iron. The cucumber adds a refreshing crunch and volume due to its high water content.

INGREDIENTS

- ¼ cup bulgur wheat, cooked
- ½ cucumber
- 1 tomato
- 4 scallions
- 1 bunch of fresh parsley
- ½ cup fresh mint leaves
- 2 tbsp olive oil
- 2 tbsp lime juice

METHOD

1. Chop cucumber, tomato, scallions, mint, and parsley. Add cooked bulgur wheat and mix.
2. Dress with lime juice and olive oil.
3. Stir to combine well. Keep refrigerated for up to 1 week.

THE LEAN BODY SOLUTION

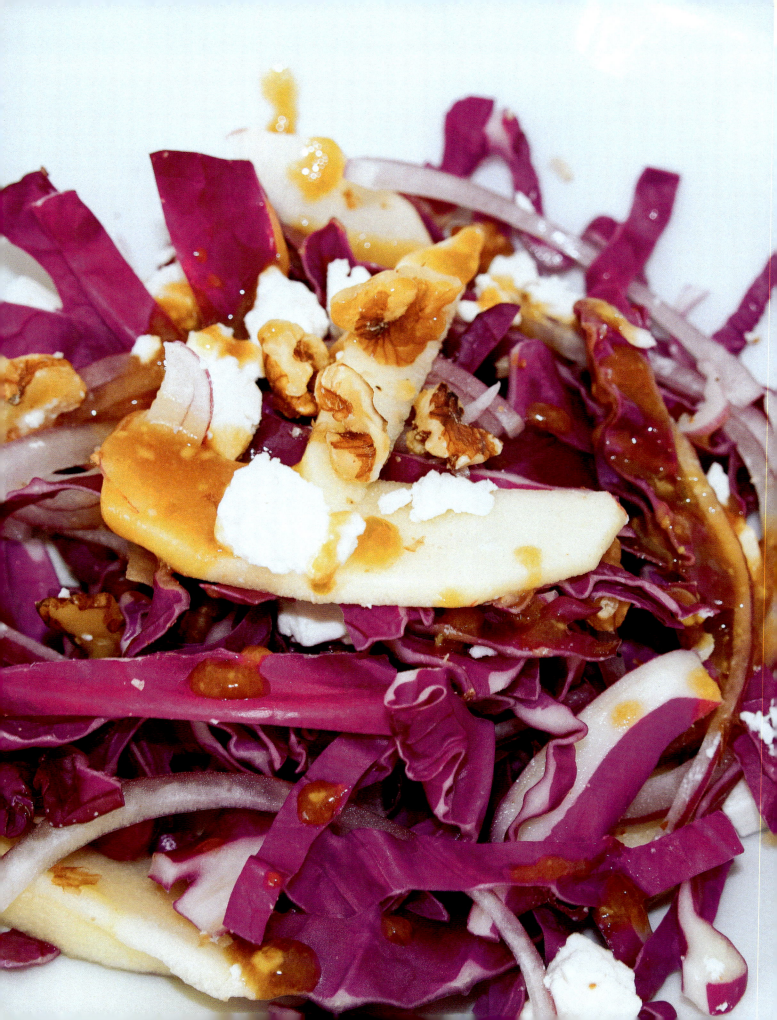

SIDES

Crunchy Apple-Walnut Salad (V)

SERVINGS: 8 (1 CUP)

MACRO BREAKDOWN
(per serve: 1 cup)

FAT: 10G

PROTEIN: 2G

CARBS: 5G

RECIPE HIGHLIGHTS

This salad not only provides you with a tasty side dish, but it also contains plant-based omega-3s from the walnuts, along with bone-building calcium from the feta.

INGREDIENTS

- 7 cups chopped red leaf lettuce (roughly 1 large head)
- 1 medium apple, cored and thinly sliced
- ½ cup walnuts, roughly chopped and toasted
- ¼ cup red onions, thinly sliced
- ¼ cup crumbled low-fat feta cheese

METHOD

1. Place all ingredients in a large salad bowl or mixer and toss until well combined.
2. Refrigerate in an airtight container for up to 1 week. Pairs well with 'Better Balsamic Vinaigrette' (see below).

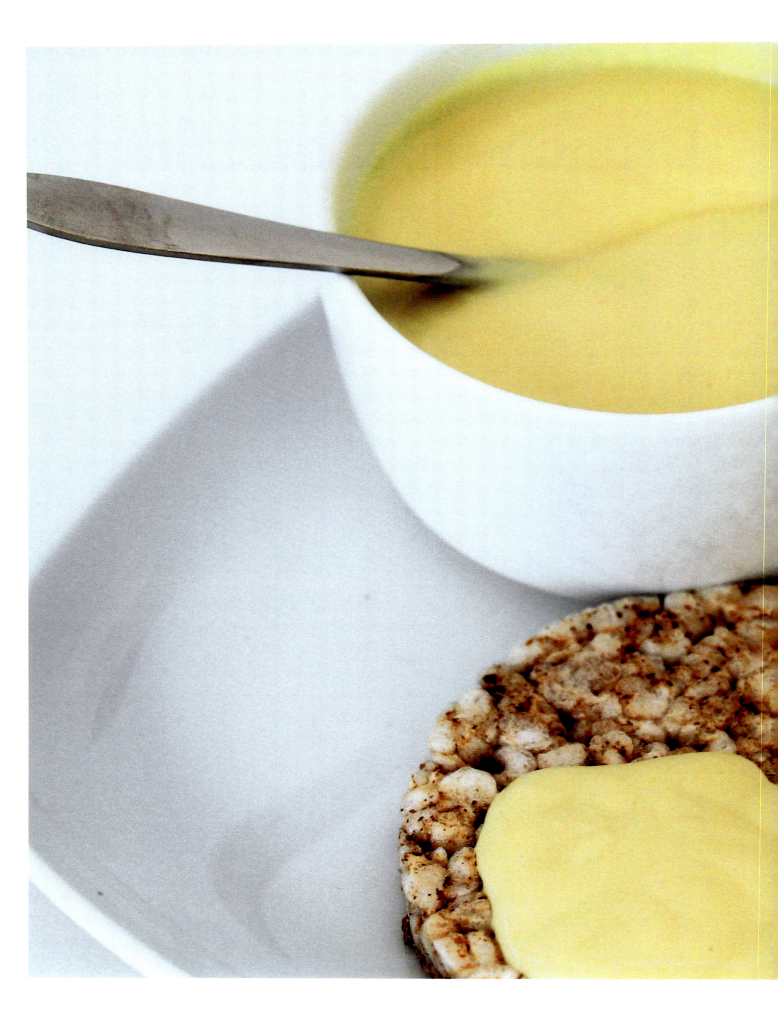

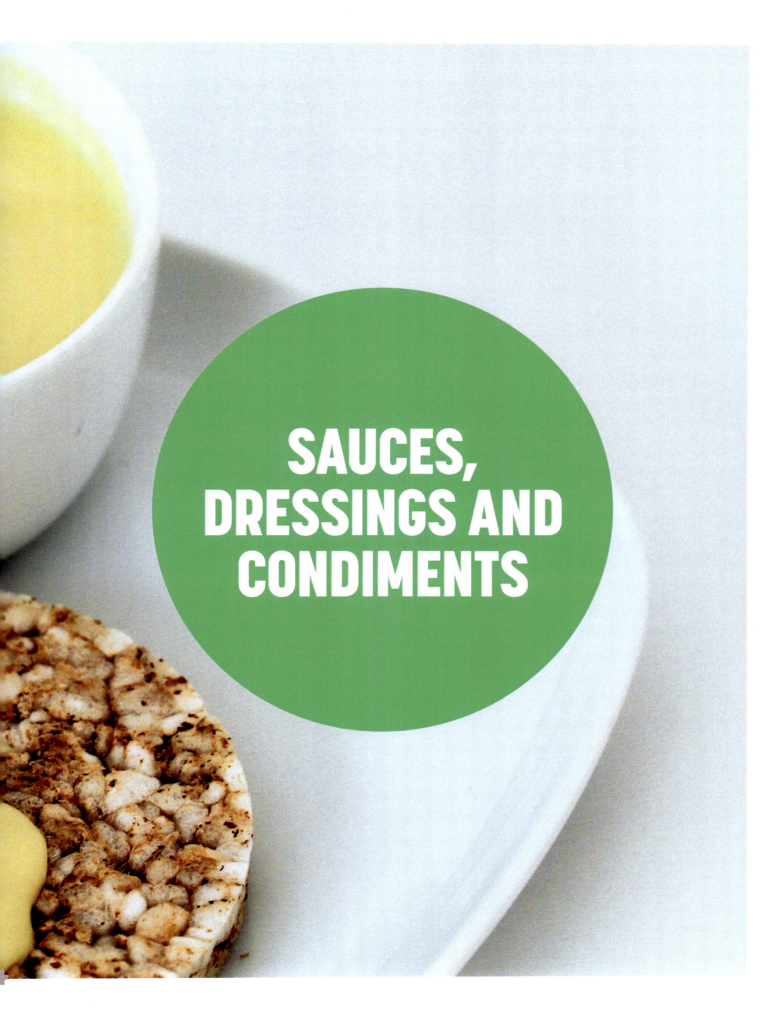

SAUCES, DRESSINGS AND CONDIMENTS

SAUCES, DRESSINGS AND CONDIMENTS

Sweet Citrus-Apple Vinaigrette (V)

SERVINGS: 4 (1.5 TBSP)

RECIPE HIGHLIGHTS

This vinaigrette boasts a unique spicy and sweet flavour. The cinnamon and allspice add warmth and depth (along with antioxidant properties). The orange zest adds a citrus aroma and imparts a burst of flavour. And the agave nectar adds a touch of sweetness without the need for refined sugars.

MACRO BREAKDOWN
(per serve: 1.5 tbsp) *with walnut oil*

FAT: 0G		**FAT: 7G**
PROTEIN: 0G		**PROTEIN: 0G**
CARBS: 8G		**CARBS: 7G**

INGREDIENTS

- 1 gala apple, cored and sliced
- 1 tbsp lemon juice
- 1 tsp cinnamon
- ¼ tsp ground allspice
- 1 tbsp orange zest
- 2 tsp agave nectar
- 1–2 tbsp walnut oil (optional)

METHOD

1. Place all ingredients in a blender or food processor and blend on low speed to start for 20–30 seconds.
2. To make thinner, add slightly more lemon juice.
3. Store in airtight container in the fridge for 4–5 days.

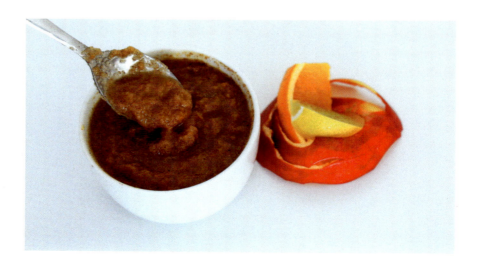

SAUCES, DRESSINGS AND CONDIMENTS

Healthier Honey-Mustard Dressing (V)

SERVINGS: 6 (2 TBSP)

MACRO BREAKDOWN
(per serve: 2 tbsp)

FAT: 9.5G

PROTEIN: 4G

CARBS: 7G

RECIPE HIGHLIGHTS

This dressing delivers a sweet and tangy taste. The Dijon mustard flavour is sharp but balanced with a small addition of honey. The plain low-fat yoghurt used as the base of the dressing adds a creamy texture along with beneficial bacteria to support gut health.

INGREDIENTS

- ½ cup plain low-fat yoghurt
- 1 tbsp olive oil
- 1 tbsp Dijon mustard
- 1 tbsp lemon juice
- 1 tsp honey

METHOD

Combine all ingredients in a small bowl and whisk with fork until well incorporated. Use within 1–3 days.

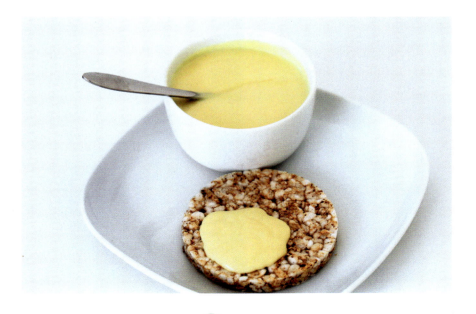

SAUCES, DRESSINGS AND CONDIMENTS

Easy and Tasty Fiesta Sauce (V)

SERVINGS: 9 (1 TBSP)

MACRO BREAKDOWN
(per serve: 1 tbsp)

RECIPE HIGHLIGHTS

This dressing will add fibre to a meal, and with the addition of the avocado oil, it will also provide a good dose of healthy monounsaturated fats. It's perfect for combining with greens or root vegetables, as the fat will help absorb vital nutrients like Vitamin A and Vitamin E.

FAT: 2.5G

PROTEIN: 1.5G

CARBS: 1.5G

INGREDIENTS

- *equal parts hummus and salsa (e.g. ¼ cup of each)*
- *1 tbsp avocado oil*
- *Salt and pepper to taste*
- *½ tsp cayenne pepper, for spiciness (optional)*

METHOD

This is the easiest sauce to make in minutes right before a meal. This can be done with a wide variety of flavours of hummus and salsa. It goes great on burritos, on top of rice, and as a vegetable dip, too.

1. In a small bowl, mix together hummus and salsa.
2. Add the avocado oil, along with salt and pepper to taste.
3. For extra kick, add in some cayenne pepper.

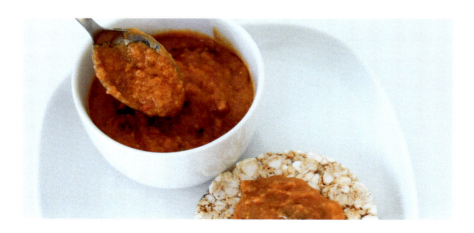

SAUCES, DRESSINGS AND CONDIMENTS

Better Balsamic Vinaigrette (V)

SERVINGS: ~11 (1 TBSP)

MACRO BREAKDOWN
(per serve: 1 tbsp)

FAT: 1.5G

PROTEIN: 1G

CARBS: 4G

RECIPE HIGHLIGHTS

Balsamic vinegar improves circulation and slows down digestion of a meal. Combine this with savoury seasonings and garlic and you get a vinaigrette with plenty of antioxidants and immune-boosting properties.

INGREDIENTS

- ¼ cup extra-virgin olive oil
- 1 tbsp Dijon mustard
- 2 garlic cloves, finely minced
- ¼ cup balsamic vinegar
- 1 tsp dried basil
- 1 tsp dried oregano
- Salt and pepper to taste

METHOD

Simply mix all ingredients together. Allow the garlic to marinate longer for extra flavour. Store in a dressing bottle for up to 2 weeks.

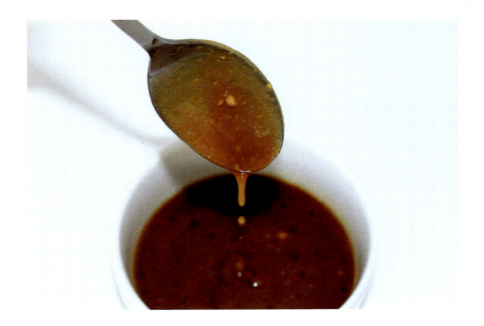

SAUCES, DRESSINGS AND CONDIMENTS

Creamy Almond Asian Dressing (V)

SERVINGS: ~12 (1 TBSP)

MACRO BREAKDOWN
(per serve: 1 tbsp)

FAT: 1G

PROTEIN: 0.5G

CARBS: 0.5G

RECIPE HIGHLIGHTS

Although this dressing is good all year round, the ginger and hot pepper oil is a great defence against a cold, as well as a natural remedy to reduce symptoms like congestion and a runny nose.

INGREDIENTS

- ⅓ cup water
- ¼ cup almond butter
- 1½ tablespoons soy sauce
- 1–2 tsp hot pepper oil (adjust based on preferred spiciness)
- 1 tablespoon rice vinegar
- 2 teaspoons maple syrup
- 1x 3 cm ginger root finely grated

METHOD

1. In a saucepan, combine all ingredients and cook over low heat.
2. Once simmering, cook for an additional 3–4 minutes.
3. Allow the mixture to cool. Serve immediately over grains, beans, vegetables, or fish.

This sauce can be stored in the fridge for 1–3 days. Before serving, add water and reheat to thin it out, as it will thicken.

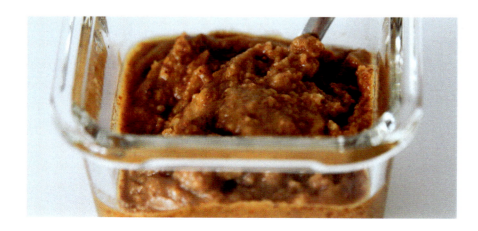

THE LEAN BODY SOLUTION

SAUCES, DRESSINGS AND CONDIMENTS

Sweet Pepper Relish (V)

SERVINGS: ~21 (1 TBSP)

MACRO BREAKDOWN
(per serve: 1 tbsp)

FAT: 0G

PROTEIN: 0G

CARBS: 1G

RECIPE HIGHLIGHTS

The capsicum adds a crisp peppery taste to the relish along with the jalapeño, which adds depth of flavour. The unfiltered apple cider vinegar balances the flavours and brings tanginess and acidity to the relish.

INGREDIENTS

- 1 cup finely diced capsicum (red, orange, or yellow)
- 1 jalapeño, finely diced
- 1½ tablespoons honey
- 3 tablespoons unfiltered apple cider vinegar
- Pinch of sea salt

METHOD

In a storage jar, combine all ingredients and allow them to marinate for at least 30 minutes before serving. The relish works well on sandwiches and burgers. It can also be pureed for more desirable consistency if required and will keep refrigerated for around one week.

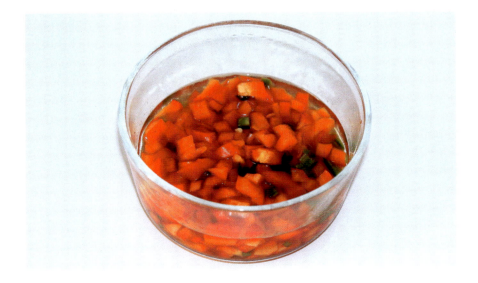

SAUCES, DRESSINGS AND CONDIMENTS

Classic Tzatziki Sauce

SERVINGS: ~23 (1 TBSP)

MACRO BREAKDOWN
(per serve: 1 tbsp)

RECIPE HIGHLIGHTS
Combining garlic with creamy yoghurt provides gut probiotics to support healthy digestion, as well as enhancing immunity.

FAT: 0.5G

PROTEIN: 3.7G

CARBS: 0.5G

INGREDIENTS
- 3 to 4 large garlic cloves, minced
- ¼ of a large cucumber, peeled, sliced, and diced
- 1 cup plain low-fat yoghurt
- 1 tbsp olive oil
- 2 tbsp fresh Italian parsley
- Sea salt to taste

METHOD
1. In a small bowl, combine all ingredients.
2. Chill for at least 30 minutes or overnight. The flavours will get more pronounced with more time.
3. Serve over Greek dishes or as a great vegetable dip. Store in the fridge for up to 1 week.

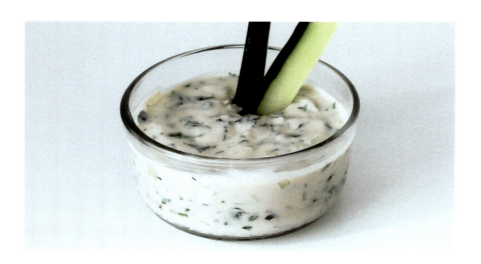

Creamy Ginger-Garlic Dressing (V)

SERVINGS: ~16 (1 TBSP)

MACRO BREAKDOWN
(per serve: 1 tbsp)

FAT: 1G

PROTEIN: 1G

CARBS: 0.5G

RECIPE HIGHLIGHTS

The tofu in this dressing provides iron, calcium, and other minerals. The tahini contributes creaminess and flavour to the dressing while also contributing a good amount of healthy fat. Ginger root has potential anti-inflammatory and digestive benefits, and it adds a zesty kick and a refreshing element to the dressing.

INGREDIENTS

- 100 g silken tofu
- ¼ cup water (more/less for texture)
- 1½ tbsp tahini
- 1½ tbsp lime juice
- 2 tsp soy sauce
- 1 tsp grated ginger root
- 2 cloves garlic minced

METHOD

1. Put all ingredients in a high-speed blender and puree until smooth. You can adjust water for a thicker or thinner dressing.
2. Store for 1–2 days in the refrigerator.

This delicious dressing is a perfect and healthy way to add extra protein to dishes, especially for vegans or vegetarians.

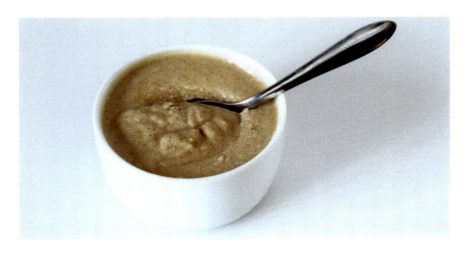

SAUCES, DRESSINGS AND CONDIMENTS

Ultimate Homemade Aioli Spread (V)

SERVINGS: ~17 (1 TBSP)

MACRO BREAKDOWN
(per serve: 1 tbsp)

FAT: 0G

PROTEIN: 1.5G

CARBS: 0.5G

RECIPE HIGHLIGHTS

This aioli spread is much lower in additives and preservatives compared to most aioli spreads on the market. It's also far more nutritious and the use of Greek yoghurt introduces more beneficial probiotics, calcium, vitamin B12, and other essential nutrients.

INGREDIENTS

- 1 cup fat-free, plain Greek yoghurt
- 2 small cloves garlic
- 1 tsp lemon juice
- ¾ tsp dried dill
- ¼ tsp sea salt
- Fresh ground black pepper to taste

METHOD

1. Place all ingredients in a blender or food processor and blend on low speed to start for 20–30 seconds.
2. To make thinner, add slightly more lemon juice. To thicken, add more yoghurt. The resulting mixture should be a thick and creamy, healthy mayo alternative.
3. Store in airtight container in the fridge for 4–5 days.

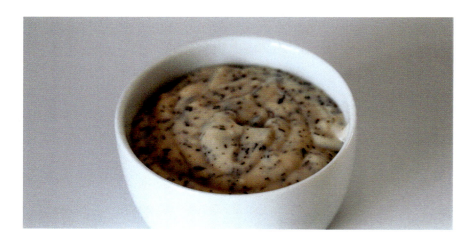

SAUCES, DRESSINGS AND CONDIMENTS

Green Chimichurri Savoury Sauce (V)

SERVINGS: 16 (¼ CUP)

MACRO BREAKDOWN
(per serve: ¼ cup)

RECIPE HIGHLIGHTS

This tasty savoury sauce is rich in vitamins A, C, and K (parsley and coriander). The garlic provides both pungent flavour and immune benefits, while the extra-virgin olive oil is a great source of monounsaturated fat.

FAT: 2G

PROTEIN: 0.5G

CARBS: 0.5G

INGREDIENTS

- 2 cups parsley
- 2 cups coriander
- 2 garlic cloves
- 2 tbsp lemon juice
- 4 tbsp extra-virgin olive oil
- ⅓ cup water
- 1 tsp sea salt
- ½ tsp black pepper
- ½ tsp red pepper

METHOD

1. In a food processor, put the garlic cloves in and blend until it is well diced.
2. Add the remaining ingredients and blend on high until the mixture is creamy.
3. Serve immediately or keep in an airtight container in the fridge for 4–5 days.

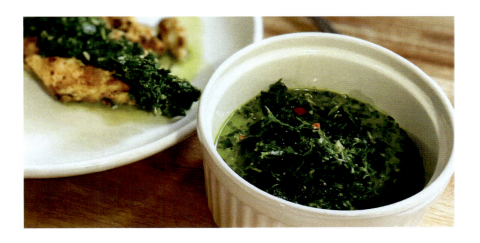

THE LEAN BODY SOLUTION

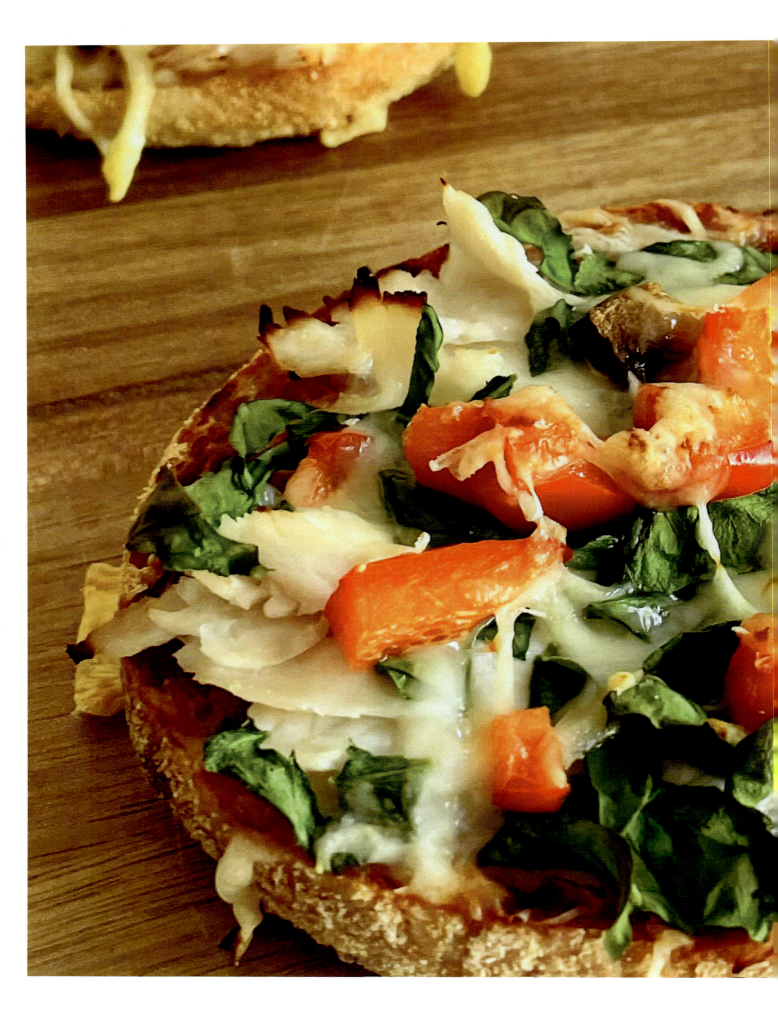

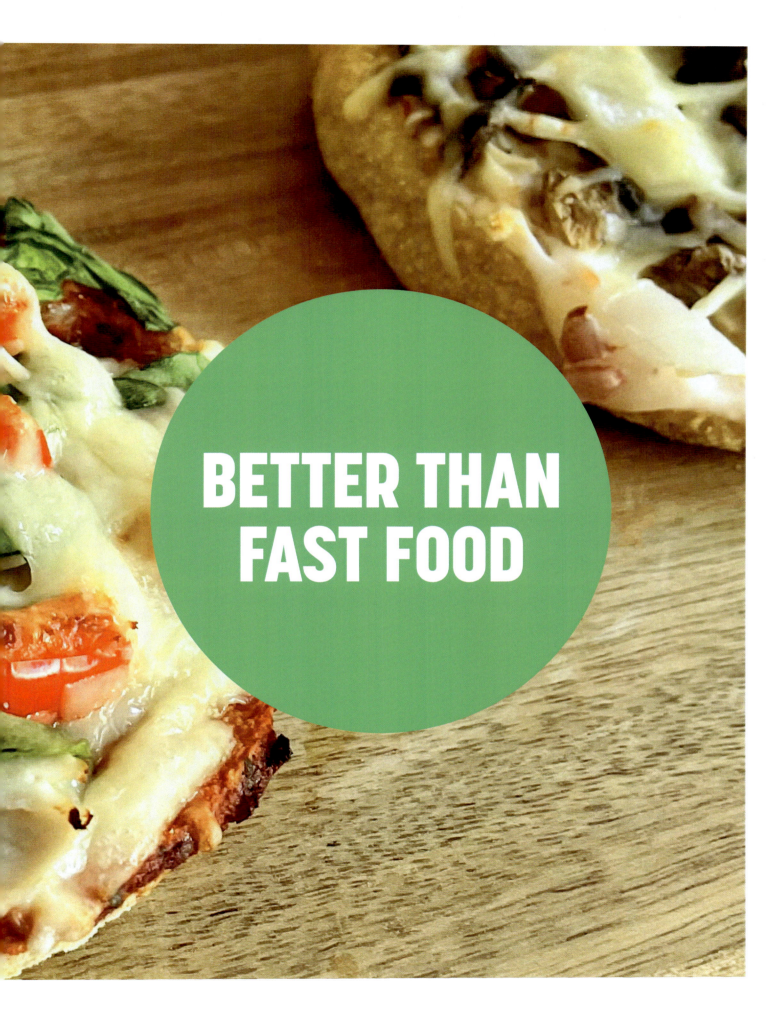

BETTER THAN FAST FOOD

"THE GREATEST VICTORY IS THAT WHICH REQUIRES NO BATTLE".
SUN TZU

In today's modern world, the temptation to indulge in innately bad food is a battle many face daily. Fast-food advertising is everywhere, and restaurants are abundantly placed in high-traffic areas. Add to this the meal delivery apps and speedy drive-thrus, and you can get any craving conveniently satisfied in minutes. What often starts out as an excuse after a long day or a lack of planning and prioritisation of one's meals soon becomes a convenient crutch that is relied upon.

However, convenience costs—especially when it comes to your body and your health.

Many people try to counter this battle and fight their cravings for fast food by looking over menu options and comparing 'Calories'. However, this is a battle one cannot ultimately win. Remember that crap food is still crap food, regardless of how many 'Calories' it contains. Put in other words: you cannot polish a turd. We're sorry, but fast-food and beverage companies do not have your health or body-composition goals at heart. Profits are the main concern, and they don't decide on healthier ingredients for some products and unhealthier ingredients for others—its either a little or a lot of the same unhealthy ingredients (usually the latter).

Hence, to wean a person off fast food, it's best not to win the battle, but instead not fight the battle at all.

The following ten pointers are included in all the recipes that follow, giving you insights for creating your own leaner and healthier versions of common fast foods. Deploy these tips whenever you have a fast-food craving and you will be surprised with how you can make it go away… along with the protruding waistline.

BETTER THAN FAST FOOD

10 Better Than Fast Food Pointers

1. CHOOSE QUALITY PROTEINS

Opt for higher-quality protein sources like beef, grilled chicken breast, turkey, and fish instead of processed meats.

2. USE LEANER COOKING METHODS

Explore cooking methods that require less oil, such as steaming, stir-frying, or sautéing with minimal oil, or using non-stick pans. This helps reduce the propensity to consume excess fat. You can also bake, grill, or air-fry foods instead of deep-frying them. This significantly reduces the amount of added fat while still maintaining the flavour and texture of the food.

3. SWAP BREADS AND GRAINS

Choose whole grain or protein-based alternatives wherever possible. Whole-wheat buns, wraps, breads, pitas, and tortillas can be used instead of processed white-flour alternatives. Protein and seed-based breads are also another good option and work well for foods like toasties. These alternatives can greatly enhance the nutrient quality and are also far more satiating.

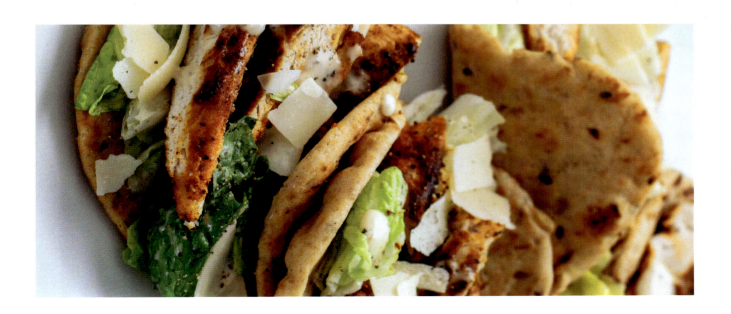

THE LEAN BODY SOLUTION

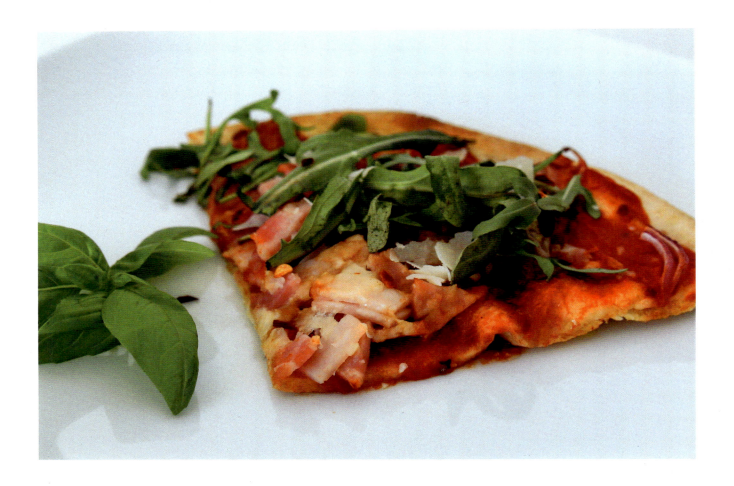

4. OPT FOR BETTER PORTION SIZES

Create smaller servings of foods like pizza, burgers, and toasties to better satisfy cravings without overindulging. Opting for smaller-sized and healthier versions like mini pizzas, sliders, and toasties using protein-based or wholewheat breads and tortillas can make a big difference to your waistline over time. The toppings and fillings can also be made with far leaner and tastier ingredients this way too.

5. INCREASE VEGETABLE CONTENT

Most fast foods are seriously lacking or even deplete of any vegetables. Making your own alternatives can enable you rectify this situation while also adding fresher and tastier ingredients. Lettuce, tomatoes, onions, peppers, pickles, cucumbers, and other nutritious toppings boost micronutrients, fibre, and flavour!

6. CREATE HEALTHIER SAUCES, DRESSINGS, AND CONDIMENTS

Prepare your own sauces, condiments, and dressings to control the ingredients and reduce added sugars, unhealthy fats, harmful additives, and preservatives. Relying on commonly used flavour enhancers such as homemade ketchup and salad dressings using fresh ingredients can really curtail your intake of unnecessary nutrients. See the 'Sauces, Dressings, and Condiments' section for better alternatives.

7. SUBSTITUTE SUGAR

Using natural sweeteners like stevia, monk fruit, xylitol, and erythritol to enhance flavour in place of sugar can make a profound difference to your waistline over time. Sugar is often hidden everywhere in today's foods (and beverages!). You will be amazed by how much excess body fat you can strip away by making this simple substitution wherever possible.

8. CONSIDER HEALTHIER SPREADS AND FILLINGS

Healthier alternatives have better nutritional value. For example, use Greek yoghurt instead of sour cream, avocado instead of processed cheese, or hummus instead of unhealthy mayonnaises.

9. CHOOSE OVEN-BAKED SIDES INSTEAD OF FRIED

Chicken nuggets can be replaced with baked chicken tenders, French fries can be easily swapped for baked protein wedges. These alternatives require less crumbed coatings and significantly reduce the amount of unwarranted fat.

10. DIY SHAKES AND SMOOTHIES

Skip the sugary milkshakes and smoothies and make your own leaner versions that actually include protein and nutritious ingredients.

These 10 pointers will enable you to get leaner and healthier by enabling you to better control your portions, employ smarter cooking techniques, and substitute with leaner and more nutritious ingredients. To help you kick the fast-food habit, here are some recipes to get you going.

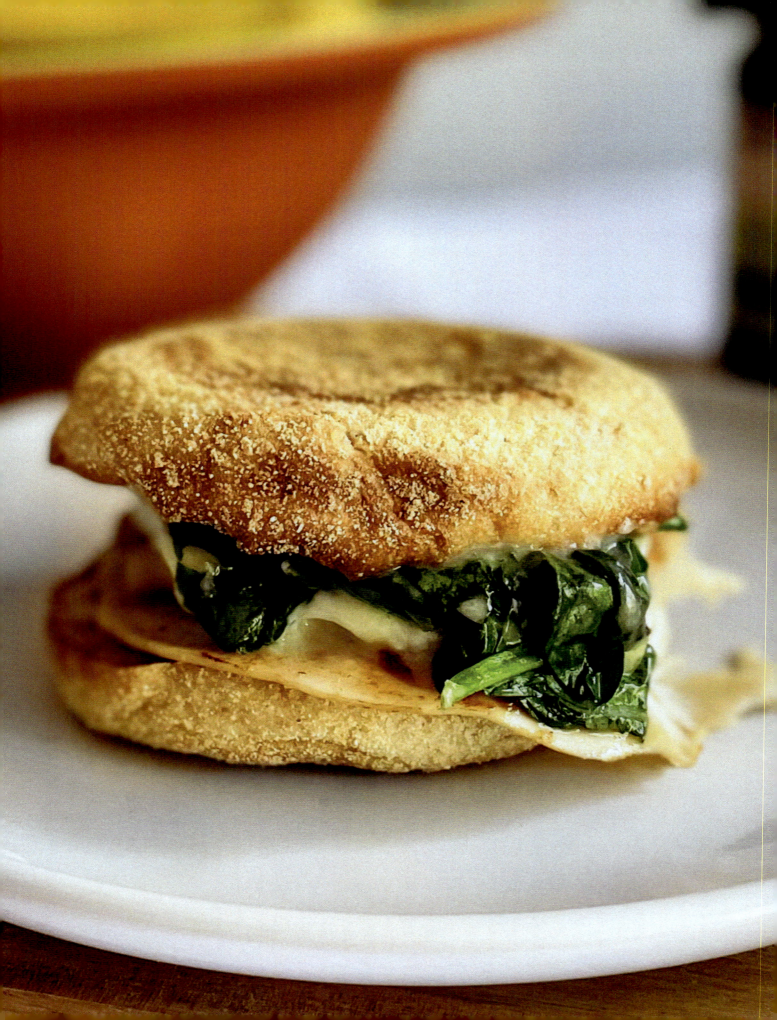

BETTER THAN FAST FOOD

Turkey and Egg White Protein Muffin

SERVINGS: 1

RECIPE HIGHLIGHTS

The combination of ingredients make this meal rich in Niacin (vitamin B3), magnesium, folate, vitamin A, and selenium. The wholemeal muffin offers more fibre and is far more filling than a typical white bread muffin.

MACRO BREAKDOWN (per serve)

FAT: 7G

PROTEIN: 31G

CARBS: 31G

INGREDIENTS

- *1 wholemeal English muffin, halved*
- *70 g egg whites (2 egg whites)*
- *50 g roast turkey breast*
- *½ cup baby spinach*
- *20 g low-fat, higher-protein cheese, grated*
- *2 tbsp onion relish*

METHOD

1. Heat a non-stick pan on high heat. Grease with cooking spray if required.
2. Fill an egg ring with egg whites on the heated pan.
3. When the egg is half cooked through, sprinkle it with cheese. Add spinach and turkey to the pan, and place the lid on to cook.
4. Meanwhile, toast an English muffin.
5. When egg white is cooked through, spinach is wilted, and turkey is slightly browned, removed from heat.
6. Spread onion relish on English muffin halves, then top with turkey, egg, and spinach.

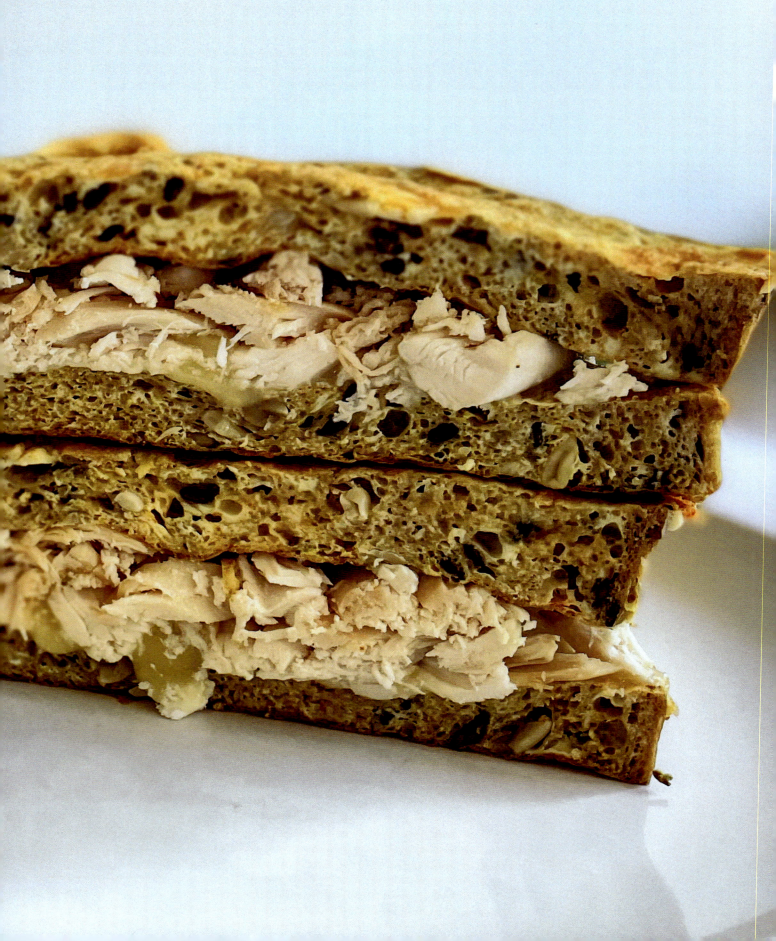

Chicken and Cheese French Toast Sandwich

SERVINGS: 1

MACRO BREAKDOWN (per serve)

FAT: 28G

PROTEIN: 64G

CARBS: 6G

RECIPE HIGHLIGHTS

If your diet calls for a filling, low-carb meal, this sandwich takes 5 minutes to make, and is packed with protein and fibre. The cheese also provides plenty of calcium to support bone health.

INGREDIENTS

- *2 slices of soy and linseed bread or similar wholegrain, higher-protein bread*
- *100 g egg whites*
- *40 g low-fat, higher-protein cheese*
- *80 g roast chicken breast*

METHOD

1. Whisk egg whites slightly, adding salt and pepper to taste.
2. Heat a sandwich press or pan over high heat; grease with cooking spray if required.
3. Soak bread in the egg white mixture, and then add to the press/pan.
4. Cook bread each side until slightly golden brown, then top 1 slice with chicken and cheese. Place the remaining bread slice on top.
5. Cook a further 1–2 minutes until cheese has melted.
6. Remove sandwich from press/pan and ENJOY!

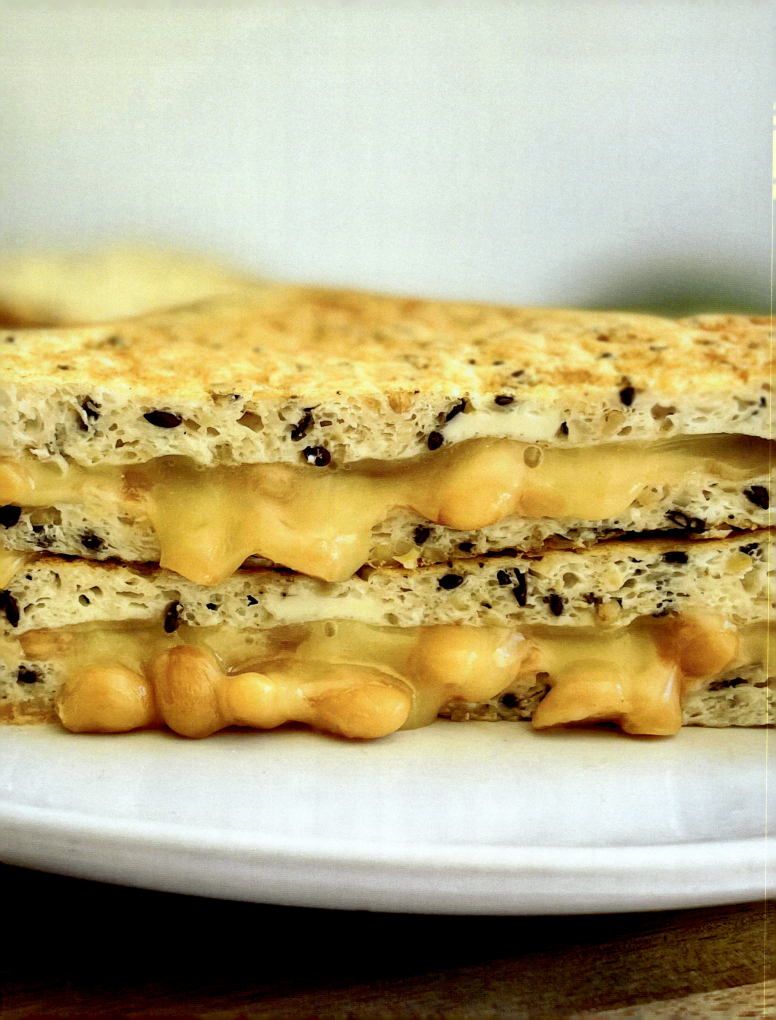

BETTER THAN FAST FOOD

Beans and Cheese French Toast Sandwich (V)

SERVINGS: 1

RECIPE HIGHLIGHTS

If you're looking for a hot sandwich that will keep you full for longer—this is the answer! It's high in protein and fibre, and it's a great nutritious alternative to typical baked beans on toast.

MACRO BREAKDOWN (per serve)

FAT: 12G

PROTEIN: 40G

CARBS: 28G

INGREDIENTS

- *2 slices of soy and linseed bread or similar wholegrain, higher-protein bread*
- *100 g egg whites*
- *40 g low-fat, higher-protein cheese*
- *100 g salt-reduced baked beans*
- *salt and pepper to season*

METHOD

1. Whisk egg whites slightly, adding salt and pepper to taste.
2. Heat a sandwich press or pan over high heat, and grease with cooking spray if required.
3. Soak bread in the egg white mixture, and then add to the press/pan.
4. Cook bread each side until slightly golden brown, then top 1 slice with beans and cheese. Place the remaining bread slice on top.
5. Cook a further 1–2 minutes until the cheese has melted.
6. Remove sandwich from press/pan and ENJOY!

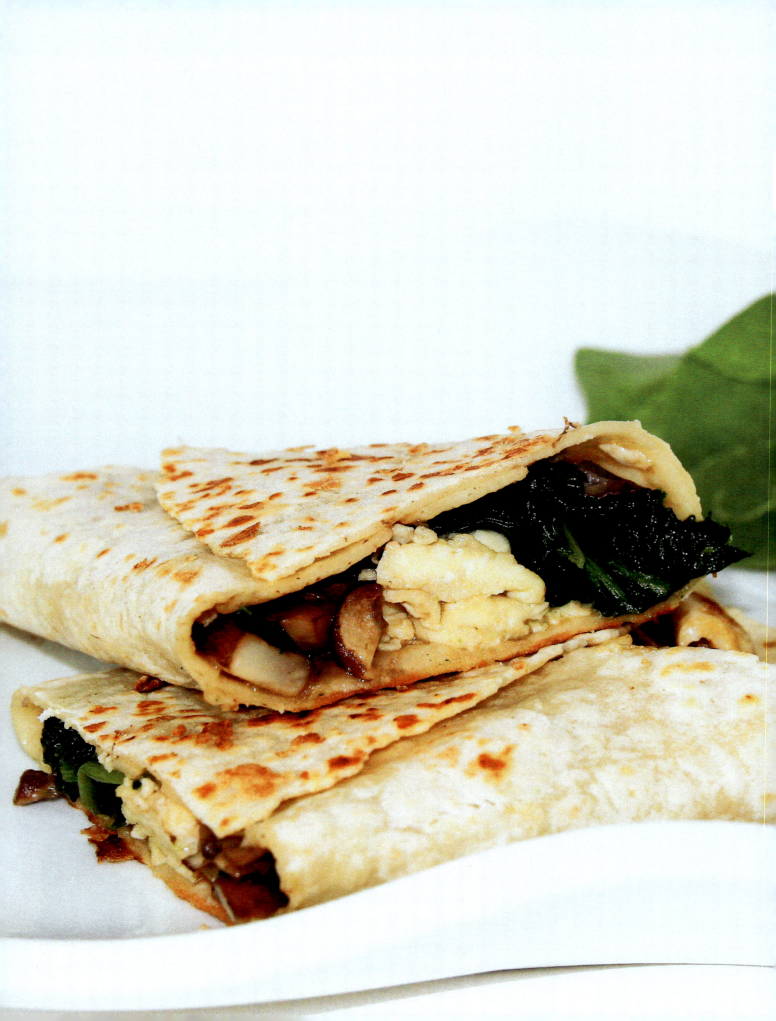

Protein-Packed Breakfast Wrap (V)

SERVINGS: 1

RECIPE HIGHLIGHTS

Egg yolks are one of the most nutrient-dense foods with multiple micronutrients such as vitamins A, B2, B12, D, and E, as well as minerals such as choline, selenium, iron, and iodine. Combine this with the high protein of egg whites and a protein wrap and you have a very nutritious breakfast.

MACRO BREAKDOWN (per serve)

FAT: 16G

PROTEIN: 24G

CARBS: 23G

INGREDIENTS

- 1 large high-protein wrap (~70 g wrap)
- 1 egg
- 2 egg whites (~70 g egg whites)
- 1 cup baby spinach
- 3 mushrooms (~60 g mushroom), sliced
- 1 tbsp sweet onion relish
- salt and pepper

METHOD

1. Preheat a sandwich press.
2. Spray a frying pan with cooking spray over medium-high heat.
3. Add sliced mushrooms and sauté for 3–4 minutes, or until mostly cooked though.
4. Add spinach to the pan and cook with mushrooms for a further minute, until spinach is wilted and mushrooms are cooked through.
5. Remove vegetables from the pan; set aside. Respray pan with cooking oil and return to the heat.
6. Whisk together egg and egg whites. Add to the pan, folding over a few times as the cook. When cooked to your desired consistency, remove from the heat.
7. Spread wrap with onion relish, then add the eggs and vegetables. Fold the wrap over the filling like a burrito, and then toast in the sandwich press for 1–2 minutes, until the wrap is cooked and crispy.
8. Remove from press and ENJOY.

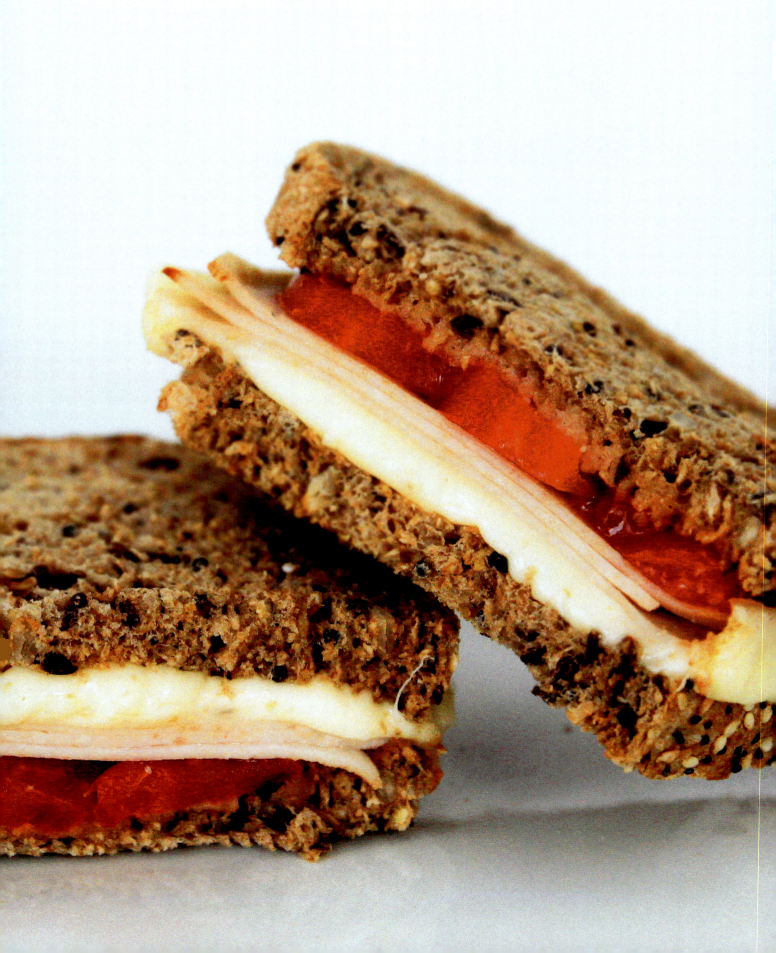

BETTER THAN FAST FOOD

Turkey, Tomato, and Cheese French Toast Sandwich

SERVINGS: 1

MACRO BREAKDOWN (per serve)

FAT: 23G

PROTEIN: 59G

CARBS: 7G

RECIPE HIGHLIGHTS

If you're struggling to meet your daily protein requirements, then this high-protein breakfast will put you on the front foot. It's low in carbs and has a good amount of fat so you can have sustained energy as you go about your day.

INGREDIENTS

- 100 g egg whites
- 70 g shaved turkey breast
- 1 medium tomato, sliced
- 40 g of 50% lower-fat cheese, sliced
- 2 slices of high-protein bread
- Salt and pepper

METHOD

1. Whisk egg whites slightly, adding salt and pepper to taste.
2. Heat a pan over high heat, and grease with cooking spray.
3. Soak bread in the egg white mixture; add to the pan.
4. Cook bread each side until slightly golden brown, then top 1 slice with cheese, tomato, and turkey. Place the remaining bread slice on top.
5. Cover pan, reduce to low heat and cook for a further 1–2 minutes.
6. Remove sandwich from the pan and ENJOY!

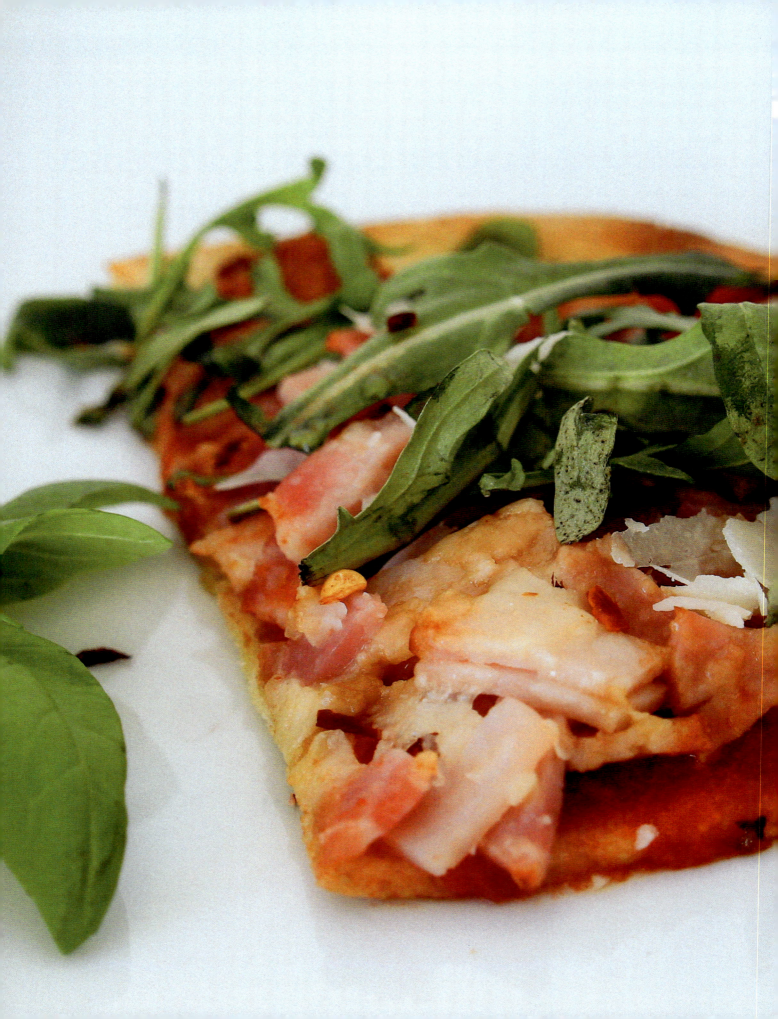

BETTER THAN FAST FOOD

Bacon, Parmesan & Basil Mini Pizzas

SERVINGS: 4 MINI PIZZAS

RECIPE HIGHLIGHTS

This recipe is a great way to enjoy pizza without the excessively high fat and carb content of typical varieties. The more fibrous base will also leave one feeling fuller for longer.

MACRO BREAKDOWN (per serve)

FAT: 21G		
PROTEIN: 26G		
CARBS: 48G		

INGREDIENTS

- ¼ red onion
- 200 g shortcut (back) bacon
- 100 g parmesan cheese
- 2 tbsp olive oil
- 5 tbsp pizza sauce
- 2 tbsp glaze vinegar
- 1 tsp chilli flakes
- 1 cup rocket (arugula) leaves
- 4 whole-wheat flatbread pitas

METHOD

1. Preheat oven to 200 °C.
2. Slice the onion and dice the bacon.
3. Place 4 large pitas on a flat oven sheet/s. Top your pitas with pizza sauce.
4. Top with chilli flakes, parmesan cheese, and diced shortcut (back) bacon, and olive oil.
5. Place the pitas in the oven for 10–15 minutes.
6. Check the pizzas to make sure the topping is cooked and edges of the pita are slightly browned (not burnt). Cooking times will vary based on ovens.
7. Once cooked to the desired texture, take out of the oven; top with rocket (arugula) and glaze vinegar. Serve immediately while hot. Each pita can be cut into 4 pizza-shaped slices.

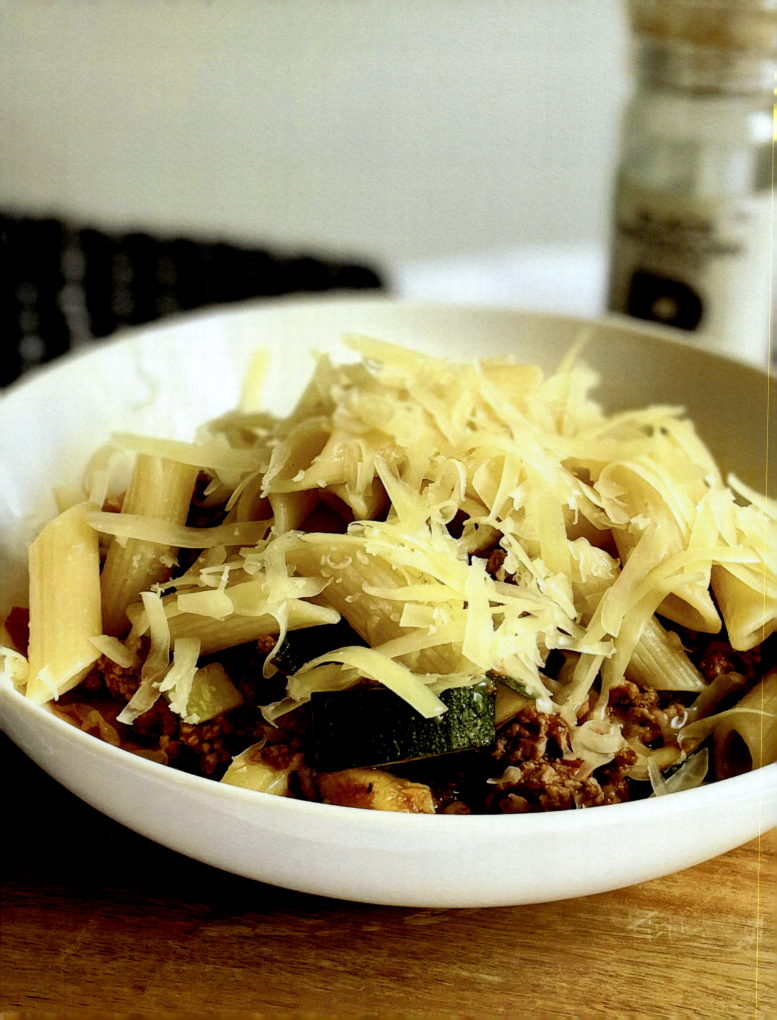

BETTER THAN FAST FOOD

Protein-Packed Pasta with Beef Bolognese

SERVINGS: 4

MACRO BREAKDOWN (per serve)

FAT: 13G

PROTEIN: 50G

CARBS: 30G

RECIPE HIGHLIGHTS

Regular pasta contains lots of bad carbohydrates and fat, and very little protein. On the other hand, this high-protein pasta provides a substantial amount of protein compared to regular pasta, to help promote satiety and lean mass. The inclusion of vegetables like zucchini and mushrooms also adds fibre, vitamins, and minerals to this dish.

INGREDIENTS

- 1 cup (~170 g) dry weight of high-protein pasta (we recommend: Vetta Smart Protein Penne)
- 1 tbsp extra-virgin olive oil
- 500 g extra-lean (95%) beef mince
- 1 large brown onion, diced
- 3 cloves garlic, crushed and chopped
- 1 large zucchini, diced
- 50 g mushrooms, chopped
- 1x 400 g canned crushed tomatoes
- ½ cup water
- 1 tbsp Italian mixed herbs
- salt and pepper
- 80 g low-fat, higher-protein cheese, grated (we recommend: Bega Light Tasty 50% Less Fat Cheese)

METHOD

1. Heat olive oil in a pan over high heat. On another hot plate, place a pot of water on high heat to bring to the boil.
2. In the pan, add onion and garlic and sauté until onion is translucent.
3. Add beef mince to the pan and stir well.
4. The pot of water should be boiling; add the pasta and cook for 10–12 minutes.
5. When the beef mince is browned and nearly cooked through, add remaining vegetables, canned tomatoes, herbs and salt and pepper to taste. Use ½ cup of water to rinse the tomato can and add to the Bolognese. Stir well to combine and cover with a lid. Reduce heat to medium. Leave to simmer, stirring occasionally.
6. When pasta is cooked, drain, and set aside.
7. The Bolognese sauce should also be ready at this stage; check that the meat is fully cooked and vegetables are cooked to your liking. Remove from the heat, and serve evenly into 4 bowls*, topping each with an even portion of pasta and sprinkling with grated cheese.

*For 4 serves, this will be approximately 85 g cooked weight of pasta, 360 g of Bolognese, and 20 g grated cheese.

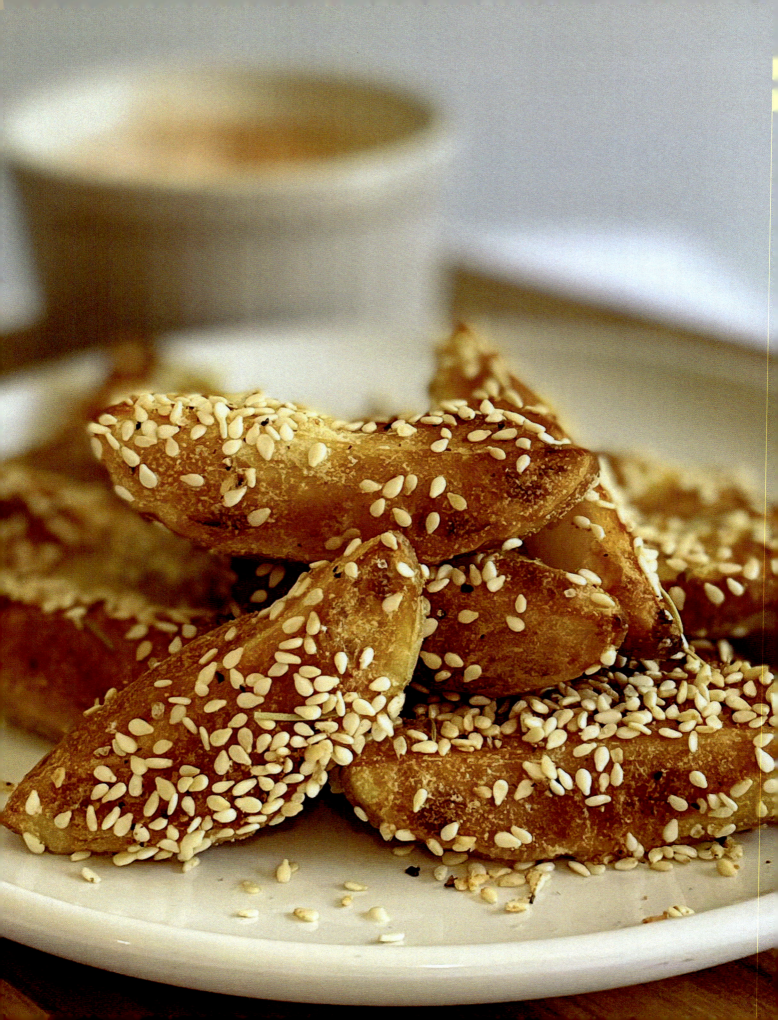

BETTER THAN FAST FOOD

Crispy Protein Wedges (V)

SERVINGS: 2

MACRO BREAKDOWN (per serve)

FAT: 5G

PROTEIN: 11G

CARBS: 23G

RECIPE HIGHLIGHTS

- These wedges provide a satisfying balance of macronutrients compared to typical take-out and fast-food alternatives.
- They include more protein, a reasonable carbohydrate content, and no unnecessary bad fats.
- The sesame seeds, garlic powder, and dried rosemary also give this recipe a salivating flavour.

INGREDIENTS

- *500 g Spud Lite baby potatoes, quartered and with skins intact*
- *100 g egg whites*
- *1 tsp garlic powder*
- *2 tbsp sesame seeds*
- *½ tsp salt*
- *½ tsp pepper*
- *1 tbsp dried rosemary*

METHOD

1. If baking in an oven, preheat to 230 °C.
2. Quarter potatoes into wedges and set aside.
3. In a bowl, add egg whites and beat until foamy.
4. In a separate bowl, combine herbs, spices, salt, pepper, and sesame seeds.
5. Coat each potato wedge in egg white and place on a lined baking tray, or in a greased air fryer basket, skin side down.
6. Once all potatoes are coated, sprinkle heavily with the seasoning mix.
7. Bake for 30 minutes at 230 °C, until potatoes are cooked through and crispy.
8. Serve immediately.

*Pairs well with homemade high-protein sweet chilli mayo. Combine ¼ cup high-protein Greek yoghurt with 2 tbsp sweet chilli sauce.

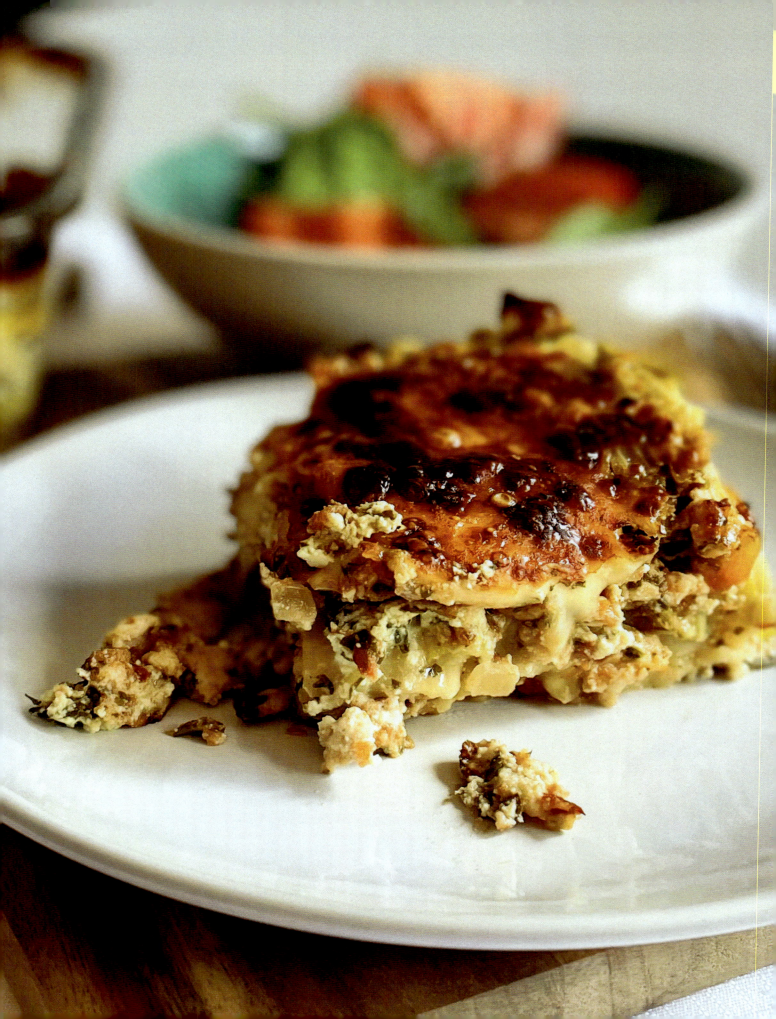

BETTER THAN FAST FOOD

Leaner Lasagne (V)

SERVINGS: 6

MACRO BREAKDOWN (per serve)

FAT: 7G

PROTEIN: 38G

CARBS: 22G

RECIPE HIGHLIGHTS

Traditional lasagnas are easy to overeat and contain a lot of simple carbs and unwarranted fat. This lean protein version will still fill you up without sacrificing the flavour.

INGREDIENTS

- 1 large brown onion, diced
- 3 cloves garlic, crushed and chopped
- 400 g lean turkey mince (98% fat-free)*
- 2 medium green zucchini's, sliced thinly length ways
- 100 g lasagne sheets
- 375 g reduced-fat ricotta cheese
- 1 cup baby spinach, chopped finely
- 100 g low-fat, higher-protein cheese, grated

*Vegetarians: substitute 200 g dry weight textured vegetable protein (TVP), rehydrated as per packet instructions.

Homemade Bolognese sauce
- 400 g tomato
- 2 cups baby spinach
- 4 cloves minced garlic
- 4 tbsp tomato paste
- 1 tbsp mixed Italian herbs
- Salt and pepper, to taste
- Mixed leaf garden salad, to serve

METHOD

1. Pre-heat oven to 200 °C.
2. Prepare your Bolognese sauce by adding all ingredients to a blender or food processor, and processing until well combined.
3. Grease a pan with cooking spray, and sauté garlic and onions over medium-high heat until golden brown. Add the turkey mince and cook through, then mix in the Bolognese sauce. Stir until well combined, then set aside.
4. In a separate bowl, mix the ricotta cheese and finely chopped spinach.
5. Spray a casserole dish with cooking spray and spread ¼ of the turkey sauce on the bottom of the casserole dish. Place ½ of the lasagne sheets evenly over the sauce. Lay ½ of the zucchini slices on top of the sheets. Spread ½ of the ricotta cheese/spinach mix on top of the zucchini and then spread ½ of the turkey mix over the ricotta. Repeat with another layer or lasagne sheets, zucchini, then ricotta, then the remaining ¼ of the turkey mince mixture on top. Sprinkle the low-free cheddar cheese evenly on top.
6. Cover with foil; place in the oven for 30 minutes. Remove the foil and bake for a further 30 minutes.
7. Allow to cool. Cut lasagne into 6 squares, and serve with a mixed-leaf garden salad.

THE LEAN BODY SOLUTION

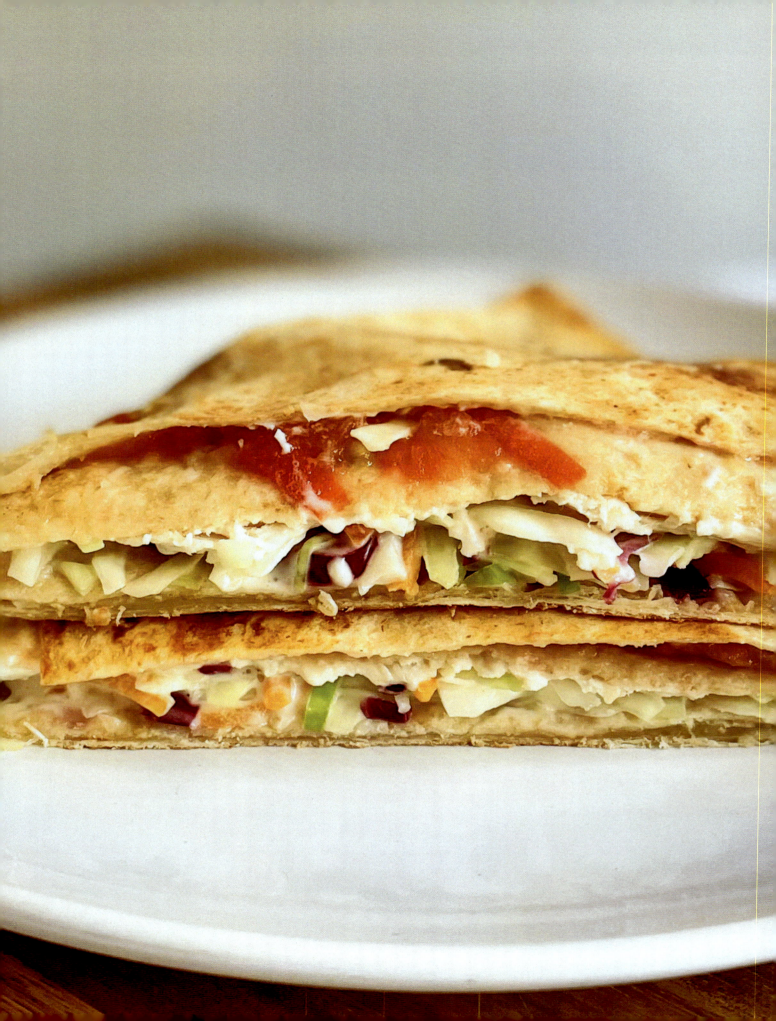

BETTER THAN FAST FOOD

Crunchy Chicken Salad Wrap

SERVINGS: 1

MACRO BREAKDOWN (per serve)

RECIPE HIGHLIGHTS

This high-protein wrap will hit the spot and leave you fuller for longer. It also makes great use of cabbage, which contains the naturally occurring antioxidants anthocyanins.

FAT: 8G

PROTEIN: 35G

CARBS: 22G

INGREDIENTS

- 1 large high-protein wrap (~70 g wrap)
- ¼ cup shredded cabbage or slaw mix
- 1 tbsp fat-free mayonnaise
- ½ medium tomato, sliced
- 80 g roast chicken breast, shredded
- 20 g low-fat cheese

METHOD

1. Preheat a sandwich press.
2. Combine cabbage/slaw in a bowl with mayonnaise.
3. Lay tortilla out on a cutting board. Use a knife to make a cut from the middle of the tortilla down to the edge.
4. Spread chicken, cabbage/slaw, tomato, and cheese each in a separate quarter of the wrap.
5. Fold the wrap up, starting from the bottom left quarter, folding it up over the top left, then folding it over to the top right, then folding it down to the bottom right.
6. Toast in the sandwich press for 1–2 mins, until golden brown and cheese is melted.

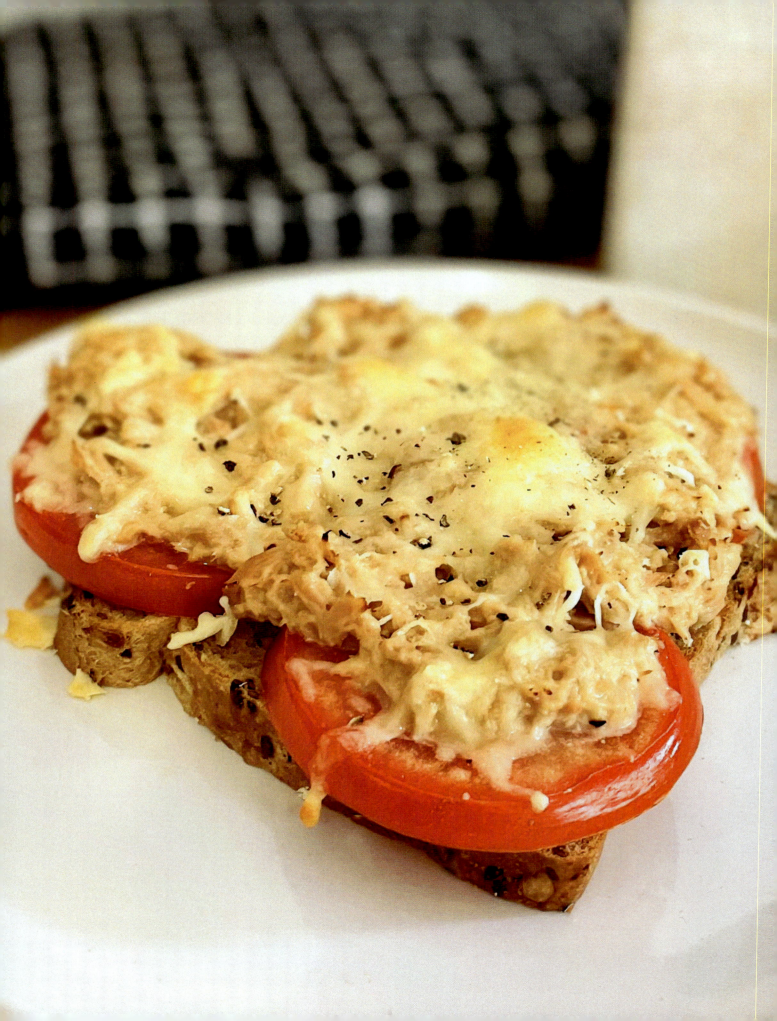

BETTER THAN FAST FOOD

Grilled Tuna Melts

SERVINGS: 1

RECIPE HIGHLIGHTS

Unlike conventional melts, this version is very lean. It's high in protein and low in carbs, and can be prepared in no time at all!

MACRO BREAKDOWN (per serve)

FAT: 10G

PROTEIN: 39G

CARBS: 11G

INGREDIENTS

- *1 slice high-protein bread*
- *1 can tuna in spring water*
- *1 tbsp fat-free mayonnaise*
- *1 tsp Worcestershire sauce*
- *1 tomato, sliced*
- *20 g low-fat cheese, grated*

METHOD

1. Preheat the oven to 180 °C with the grill function on.
2. Combine tuna in a bowl with the mayonnaise and Worcestershire sauce.
3. Place bread on a baking tray, and top with sliced tomato, tuna, and grated cheese.
4. Toast under the grill for 3–4 minutes until the cheese is melted and golden brown.

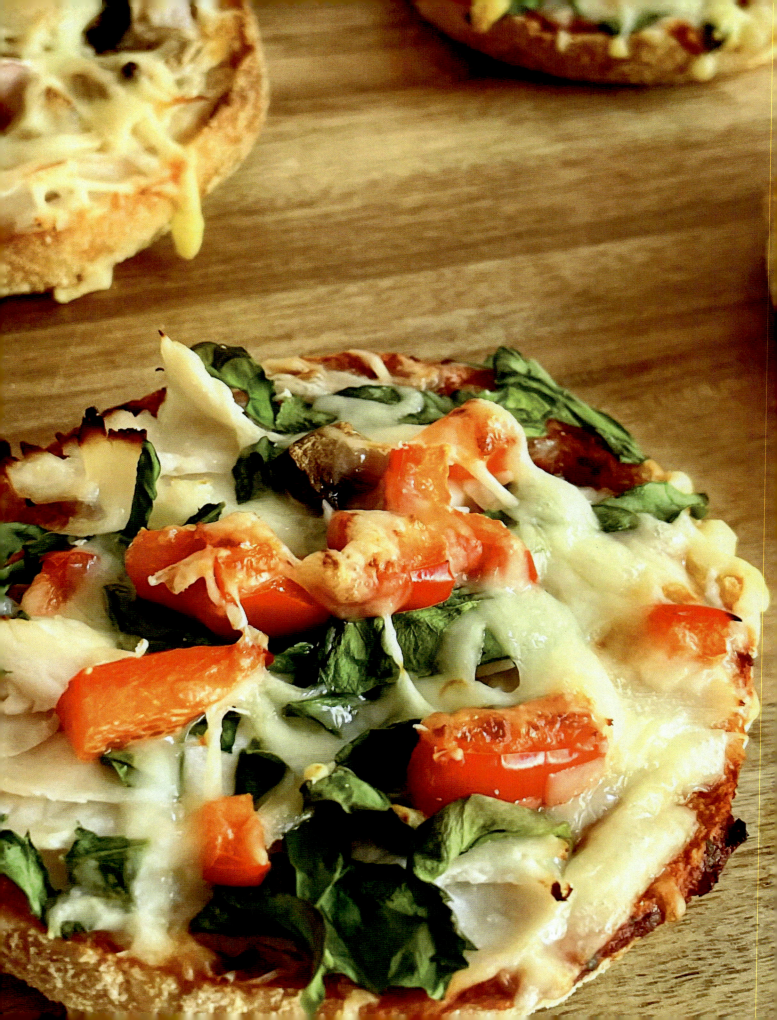

BETTER THAN FAST FOOD

English Muffin Mini Pizzas

SERVINGS: 1

RECIPE HIGHLIGHTS

These pizzas are higher in protein and veggies than most. They also pack more fibre and less cheese. Don't be fooled by the size; due to the ingredients used these pizzas are very satiating.

MACRO BREAKDOWN (per serve)

Chicken, red onion and mushroom with creamy base version	*Turkey, spinach and capsicum with tomato base version*
FAT: 6.5G	**FAT: 8G**
PROTEIN: 31G	**PROTEIN: 23G**
CARBS: 33G	**CARBS: 24G**

INGREDIENTS

Chicken, red onion and mushroom with creamy base version
- 1 wholemeal English muffin, halved
- 2 tbsp high-protein Greek yoghurt
- 1 tbsp sweet chilli sauce
- 50 g chicken breast, shredded
- 2 tbsp red onion, diced
- 2 tbsp mushroom, diced
- 20 g low-fat, higher-protein cheese, grated

Turkey, spinach and capsicum with tomato base version
- 1 wholemeal English muffin, halved
- 2 tbsp tomato paste
- 50 g shaved turkey breast, shredded
- 2 tbsp baby spinach, chopped
- 2 tbsp red capsicum, diced
- 20 g low-fat, higher-protein cheese, grated

METHOD

Chicken, red onion and mushroom with creamy base version

1. Preheat the oven to 150 °C, with the grill setting on.
2. Prepare topping ingredients.
3. In a small bowl, mix together yoghurt and sweet chilli sauce, then spread on the English muffin slices.
4. Top with chicken, mushroom, red onion, and cheese.
5. Place pizza muffins on an oven tray lined with baking paper. Cook under the grill for 5 minutes, or until the cheese is melted and the muffin is toasted.

Turkey, spinach and capsicum with tomato base version

6. Preheat the oven to 150 °C, with the grill setting on.
7. Prepare topping ingredients.
8. Spread tomato paste evenly on the English muffin slices. Top with turkey, spinach, red capsicum and cheese.
9. Place pizza muffins on an oven tray lined with baking paper. Cook under the grill for 5 minutes, or until the cheese is melted and the muffin is toasted.

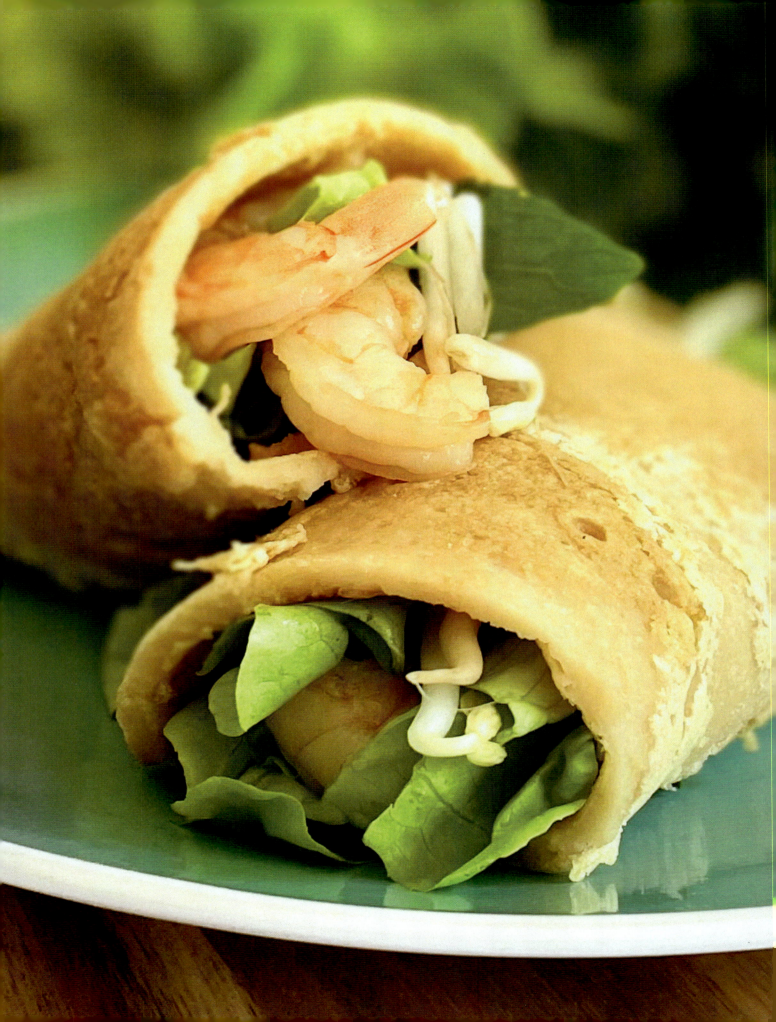

BETTER THAN FAST FOOD

Vietnamese Prawn Salad Red Lentil Wrap

SERVINGS: 6

MACRO BREAKDOWN (per wrap)

FAT: 3G

PROTEIN: 27G

CARBS: 23G

RECIPE HIGHLIGHTS

These deliciously fresh, protein-packed wraps are very easy to make! The use of red lentil wraps results in more fibre and better nutritional quality. The prawns add an array of nutrients crucial for thyroid health, including iodine, selenium, and zinc.

INGREDIENTS

For wraps
- 200 g red lentils, soaked overnight and rinsed well
- 2 cups water

For filling
- 480 g prawns
- Mint
- Bean shoots
- Butter lettuce

For Vietnamese style dressing
- 1 tbsp fish sauce
- ¼ cup rice vinegar
- 1 tbsp honey
- 1 tsp garlic
- 1 tbsp lime juice
- 1 tsp chopped chilli (optional)

METHOD

1. Soak red lentils overnight and then rinse them well.
2. Prepare dressing by combining all ingredients.
3. Blend the lentils and water in a blender or food processor until smooth. It should have a pancake batter consistency. Add a bit more water if needed.
4. Lightly grease a frying pan with cooking spray and heat over high heat. Pour some batter into the pan as you would a crepe. Fry the lentil wraps for a couple of minutes and flip once bubbles form and the wrap is coming up slightly at the side. Fry for another couple of minutes or until appropriately cooked through. Make a total of 6 wraps.
5. Top wrap with lettuce, mint, bean shoots, prawns, and drizzle with your dressing. Serve immediately.

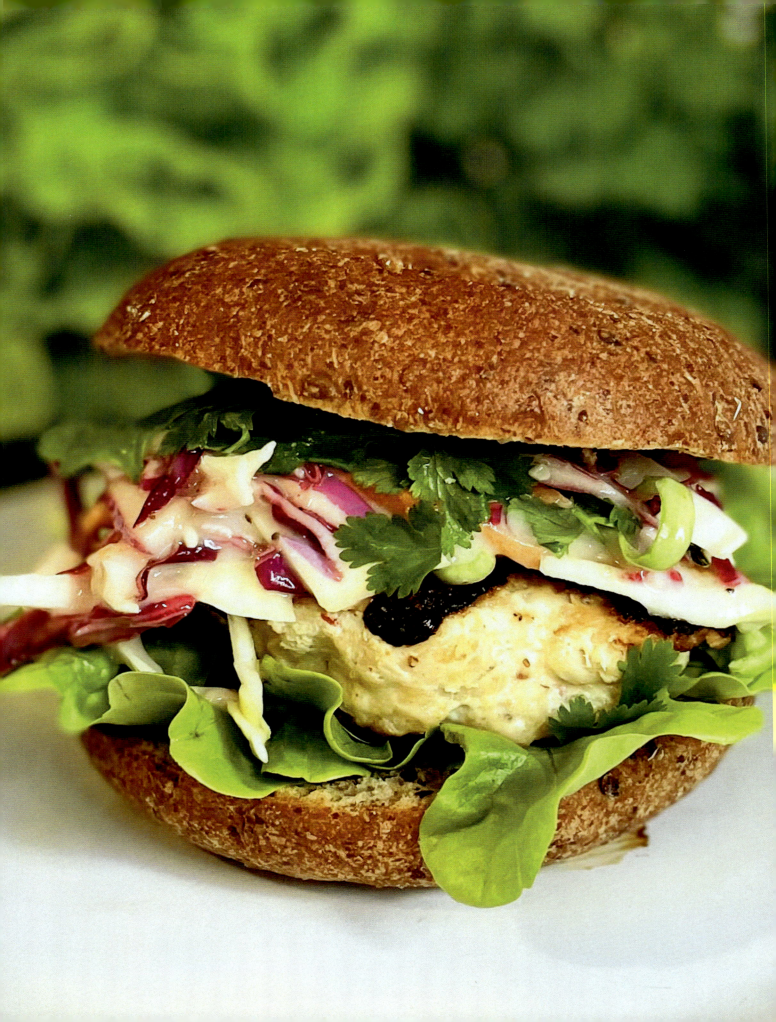

Sweet Chilli Chicken Burgers with Lime-Pepper Slaw

SERVINGS: 6

RECIPE HIGHLIGHTS

By incorporating lean chicken mince as well as a protein burger bun, this chicken burger comes with twice as much protein than typical alternatives. The fresh vegetables and whole food ingredients also offer more fibre and essential nutrients, while still delivering on flavour.

MACRO BREAKDOWN (per burger)

FAT: 10G

PROTEIN: 42G

CARBS: 22G

INGREDIENTS

For patties (makes 6)
- 500 g chicken mince
- 1 onion, diced
- 1 egg
- 1 tsp ground chilli
- 2 tbsp sweet chilli sauce
- 2 tbsp breadcrumbs
- salt/pepper to taste

For lime-pepper slaw (makes 6)
- ½ cup low-fat mayo
- Juice of 1 lime
- Pepper
- 2 cups shredded cabbage and carrot

For the burger (makes 1)
- Protein burger bun
- Butter lettuce
- Coriander

METHOD

1. Place all burger patty ingredients together in a large bowl; mix together well.
2. Heat a large frying pan over high heat, and spray lightly with cooking oil.
3. Split patty mixture into 6 equal portions and roll into balls. When the frying pan is hot, place patties in the pan and flatten into a burger patty shape (you may need to cook 2 batches of 3 if they do not all fit in the pan at once).
4. Cook for 8 minutes each side, or until cooked through.
5. Arrange your burger by slicing the burger bun in half and placing on the lettuce, then a burger patty, then ~1/3 cup of the slaw. Sprinkle some coriander on top, then top with the other half of the bun.

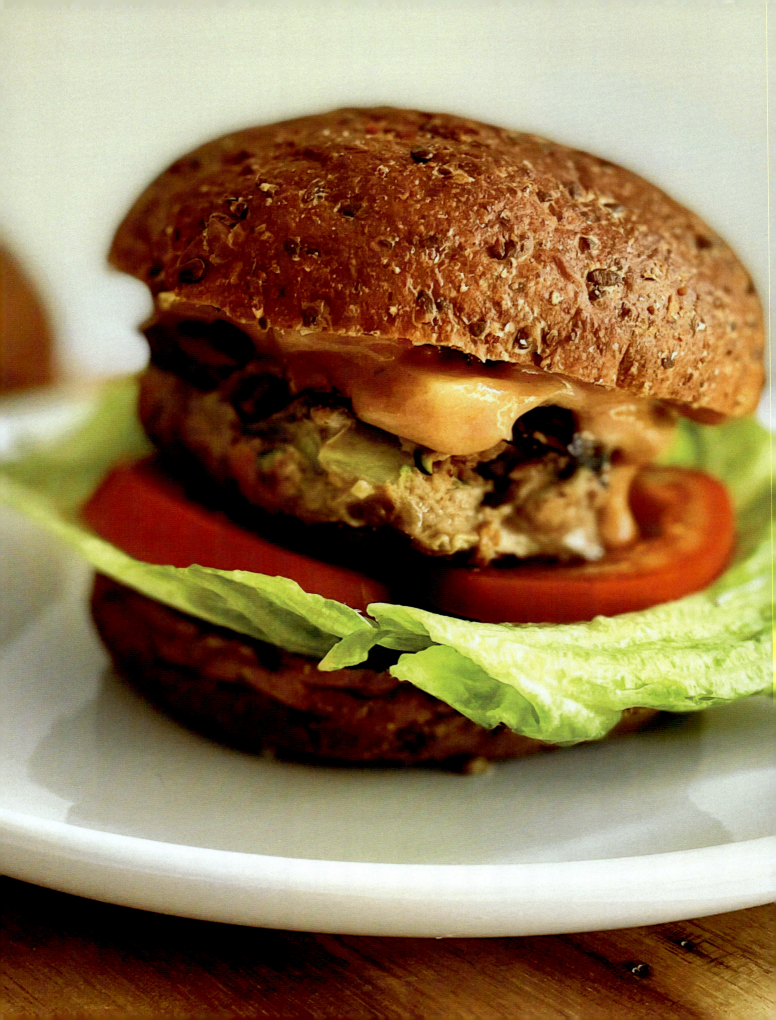

BETTER THAN FAST FOOD

Lean Beef Burgers

SERVINGS: 1

MACRO BREAKDOWN (per burger)

FAT: 13G

PROTEIN: 39G

CARBS: 15G

RECIPE HIGHLIGHTS

These deliciously juicy beef burgers take only 5 minutes to make, and boast a serve of veggies within each patty. There is no excess carbohydrate and fat included, and the high-protein bun makes meeting daily protein requirements a hell of a lot easier.

INGREDIENTS

For patties (makes 8–10)
- 500 g lean beef mince
- 2 eggs
- 1 onion, diced
- 1 carrot, grated
- 1 zucchini, grated
- 1 tbsp minced garlic
- 3 tbsp breadcrumbs
- 1 tbsp Mexican seasoning
- salt and pepper

For the burger (makes 1)
- 1 beef patty
- 1 protein burger bun
- 1 large lettuce leaf
- 2–3 tomato slices
- 15 g low-fat, higher-protein cheese
- 2 tbsp homemade burger sauce

For the sauce (makes 16 serves)
- ½ cup low-fat mayonnaise
- ¼ cup tomato paste
- ¼ cup mustard
- ¼ teaspoon minced garlic
- ⅛ teaspoon white vinegar
- pepper to taste
- hot sauce to taste (optional)

METHOD

1. Place all burger patty ingredients together in a large bowl; mix together well.
2. Heat a large frying pan over high heat, and spray lightly with cooking oil.
3. Split patty mixture into 8 equal portions and roll into balls. When the frying pan is hot, place patties in the pan and flatten into a burger patty shape (you may need to cook 2 batches of 4–5 if they do not all fit in the pan at once).
4. Cook for 6–8 minutes each side, or until cooked through.
5. Arrange your burger by slicing the burger bun in half and placing on the lettuce, then tomato, then a burger patty. Place a slice of cheese on top of the patty, and spread the sauce onto the remaining burger bun half before placing that on top.

THE LEAN BODY SOLUTION

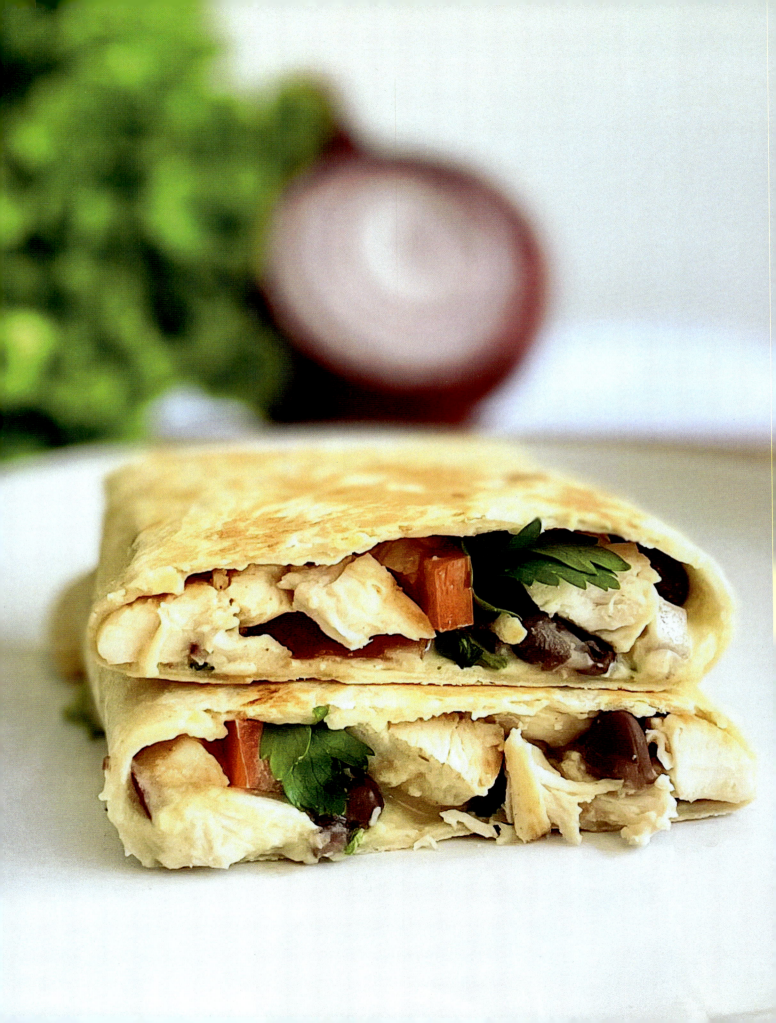

BETTER THAN FAST FOOD

Lean Chicken Salsa Wrap

SERVINGS: 1

RECIPE HIGHLIGHTS

These lean chicken wraps are packed full of nutrient rich vegetables and flavours. They also provide lots of protein in the form of chicken, cheese, black beans, and a high-protein wrap.

MACRO BREAKDOWN (per serve)

FAT: 9G

PROTEIN: 31G

CARBS: 16G

INGREDIENTS

- *High-protein tortilla (we used Simson's pantry low-carb, high-protein wrap)*
- *60 g chicken breast, grilled*
- *¼ cup lettuce, shredded*
- *25 g black beans*
- *25 g tomato, diced*
- *10 g red onion, diced*
- *Parsley*
- *10 g low-fat, high-protein cheese, shredded*

For the sauce
- *1 tbsp low-fat mayonnaise*
- *1 tsp lemon juice*
- *1 tsp Dijon mustard*
- *½ tsp minced garlic*

METHOD

1. Heat a pan and spray lightly with cooking oil.
2. Trim a chicken breast of fat and slice into strips. Add to the heated pan and grill chicken breast strips for 4–5 minutes each side, or until chicken is cooked. Cut the grilled chicken into pieces and place 60 g onto tortilla.
3. Top with tomatoes, red onion, beans, lettuce, and parsley.
4. In a small bowl, whisk together the sauce ingredients.
5. Drizzle the sauce over the tortilla fillings and grate cheese over the top.
6. Wrap the tortilla tightly, then place in a preheated sandwich press. Toast for 2–3 minutes, or until cheese is melted and the wrap is golden brown and crunchy. Serve immediately.

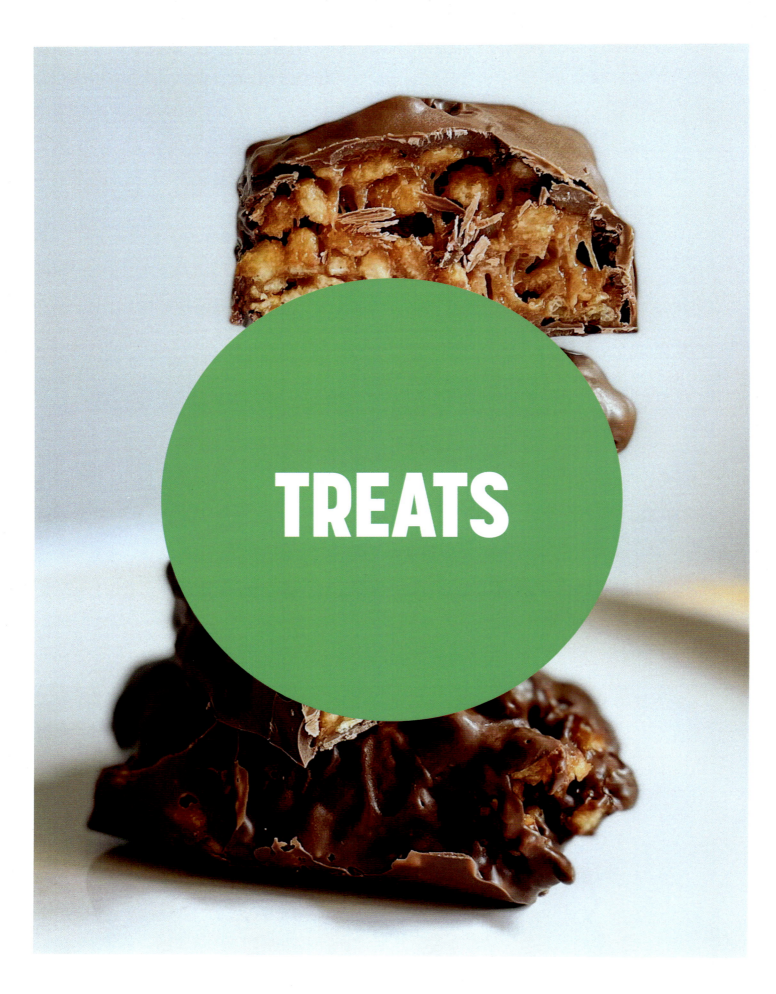

"TREAT YOURSELF AS YOU SHOULD".
ANONYMOUS

The word 'treat' as it relates to food originated from the Middle-English word 'tret' or 'tretes', which meant a small portion or reward given to someone. Many people innately know what treats are, but many have made these types of foods staples in their day to day eating. Apart from the overconsumption of pleasure foods, another problem is that many people don't treat themselves right by having silly treats.

What do we mean here? Most people choose the worst possible foods to treat themselves with when these could often be replaced with healthier, leaner, and just as tasty options. Ones that don't easily derail their progress or blow out their waistline. If you do treats right, you can also afford to have them more often. In the following section, we have included some treats for the time you may encounter the occasional sweet tooth. As a disclaimer, be warned that these are VERY delicious!

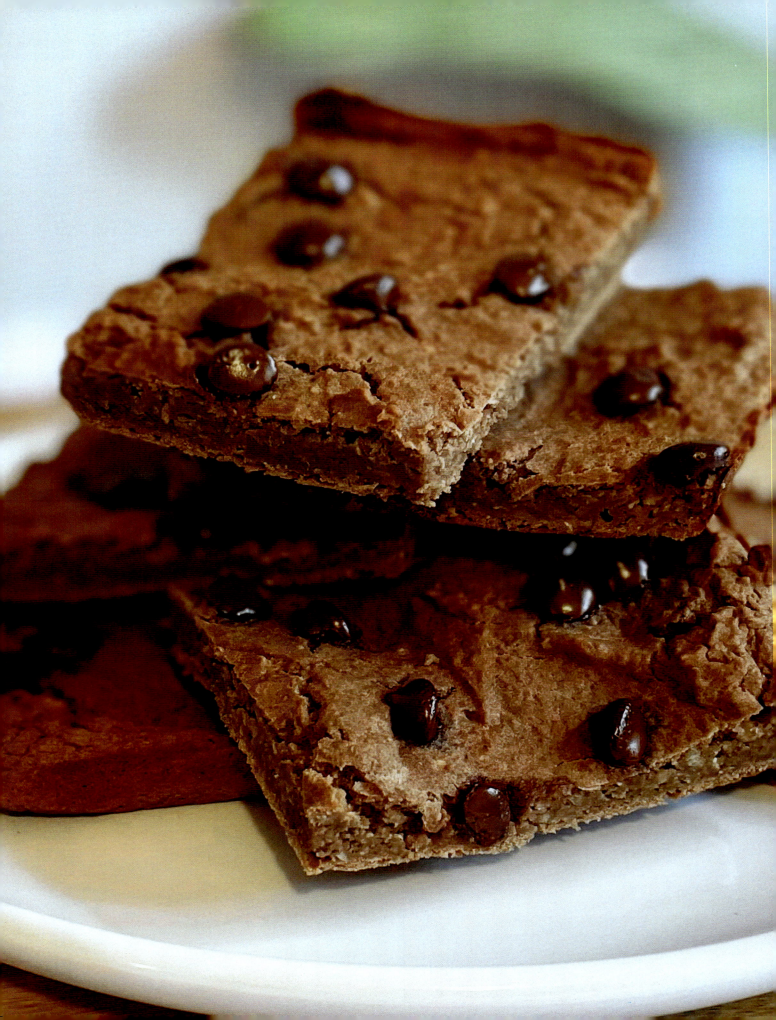

TREATS

Choc Mint Brownie Bars (V)

SERVINGS: 8 BARS

MACRO BREAKDOWN (per bar)

FAT: 2G

PROTEIN: 7G

CARBS: 7G

RECIPE HIGHLIGHTS

Perfect for a quick snack or heated up for breakfast/dessert with yoghurt and berries, these protein brownies made with chickpeas are a great source of manganese, which supports gut health, bone formation, healthy connective tissues, and recovery from injury.

INGREDIENTS

- 375 g can chickpeas, drained and rinsed
- 2 scoops (50 g) chocolate protein powder
- ¼ tsp sea salt
- ½ tsp baking powder
- ¼ cup egg whites
- ¼ cup sugar-free syrup (naturally sweetened)
- ½ tsp peppermint essence
- 2 tbsp sugar-free choc chips (naturally sweetened)

METHOD

1. Preheat oven to 180 °C and lightly grease a 9x18-inch baking dish with cooking spray.
2. In a food processor, blend together all ingredients, except the chocolate chips.
3. Fold brownie batter into the baking dish, and sprinkle with choc chips.
4. Bake for 12–15 minutes, or until a skewer comes out clean.
5. Allow to cool in the pan before removing and slicing into 8 bars.
6. Consume as is, or serve with high-protein yoghurt and berries. Store in an airtight container in a dry cool spot, or in the fridge.

THE LEAN BODY SOLUTION

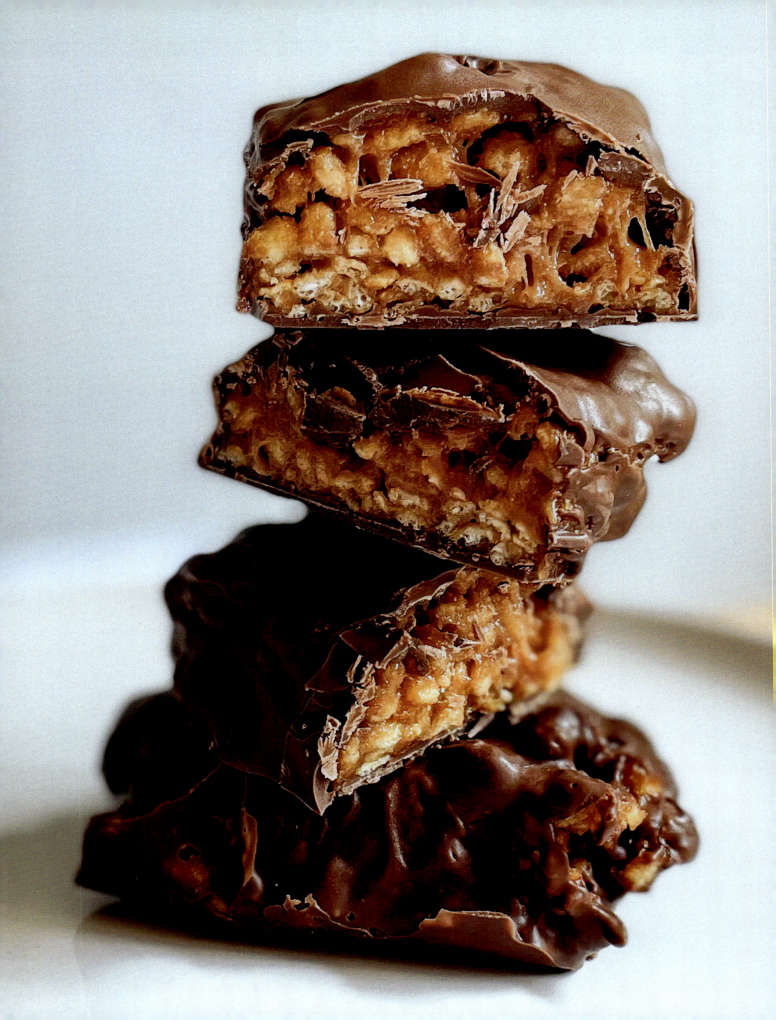

TREATS

Crunchy No-Bake Protein Bars (V)

SERVINGS: 20 BARS

MACRO BREAKDOWN (per bar)

FAT: 10G

PROTEIN: 8G

CARBS: 8.5G

RECIPE HIGHLIGHTS

Save the chocolate bar and opt for these instead. These protein bars have far less sugar, a decent amount of protein, and are filling enough to handle any sweet tooth. The best part is that they can be made in big batches without any baking.

INGREDIENTS

- 4 cups brown rice cereal
- 1 cup smooth natural peanut butter (any nut butter of choice works)
- 1 cup sugar-free maple syrup (preferably monk fruit sweetened)
- 2x 30 g scoops of protein powder of choice
- 2 cups stevia-sweetened chocolate chips

METHOD

1. Line an 8x8-inch pan or 8x10-inch pan with baking paper.
2. In a mixing bowl, mix the nut butter with the maple syrup and until well combined. Add the protein powder and mix well, then the rice cereal, ensuring everything is fully incorporated.
3. Transfer the mixture to the lined pan and press firmly in place. Refrigerate until firm.
4. Once firm, use a sharp (and slightly wet) knife to cut 20 bars.
5. Melt the chocolate chips in a microwave or on a stovetop; moving quickly, use two forks to dip and evenly coat each bar in the melted chocolate.
6. Repeat until all the bars are coated in chocolate. Refrigerate until firm.

THE LEAN BODY SOLUTION

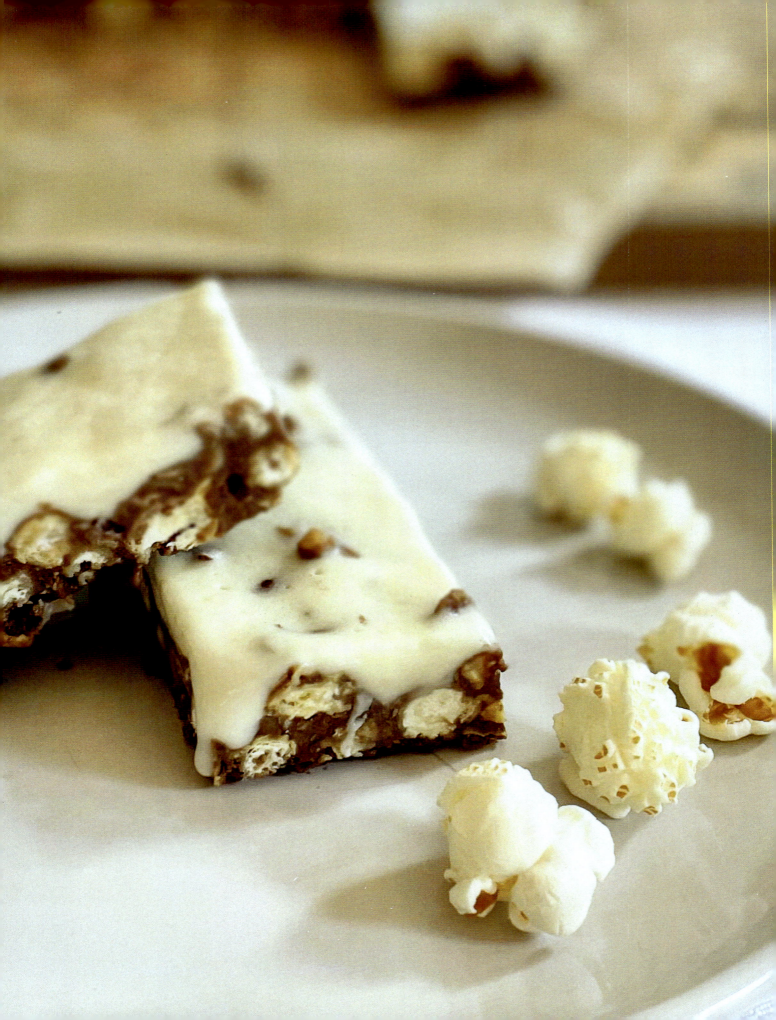

TREATS

Popcorn Protein Bars (V)

SERVINGS: 12 BARS

MACRO BREAKDOWN (per bar)

FAT: 6G

PROTEIN: 7G

CARBS: 6G

RECIPE HIGHLIGHTS

Popcorn is a great high-volume, lower-carb snack. It provides great bulk to this recipe, so you can feel fuller for longer. The popcorn flavour works amazingly well in these tasty protein bars—just be sure to use air popped popcorn without added oil/butter (either natural flavoured or lightly salted).

INGREDIENTS

- 3 tbsp coconut oil
- 2x ½ cup sugar-free maple syrup (naturally sweetened)
- 1 tbsp vanilla paste
- 100 g natural popcorn
- 1 scoop (~30 g) choc caramel protein powder
- 2 tbsp LSA
- ¼ cup unsweetened almond milk
- ½ cup low-fat, high-protein yoghurt
- 1 tbsp stevia
- 1 scoop (~30 g) vanilla protein powder

METHOD

1. To make a caramel sauce, heat a saucepan over high heat, then add coconut oil and maple syrup. Stir continuously to combine well and prevent the caramel from sticking.
2. When the sauce has thickened, remove from the heat, and stir in the vanilla paste.
3. Add the popcorn and stir to combine; ensure the caramel coats all the popcorn pieces.
4. Line a baking tray with baking paper. Spread the caramel covered popcorn into the tray.
5. In a blender or food processor, combine the remaining ingredients. Drizzle mixture evenly over the popcorn in the baking tray. Place in the freezer for 2 hours or until solid. Cut into 10 bars to serve.

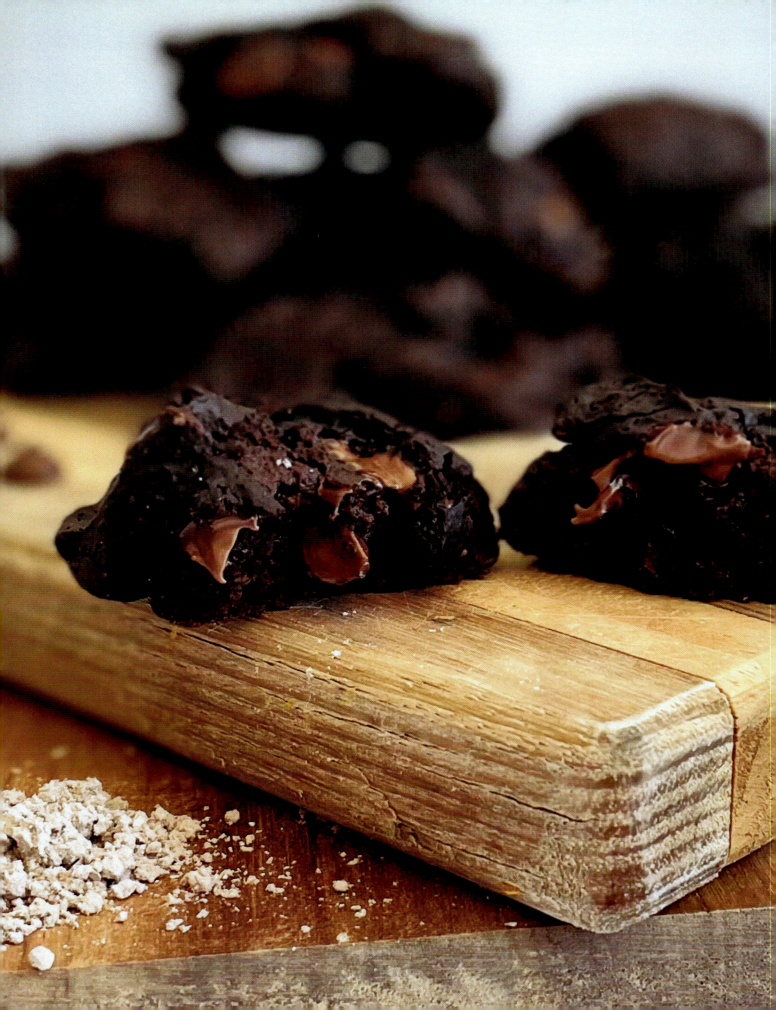

TREATS

Choc Chip Brownie Cookie Bites (V)

SERVINGS: 10 COOKIE BITES

RECIPE HIGHLIGHTS

A tasty, gooey treat that is almost completely sugar-free! Each brownie bite also has 5 g of protein! If you're craving a sweet chocolatey treat then go for these!

MACRO BREAKDOWN (per cookie bite)

FAT: 2G

PROTEIN: 5.5G

CARBS: 3G

INGREDIENTS

- *50 g (2 scoops) chocolate protein powder*
- *1 large egg*
- *2 tbsp stevia*
- *¼ cup cocoa powder*
- *1 tsp baking soda*
- *2 tbsp spelt flour*
- *1 large egg*
- *2 tbsp unsweetened almond milk*
- *1 tsp vanilla essence*
- *2 tbsp mini sugar-free chocolate chips (naturally sweetened)*

METHOD

1. Preheat oven to 160 °C.
2. Combine dry ingredients in one bowl and wet ingredients in another bowl.
3. Make a well in the dry ingredients and add wet ingredients, stirring well to combine. Add extra almond milk as needed to reach desired consistency.
4. Add chocolate chips and stir evenly through the mixture.
5. Spoon out mixture into 10* rough balls on a paper lined tray.
6. Bake for 6–8 mins; until cooked but still soft and gooey.
7. Leave cookie bites to cool on the pan, then ENJOY.

*Alternatively, you can make 4–5 larger cookies as desired.

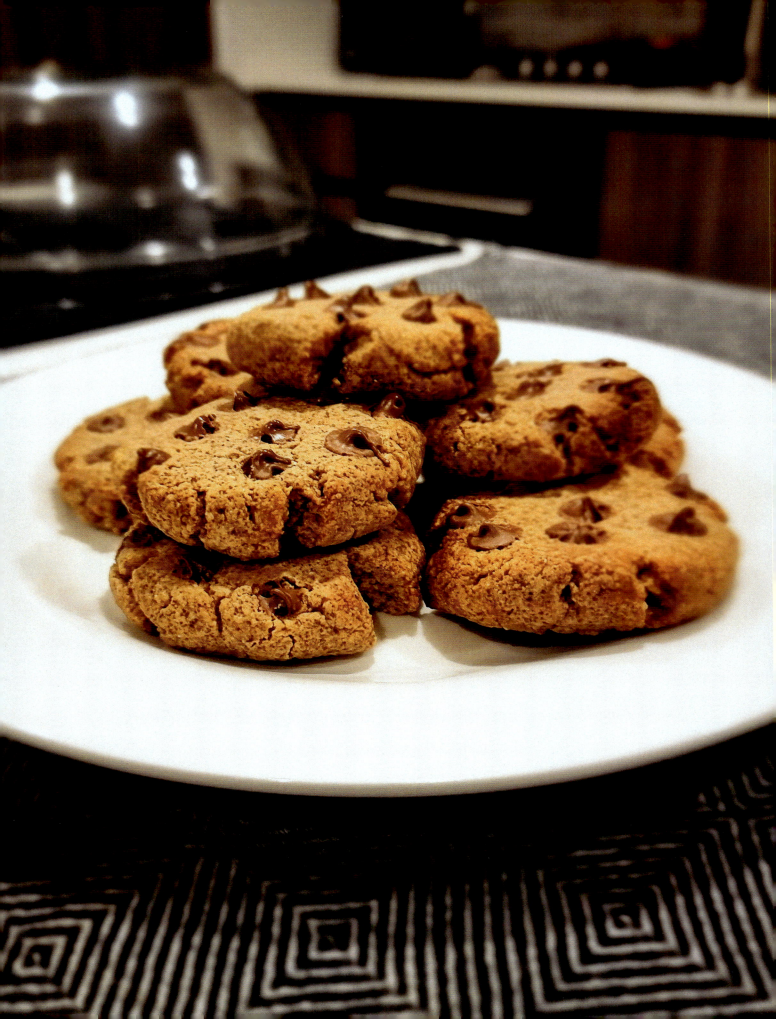

TREATS

Sugar-Free Protein Cookies (V)

SERVINGS: 12 COOKIES

MACRO BREAKDOWN (per cookie)

FAT: 12G

PROTEIN: 8G

CARBS: 3G

RECIPE HIGHLIGHTS

It's hard to find cookies that are very low in sugar and that taste great. These cookies do both of those and will also provide a decent dose of protein in the process.

INGREDIENTS

- 1 cup smooth natural peanut butter (any nut butter of choice works)
- ⅔ cup Natural Brown Sugar Sweetener (or other zero-sugar granulated brown sugar natural sweetener such as erythritol or monk fruit).
- ½ cup protein powder (use unflavoured or vanilla)
- ¼ cup stevia sweetened chocolate chips (naturally sweetened)
- 1 egg

METHOD

1. Preheat oven to 180 °C. Line a cookie or baking tray with baking paper.
2. In a small mixing bowl, combine all your ingredients until well incorporated.
3. With your hands, form 12 balls of cookie dough. Place each on the lined tray. Press down and flatten each ball into a cookie shape.
4. Bake the cookies for 10–12 minutes (or until edges begin to brown).
5. Remove from the oven and allow the cookies to cool on the tray before serving.

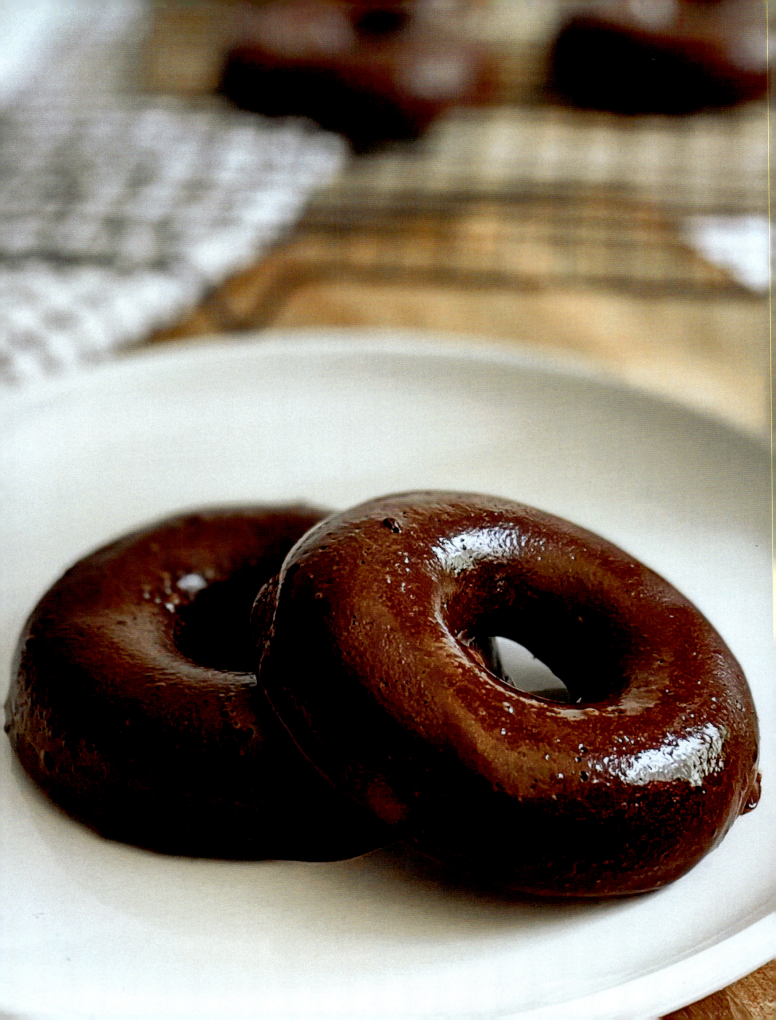

TREATS

Pronuts (Protein Donuts) (V)

SERVINGS: 6 DONUTS

MACRO BREAKDOWN (per donut)

RECIPE HIGHLIGHTS

These delicious chocolate mud cake style donuts are so simple to make, and provide 5 g more protein than any commercially bought donuts. They also have far less sugar and carbs even when compared to a regular cinnamon donut.

FAT: 6G

PROTEIN: 6G

CARBS: 8G

INGREDIENTS

- ½ cup spelt flour
- 1 scoop (30 g) chocolate protein powder
- 2 tbsp sweetener (e.g. stevia)
- 1 tsp baking powder
- ½ cup unsweetened almond milk
- 2 tbsp coconut oil

For the icing
- 2 tbsp sugar-free icing sugar substitute (naturally sweetened)
- 2 tbsp cocoa powder
- 4 tbsp almond milk

METHOD

1. Preheat oven to 220 °C.
2. In a bowl, combine the dry ingredients for the donuts.
3. Make a well in the centre and add the almond milk and coconut oil. Stir well to combine.
4. Split batter evenly into a 6-hole silicone donut mould. Bake for 12–15 mins, or until a skewer comes out clean. Remove from the oven to cool in the mould, then pop out the donuts onto a wire rack to cool completely.
5. For the icing, combine the icing sugar substitute and cocoa powder in a bowl, then slowly add the almond milk, stirring well, until you have reached your desired icing consistency.
6. Place each donut in the icing to glaze completely and then return it back onto the wire rack to set. Once set, consume immediately, or the donuts can be stored in the fridge for up to 3 days.

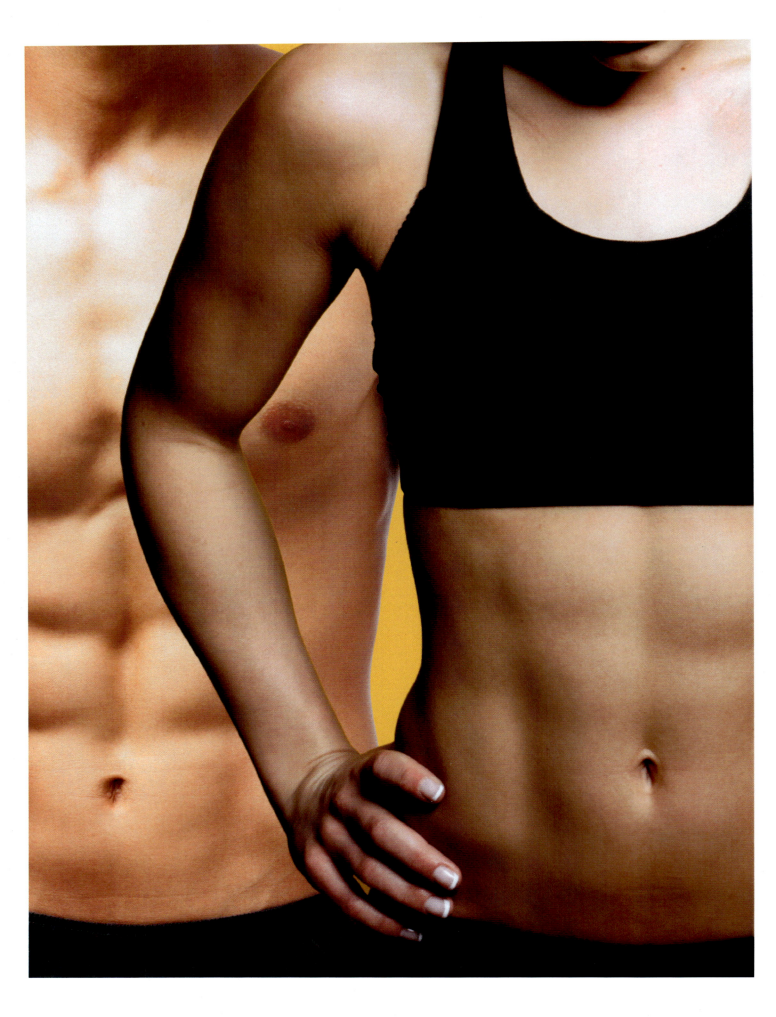

THE LEAN BODY WAY

The Great Disparity & Ensuring Your Success

> "INFORMATION IS NOT KNOWLEDGE.
> THE ONLY SOURCE OF KNOWLEDGE IS EXPERIENCE".
> ALBERT EINSTEIN

With the advent of the internet, now more than ever, there is an abundance of information, experts, and resources to help people just like you get your health and body back on track. Yet, with so much at our fingertips, most of us fail to forge a proper path. More people than ever are overfat, have dangerous health issues, and lack the physicality to function properly.

Why the lacklustre results? We have discussed the information disconnect at length in this text. There are some other reasons why so many people still struggle though—even when they have all the right information. Those other reasons are as follows:

1. IDENTITY ISSUES

Many fail to change their body because they want the outcome (leaner body, increased performance, better health), but they never really identify themselves as a lean, fit, and healthy person. To use an analogy, which person will be better at staying sober, the person who says they are "trying to get off the booze this month" or the person who says, "I'm not a drinker"?

In the same way, the person who identifies as a 'lean and healthy person' will have far greater success with their body composition and health than the person who simply 'wants to lose X amount of weight'. If you determine your identity, the outcomes will take care of themselves. Stop worrying about 'getting in shape' and instead start focusing on becoming the type of person who doesn't skip proper meals or workouts.

2. BUILT BY BAD HABITS

It's easy to become lazy in this world, and technology has made life far too comfortable. We don't walk: we catch rides. We don't cook: we order food to our doorsteps in minutes. We don't sleep: we load up on caffeine and other stimulants to get by. These are easy traps to fall into and many of us lack emotional intelligence (EQ) when it comes to food. Unless one is serious about both recognising and changing well-ingrained destructive behaviour patterns, success is very unlikely.

Nobody gains an extra 10 kg of fat overnight; it happens by stacking one bad habit on top of another over time. In the same way, losing 10 kg will require replacing one bad habit at a time with a better one. We first make our habits, then our habits make us. Just like getting stronger in the gym requires practice, so too does eating your way to a leaner and healthier body. We've provided you with great time-tested resources, but you have put in the work. It's not going to fix itself overnight.

All of our successful clients have systematically built better habits into their days and changed their physique sustainably over time. This meant starting each day with breakfast when it had been previously absent. It meant having pre-packed lean snacks every day at work instead of resorting to the vending machine. It meant adding colour to lunches and consuming a few extra serves of vegetables consistently each day. When even slightly out of shape people stack habits like these, they look and feel a hell of a lot different within a period of months (and with less effort!).

You learnt your own unhealthy eating habits in the same way, which means that you can also unlearn them and replace them with better ones in place. Habits take time to master and you're going to need to accept and start where you're at. Just resolve to be a little better every day. One of our Lean Body Program clients nicknamed OJ had terrible eating habits before he decided to lose weight. He admitted to us that when he was overfat and weighed 130 kg (over 30 kg heavier than he is now), he would eat a whole box of ice creams before training in the morning!

OJ is proof that no matter how bad your habits are, they can be changed! OJ is also proof that you can't out-train a bad diet and being honest with oneself and others regularly is a great virtue that yields outsized returns.

3. LACK OF SUPPORT

Change is hard, especially when trying to do it alone. Auto-suggestion is powerful—the environments and people we surround ourselves with have a profound influence on us (whether we are willing to admit it or not). There is a reason why incarcerated criminals are recidivist offenders and go back to jail again not long after they are released back into their community. They're often surrounded by the same people and the same triggers. We are the average of the five people we spend the most time with. This might mean that in order to get in shape, you will very likely have to put yourself in new environments and amongst people with different values.

We openly admit that this is a major contributing factor in the success of our Lean Body Program: people come for the abdominals, but they stay for the association. If you're serious about getting your health and body back on track, you will very likely fail if you're in the wrong environment. There is a harsher reality to choose, though, and that is to keep things unchanged. As professionals in this field, we can tell you emphatically from our experience that being overfat, unhealthy, and physically incapable never ends well.

The power of mentors cannot be denied either; it's a lot easier to get where you need to go if you follow the path of someone who has walked the path that lies ahead of you. This explains why more than 75 per cent of Fortune 500 companies and 100 per cent of the Fortune 50 have mentoring programs. The quickest and surest way to success is to mimic someone who has done it before you. Good mentors and coaches push you in the right direction—often faster than you ever would yourself. And not only can a good mentor or coach guide you the correct way, but they will also stand as a point of deflection and stop you from being diverted off track when things get tough (which they inevitably will).

Knowing what to do is not enough. There are a few defining factors that will determine your success regardless of whichever approach you pursue.

Due Diligence

"CIRCUMSTANCES DO NOT MAKE THE MAN; THEY REVEAL HIM".
JAMES ALLEN

At this stage, you may still feel confused, lacking in confidence, or struggling to come to terms with changing your environment. Being in the field we are in, we know these feelings all too well. If you feel you lack support and confidence in reaching your lean body goals, feel free to reach out to us at performancerevolution.com.au/#contact with your number one goal and your main struggle.

…But before you jump the gun, there are two questions you need to answer honestly:

"Do you really want to change?"
and
"Are you committed to practising to get better?"

These questions aren't answered with rhetoric either—they're answered with ACTION!

In other words "Don't tell me: show me!"

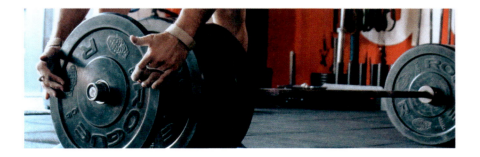

It's not enough to simply know something. The world is full of people who say those two dangerous words: "I know". These words will get you nowhere. Only after you implement something and apply it, do you truly 'know' something.

Don't put it off and tell yourself that circumstances will be better if you start 'some day' in the future. The traffic lights are rarely always green and there will never be a perfect time to get going. Time is the enemy of choices; the shorter the time, the fewer the choices. Most people are running out of time and are left with very few choices when it comes to reclaiming their body and their health—don't be one of those people. Do it now!

This is not easy; it requires due diligence. When most people hear the words 'due diligence' they think of analysing every bit of information and assessing the potential risks and benefits associated with a particular action. This is not what we mean here. We mean practising diligence (as is required) to get where you need to go. The dictionary definition of diligence is:

"Constant and earnest effort to accomplish what is undertaken; persistent exertion of body or mind".

This definition leaves no room for partiality or surrender. Rather, it requires perseverance and a willingness to overcome challenges in order to achieve the desired outcome.

We have experimented with a large number of clients over the years who have achieved amazing results. Many of these people did so in the face of circumstances and struggles that are unimaginable to most. They practised diligence and used (and are still using) the exact same information that you currently hold at your fingertips. The only thing stopping you from achieving the same great results is YOU.

And if you're worried that you don't know everything or have all the information, that's normal. Apply what you do know! If you're unsure and don't see certain things, then it's likely that we do not advocate it anyway. Go and apply as much as you can of what we have presented to you. The other minutiae can be worked out later once you've already experienced results.

To see some great testimonials of people who have used this resource to the best of their abilities and achieved remarkable results, head over to the results section of our website at **performancerevolution.com.au/#success-stories**.

Our One Request

> **"LIFE'S MOST PERSISTENT AND URGENT QUESTION IS: 'WHAT ARE YOU DOING FOR OTHERS?' PAY IT FORWARD, FOR IN LIFTING OTHERS, WE LIFT OURSELVES".**
> MARTIN LUTHER KING JR.

We have put a lot of time and effort into this resource to make it a reality. We also made it close to a steal, too! This way, anyone (no matter where they're currently at) can have access to this information and possess the proper tools to lead a leaner and healthier existence.

We're confident that you have obtained a lot of value from this resource and trust that it will be life-changing for you! In light of this, we only have one simple request for you: pay it forward. Tell your friends, work colleagues, loved ones, family members, and whoever else you know will benefit from this text. As you could agree, there are too many needlessly overfat, energy-drained, and disease-destined people out there in this world. These people could surely do with some guidance and help in getting their body and their confidence back. We want to reach as many of these people as possible and make a difference. We can't do that alone, so we ask that you generously share the experience of what you have learned with others today.

If you believe you have no one you could share this resource with, we ask the next best thing—to please leave an honest review once you finish reading this resource. We are constantly looking to improve the way we help people, and we would really appreciate your feedback. Thanks in advance.

Where to Next?

> "SEEKING HELP IS NOT A SIGN OF WEAKNESS; IT'S A SIGN OF STRENGTH. IT TAKES COURAGE TO RECOGNIZE WHEN WE NEED SUPPORT AND EVEN MORE STRENGTH TO REACH OUT FOR IT".
>
> LALAH DELIA

Need more help and further personalisation of your nutrition plan? Do you have a muscle-building goal, a shredded-physique goal, a performance or sporting goal, or even a particular health or eating condition?

Or maybe you're looking for some more guidance with your training and you're naturally curious about our Lean Body Program?

Whatever it is, in order to guide you in the right direction, send us a message to **performancerevolution.com.au/#contact** and let us know what your number one goal is right now along with your biggest struggle in achieving it. This way we can point you in the right direction.

Remember, you don't have to fight your battles alone. Getting help and clarity is a sign of courage, not cowardice.

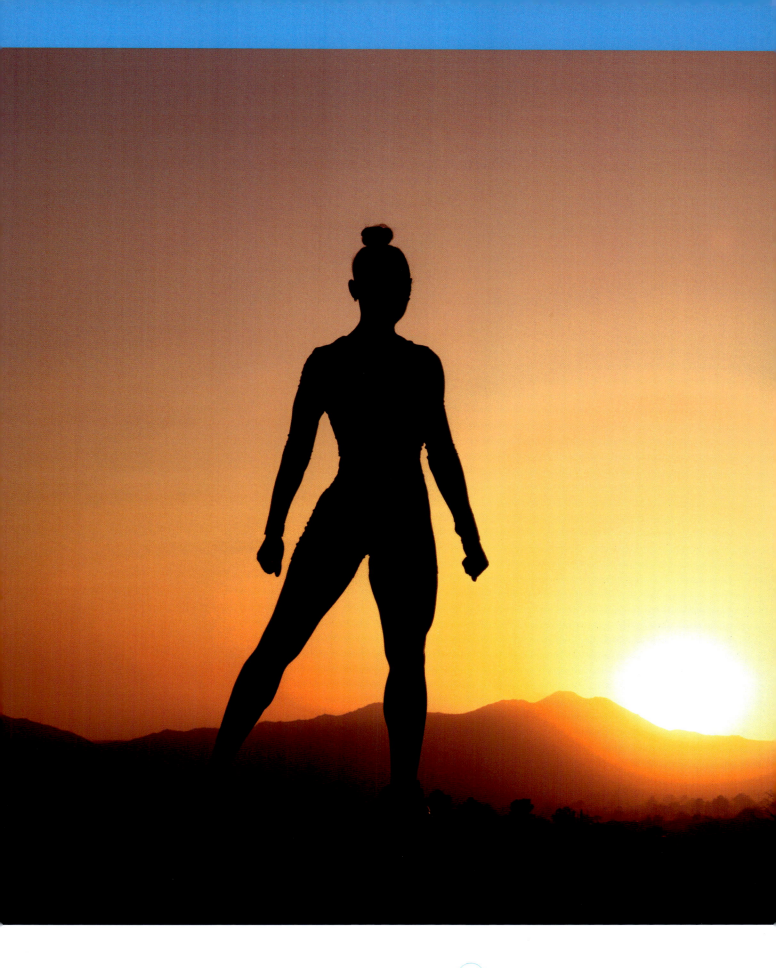

Recipe Index

Recipes marked '(V)' are suitable for vegetarians.

Almond Crusted Chicken, 195
Avocado and Egg White Tartines (V), 159

Bacon, Parmesan & Basil Mini Pizzas, 287
Banana-Protein Pancakes (V), 155
BBQ Beef Stir-Fry, 209
Beans and Cheese French Toast Sandwich (V), 281
Beefy Mushroom Chilli, 205
Better Balsamic Vinaigrette (V), 263
Better Choc Banana Protein Smoothie (V), 173
Breakfast Protein Muffins (V), 147

Carb Craver Choc Mint Protein Bars (V), 177
Chicken and Cheese French Toast Sandwich, 279
Choc Chip Brownie Cookie Bites (V), 317
Choc Mint Brownie Bars (V), 311
Choc Mint Protein Paddle Pops (V), 225
Choc Peanut Butter Protein Balls (V), 181
Chocolate Protein Mousse (V), 219
Classic Tzatziki Sauce (V), 266
Cocoa Black Bean Brownies (V), 221
Coconut Chicken Schnitzel, 187
Coconut Rough Protein Balls (V), 175
Creamy Almond Asian Dressing (V), 264

Creamy Ginger-Garlic Dressing (V), 267
Crispy Protein Wedges (V), 291
Crunchy Apple-Walnut Salad (V), 257
Crunchy Chicken Salad Wrap, 295
Crunchy No-Bake Protein Bars (V), 313
Curried Lentil Omelette (V), 157

Easy and Tasty Fiesta Sauce (V), 262
Easy Rocket & Steak Salad, 203
English Muffin Mini Pizzas, 299
Espresso Protein Shakes & Smoothies (V), 179

French Toast Sweet Sandwich Stack (V), 169
French Vanilla Almond Mousse (V), 217

Greek Dill Tzatziki Sauce/Dip (V), 235
Green Chimichurri Savoury Sauce (V), 269
Grilled Tuna Melts, 297
Grilled Veggie Omelette (V), 163

Healthier Honey-Mustard Dressing (V), 261
Homemade Almond Crackers with Hummus (V), 241
Homemade Sauerkraut (V), 246
Hot Smoked Salmon with Zucchini Linguine, 185

Lean Beef Burgers, 305
Lean Chicken Salsa Wrap, 307
Leaner Lasagne (V), 293
Lower-Carb Fish Tacos, 199

RECIPE INDEX

Niçoise Salad with Tasmanian Salmon, 197

Overnight Vanilla Chia Cup (V), 149

Peanut Butter and Choc Chip Brownies (V), 229
Popcorn Protein Bars (V), 315
Prawn and Avocado Omelette, 161
Pronuts (Protein Donuts) (V), 321
Protein Coconut Fruit Salad (V), 223
Protein-Packed Breakfast Wrap, 283
Protein-Packed Pasta with Beef Bolognese, 289

Quick & Warm High-Protein Muesli (V), 151

Reuben-Style Turkey Sandwich, 193
Roasted Veggie Frittata (V), 167

Seared Yellowfin Tuna with Fried Greens & Mushrooms, 201
Simple & Classic Hummus (V), 239
Simple & Spicy Pico de Gallo (V), 253
Sofrito (V), 249
Spicy Red Pepper & Tomato Soup (V), 245
Spinach, Black Bean, and Quinoa Salad (V), 213
Strawberry Breakfast Smoothie (V), 153
Sugar-Free Protein Cookies (V), 319
Sweet 'n' Sticky Pork Meatballs, 211
Sweet and Creamy No-Oats Porridge (V), 165
Sweet Chilli Chicken Burgers, 303

RECIPE INDEX

Sweet Chilli Chicken San Choy Bau, 189
Sweet Citrus-Apple Vinaigrette (V), 260
Sweet Pepper Relish (V), 265

Tasty Cauliflower Mash (V), 251
Tasty Tabouli Salad (V), 255
Turkey and Egg White Protein Muffin, 277
Turkey, Tomato, and Cheese French Toast Sandwich, 285

Ultimate Homemade Aioli Spread (V), 268

Vietnamese Prawn Salad Red Lentil Wrap, 301

White Choc Raspberry Protein Ice Cream Bars (V), 227
Wok'd Mushroom Beef Noodles, 207

Zesty Chicken and Black Bean Burritos, 191
Zesty Pesto (V), 237

About the Authors

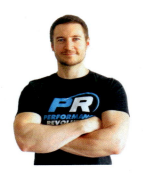

MICHAEL HERMANN
PERSONAL TRAINER + NUTRITIONIST + STRENGTH & CONDITIONING COACH

Michael Hermann is the founder and director of Performance Revolution, a company dedicated to helping people reach their physical potential. Michael began his career foremost as a strength and conditioning coach and personal trainer. At the time of this writing, he has conducted more than 28,000 'hands-on' coaching sessions in the space of 12 years. His clientele ranges from everyday people with health and body-composition goals to national-level athletes looking to enhance performance.

Michael's love for nutrition was born early on in his career and manifested itself in the outstanding results he has achieved for his clients. Michael sees the importance of growing his nutritional knowledge and application just as much as his exercise acumen and prescription.

In addition to his hands-on experience, Michael is an author and contributing writer for popular fitness magazines including *Oxygen* and *Muscle and Health*. He also uses his skills and experience to mentor and lecture other aspiring trainers at various Australian colleges and institutions.

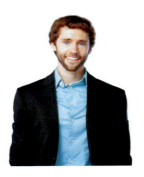

DYLAN JONES
DIETITIAN + CLINICAL EXERCISE SPECIALIST

Dylan Jones is a registered dietitian and clinical exercise specialist. His educational background includes degrees in human nutrition and exercise physiology and metabolism.

In addition to his strong educational foundation, Dylan also possesses vast practical experience in his fields—working in hospitals, weight-loss centres, medical facilities, and with competitive athletes.

Dylan is passionate about viewing food as medicine and relying on daily exercise for wellbeing, so much so that he currently runs a clinical bariatric program to provide nutritional and lifestyle solutions for diabetics. Dylan ventures well clear of the boring and impractical when it comes to healthy nutrition. His comprehensive education and expanded practical background also make him a trusted advisor when it comes to all things food.